Evaluating AIDS Prevention Programs

Expanded Edition

Susan L. Coyle, Robert F. Boruch, and
Charles F. Turner, *Editors*

PANEL ON THE EVALUATION OF AIDS INTERVENTIONS

COMMITTEE ON AIDS RESEARCH
AND THE
BEHAVIORAL, SOCIAL, AND STATISTICAL SCIENCES

COMMISSION ON THE BEHAVIORAL AND
SOCIAL SCIENCES AND EDUCATION

NATIONAL RESEARCH COUNCIL

NATIONAL ACADEMY PRESS
WASHINGTON, D.C.   1991

NATIONAL ACADEMY PRESS ● **2101 Constitution Avenue, N.W.** ● **Washington, D.C.** ● **20418**

NOTICE: The project that is the subject of this report was approved by the Governing Board of the National Research Council, whose members are drawn from the councils of the National Academy of Sciences, the National Academy of Engineering, and the Institute of Medicine. The members of the committee responsible for the report were chosen for their special competences and with regard for appropriate balance.

This report has been reviewed by a group other than the authors according to procedures approved by a Report Review Committee consisting of members of the National Academy of Sciences, the National Academy of Engineering, and the Institute of Medicine.

The National Academy of Sciences is a private, nonprofit, self-perpetuating society of distinguished scholars engaged in scientific and engineering research, dedicated to the furtherance of science and technology and to their use for the general welfare. Upon the authority of the charter granted to it by the Congress in 1863, the Academy has a mandate that requires it to advise the federal government on scientific and technical matters. Dr. Frank Press is president of the National Academy of Sciences.

The National Academy of Engineering was established in 1964, under the charter of the National Academy of Sciences, as a parallel organization of outstanding engineers. It is autonomous in its administration and in the selection of its members, sharing with the National Academy of Sciences the responsibility for advising the federal government. The National Academy of Engineering also sponsors engineering programs aimed at meeting national needs, encourages education and research, and recognizes the superior achievements of engineers. Dr. Robert M. White is president of the National Academy of Engineering.

The Institute of Medicine was established in 1970 by the National Academy of Sciences to secure the services of eminent members of appropriate professions in the examination of policy matters pertaining to the health of the public. The Institute acts under the responsibility given to the National Academy of Sciences by its congressional charter to be an adviser to the federal government and upon its own initiative, to identify issues of medical care, research, and education. Dr. Samuel O. Thier is president of the Institute of Medicine.

The National Research Council was established by the National Academy of Sciences in 1916 to associate the broad community of science and technology with the Academy's purposes of furthering knowledge and of advising the federal government. Functioning in accordance with general policies determined by the Academy, the Council has become the principal operating agency of both the National Academy of Sciences and the National Academy of Engineering in providing services to the government, the public, and the scientific and engineering communities. The Council is administered jointly by both Academies and the Institute of Medicine. Dr. Frank Press and Dr. Robert M. White are chairman and vice-chairman, respectively, of the National Research Council.

The work that provided the basis for this volume was supported by a contract from the U.S. Public Health Service.

Library of Congress Cataloging-in-Publication Data

Evaluating AIDS prevention programs / Susan L. Coyle, Robert F. Boruch, and Charles F. Turner, editors; Panel on the Evaluation of AIDS Interventions, Committee on AIDS Research and the Behavioral, Social and Statistical Sciences, National Research Council. – Expanded ed.
    p.   cm.
    Includes bibliographical references and index.
    ISBN 0-309-04281-X (paper). – ISBN 0-309-04288-7 (cloth)
    1. AIDS (Disease)–Prevention–Evaluation–Methodology. I. Coyle, Susan L. II. Boruch, Robert F. III. Turner, Charles F. IV. Title.
    [DNLM: 1. Acquired Immunodeficiency Syndrome–prevention & control. 2. Program Evaluation. WD 308 N27725e] RA644.A25N27 1991
    614.5'993–dc20
DNLM/DLC
for Library of Congress   90-13649
                                                      CIP

Panel on the Evaluation of AIDS Interventions

Liaison Representatives to the Panel from the
U.S. Public Health Service

ZILI AMSEL, National Institute on Drug Abuse
G. STEPHEN BOWEN, Centers for Disease Control
DAVID BROWNELL, Centers for Disease Control
ISABEL FERNANDEZ, Centers for Disease Control
JACOB GAYLE, Centers for Disease Control
JANINE JASON, Centers for Disease Control
C. FREDERIC KROGER, Centers for Disease Control
SUSAN MIDDLESTADT, Centers for Disease Control
KEVIN O'REILLY, Centers for Disease Control
DEBORAH L. RUGG, Centers for Disease Control
ELLEN STOVER, National Institute of Mental Health
RONALD W. WILSON, National Center for Health Statistics, Centers for
    Disease Control

Consultants

MICHAEL L. COHEN, School of Public Affairs, University of Maryland
SAHR J. KPUNDEH, Department of Political Science, Howard University
LEAH MAZADE, National Academy Press
LAURA RUDKIN-MINIOT, Department of Sociology, Princeton University
MICHAEL A. STOTO, Division of Health Promotion and Disease Prevention,
    Institute of Medicine

Preface

As the second decade of the epidemic of acquired immune deficiency syndrome (AIDS) begins, behavioral change remains our primary weapon in the fight against the spread of the human immunodeficiency virus (HIV) and AIDS. It is unfortunate, however, that we know relatively little as scientists about the comparative effectiveness of different strategies intended to encourage and facilitate protective behavioral change among persons who are at risk of HIV transmission.

It is our strong belief that such knowledge is an urgent national priority and that it will require a long-term commitment to a course of rigorous (and selective) research assessing current and future AIDS prevention programs. Such research will enable us to learn from both our failures and our successes in inducing protective changes in sexual and drug-using behaviors.

The present report provides a blueprint for action. It has been undertaken at the behest of the U.S. Public Health Service, which requested assistance in developing strategies for evaluating the three major AIDS prevention programs sponsored by the Centers for Disease Control. This report[1] was prepared by the Panel on the Evaluation of AIDS Interventions, which was convened by the National Research Council Committee on AIDS Research and the Behavioral, Social, and Statistical Sciences. The panel's work extends the committee's previous assessment of intervention needs, reported in *AIDS, Sexual Behavior, and Intravenous Drug Use* (Turner, Miller, and Moses, 1989). That report argued strongly for a national commitment to the careful design and evaluation of AIDS intervention strategies.

We recognize that the high quality evaluation research recommended in this report will be costly, but we believe that uncertainty about program effectiveness is even more costly. The price of continued ignorance will be measured both in dollars spent on ineffective programs and in deaths and disease that might have been prevented. A commitment to

---

[1]The present volume is an expanded edition of the Panel's 1989 report. This edition incorporates new sections on nonexperimental approaches to intervention (Chapter 6 and Appendix F) and methodological issues in mounting evaluations (Appendixes C–E).

well-conducted evaluation research must be made now, and it must be maintained if we are to improve our understanding of how to control this deadly epidemic.

There is good reason to believe that this nation can and will do a better job in the future in determining which AIDS prevention programs do change behavior and which do not. Federal officials and people who have been on the front lines of AIDS prevention activities since the early days of the epidemic all express a considerable desire for evaluation of their work. The paucity of rigorous evaluations conducted to date is not due to individuals' unwillingness to undertake the research but to a lack of resources and expertise. It is evident that past links between those who provide services and manage programs, on the one hand, and those who conduct research and evaluation, on the other, have not been strong.

It is our hope that this volume will foster such collaboration and thereby advance our understanding of and ability to facilitate the behavioral changes required to retard the spread of HIV in the future.

SUSAN L. COYLE, *Study Director*
ROBERT F. BORUCH, *Chair*
Panel on the Evaluation of AIDS Interventions

CHARLES F. TURNER, *Director*
Committee on AIDS Research and the Behavioral, Social, and Statistical Sciences

Acknowledgments

During the course of this study, the panel was assisted by a number of scientists who took time to share their insights and expertise. To those who assisted us in our work, the panel extends its sincere thanks and appreciation. The panel's work was supported by the U.S. Public Health Service.

Note on Contributions

This report is the collective product of panel members and staff. The content of this report reflects the deliberations of the panel, and the report presents the panel's recommendations. The list below identifies the persons who shared major responsibility for preparing initial drafts of materials for each chapter in this report. The panel reviewed all contributions, and they have been revised and edited in light of the panel's discussions and the comments of outside reviewers. The purpose of the following alphabetical list, therefore, is to give credit to individuals but not to assign final responsibility for the published text. It should also be noted that, although the list covers major sections of this volume, these sections frequently contain additional paragraphs or pages from other hands.

SUMMARY: Coyle, Turner

CHAPTER 1: Boruch, Coates, Coyle, Laird, Moses, Turner

CHAPTER 2: Martin, with Coyle

CHAPTER 3: Flay and Kessler, with Utts

CHAPTER 4: Boruch, Hubbard, Turner, Waller

CHAPTER 5: Boruch, Coates, Coyle, Davis, Hubbard, Martin, Turner

CHAPTER 6: Coyle, Moses, and Turner, with Boruch, Cohen, Hubbard, Laird

APPENDIX A: Waller

APPENDIX B: Boruch

APPENDIX C: reprinted from Miller, Turner, and Moses (1990), contributors—S. Lindenbaum, J. Sorensen, C. Turner, J. Wiley, with P. Blumstein, R. Dawes, L. Rudkin-Miniot

Contents

Appendixes

Evaluating AIDS Prevention Programs

Expanded Edition

Summary

In early 1989, the Public Health Service requested that a panel be established to recommend strategies for evaluating three of the major AIDS prevention programs sponsored by the Centers for Disease Control (CDC). To that end, the Panel on the Evaluation of AIDS Interventions was formed–and delivered the first of two reports, *Evaluating AIDS Prevention Programs,* in August 1989. In the initial report, the panel recommended randomized experiments as the primary strategy for evaluating program effectiveness. In addition, the panel proposed to discuss nonexperimental strategies in more depth in our next report. This we do now in *Evaluating AIDS Prevention Programs, Expanded Edition.* This second volume retains the original Chapters 1-5 and Appendices A-B from the first report and offers new material in Chapter 6 and Appendices C-F on nonexperimental methods and other evaluation issues.

BACKGROUND

CDC is the principal public health agency responsible for AIDS education and prevention. Each of the programs CDC selected for the panel's review was designed to intervene at a different level of society: (1) the multiphase national AIDS media campaign is directed at the general population of the United States as well as at more specific audiences; (2) projects of community-based organizations, primarily health education and risk reduction interventions, focus on small groups or specific populations; and (3) a network of counseling and testing projects is targeted to individual clients.

The first designated intervention, the national AIDS media campaign, was established in April 1987 by CDC's National AIDS Information and Education Program. Shortly afterward, the advertising and public relations firm of Ogilvy & Mather was selected by competitive bid to develop the multiphase campaign of public service announcements, the

1

most visible component of the program. The media campaign is intended not only to provide information about how HIV is spread and how that spread can be prevented, but also to generate social support for infected individuals. The campaign uses a variety of media in addition to the public service announcements to deliver information to the general public as well as to specific populations.

The second program, the AIDS prevention projects of community-based organizations (CBOs), channels health education and risk reduction information to selected populations that are at high risk for HIV infection. CBOs are uniquely positioned to reach hard-to-reach groups such as gay men or intravenous drug users. CDC's Center for Prevention Services funds these organizations through three mechanisms: cooperative agreements with state and local health agencies who oversee the community organizations; a cooperative agreement with the U.S. Conference of Mayors to provide "seed money" to local minority organizations; and a direct funding initiative for community-based organizations.

The third program offers individual clients (and occasionally their partners) testing for HIV infection in conjunction with pretest and posttest counseling. A typical delivery setting is a local health department or other health services facility (such as a clinic for sexually transmitted diseases) that receives indirect CDC funding channeled through the state health department. CDC also provides guidelines for the content and conduct of the counseling component of these programs. CDC began funding counseling and testing sites in fiscal 1985 through its Center for Prevention Services. Resources are distributed to over 5,000 sites in the form of cooperative agreements with 64 state and local agencies.

The panel's findings, conclusions, and general recommendations are presented in the next several sections of this summary, following the structure of the expanded report. We first consider general evaluation and outcome measurement issues (Chapters 1 and 2). We then present issues specific to the three types of AIDS prevention programs: the national media campaign (Chapter 3); CBO health education/risk reduction projects (Chapter 4); and the HIV testing and counseling program (Chapter 5). In this edition, the panel also reviews a number of nonexperimental strategies that researchers have used to evaluate other social programs (Chapter 6). The last section of the summary presents the panel's specific recommendations.

EVALUATION: NEEDS AND IMPLEMENTATION

Program evaluation in the context of AIDS prevention is as difficult as program implementation itself, and as necessary. To educate the public about what is essentially a health emergency, states and cities have rapidly implemented prevention programs, often without the necessary staff or plans for evaluating their effectiveness. The panel believes that future AIDS prevention efforts should plan and allocate sufficient resources to obtain sound evidence about what works best to alter those behaviors that are known to transmit HIV.

The evaluation policy proposed in Chapter 1 hinges on a framework of three questions:

- What interventions are actually delivered?
- Do the interventions make a difference?
- What interventions or variations work better?

Each of these evaluative questions engenders further questions that bear on how credible evidence can be produced, the resources required to produce that evidence, and the methodological problems that affect evidence quality.

The evaluation of AIDS intervention programs is not an easy task: it will take time, and it will also require a long-term commitment of effort and resources. Because the environment in which these programs are implemented is constantly changing, and because prevention may require life-long behavioral changes, it is inappropriate to view program design, implementation, and evaluation as short-term or one-time events. Given the seriousness of the disease and the benefits associated with prevention, commitment of adequate resources for careful evaluations of the effectiveness of AIDS prevention programs should be viewed as a wise investment in the future.

The panel's aim is to be realistic–not discouraging–when it also notes that the difficulties and costs of program evaluation should not be underestimated. Many of the research strategies proposed in this report will require major investments of talent, time, and financial support, as well as a substantial amount of planning. Once these investments have been made, however, and a body of findings and practical experience has accumulated, subsequent evaluations should be easier and less costly to conduct. The panel notes, however, that because some of the major CDC intervention programs are likely to continue indefinitely, periodic reassessments are warranted to ensure that intervention components continue to be delivered as specified in the program protocol or standards.

The nature of the HIV/AIDS epidemic demands an unwavering commitment to prevention programs, and ongoing prevention programs require a similar commitment to their evaluation. A full complement of sustained evaluation research is needed. The panel endorses the appropriate use of formative, process, and outcome evaluation and urges that evaluation be a part of intervention program design.

Formative evaluation involves a small-scale effort to identify and resolve intervention and evaluation issues systematically before a program is widely implemented. This type of evaluation might be used to provide tentative answers to any of the three evaluation questions, but in this report it is formally recommended only for the media campaign, for which "What works better?" is the salient question for formative evaluation. For example, before implementing a full-scale media campaign of public service announcements, researchers can randomly assign participants to view different preliminary advertising layouts, and self-reported knowledge, attitudes, and behavioral intentions can then be compared for the different versions. Even when done on a small-scale, however, formative evaluation requires financial resources and trained staff.

Process evaluation involves finding answers to the question "What services are actually delivered?" and it is appropriate for all three of the major AIDS intervention programs. Process evaluation generally requires few additional program resources. For example, evaluations of who receives HIV testing and counseling could be conducted by gathering and systematically reporting information on the clientele served by the testing sites. The costs associated with such a strategy are not large relative to the costs of the program.

A major shortcoming of process evaluation, however, is that it cannot demonstrate whether programs are effective. Process evaluation can yield important data on the number of individuals reached by a message or program, and it can document client flow or illuminate program accessibility. What it cannot do is provide information on whether the program changed the knowledge, beliefs, intentions, or behaviors of the individuals it served. Process evaluation, therefore, is necessary but not sufficient to determine project results.

Outcome evaluation assesses the effectiveness of an intervention program and can be used to answer the questions "Do the interventions make a difference?" and "What works better?" The panel endorses randomized field experiments–when feasible and appropriate–to test the effects of the media campaign and the health education/risk reduction projects of CBOs and thus answer the question, "Do the interventions make a difference?" When properly executed, randomization ensures that the observed differences in outcomes between treatment and control groups do not arise from biased assignment of persons to these groups. Because randomization leads to unbiased estimates, it thereby permits a fair assessment of the absolute size as well as comparative level of treatment effects and provides a statistically legitimate statement about the level of confidence that may be placed in that assessment.

The value and benefits of randomized experiments must be weighed against their drawbacks. They can be difficult to deploy, both practically and politically, and they require significant investments of time, expertise, and financial support, as well as cooperation from and coordination among projects, federal agencies, and research teams. The panel estimates, for example, that an adequate evaluation of the impact of some set of CBO projects would take at least 3 years to complete and that a formative evaluation using a randomized experiment to test effects of different media campaigns would cost at least $200,000.

Although we are persuaded that the randomized controlled experiment should form the backbone of CDC's strategy for outcome evaluation, we also recognize the value of nonexperimental approaches when it is not possible to conduct a randomized trial. Alternative approaches should be investigated, for example, in the case of testing and counseling projects, for which we cannot recommend randomized experiments with no-treatment control groups because it is neither ethical nor possible to direct individuals to a group that is denied testing.

To assess the relative effectiveness of different program options in order to determine "what works better," the panel recommends using randomized experiments with alternative-treatment controls for each of the three major AIDS intervention programs. Because such experiments test alternative or enhanced treatments rather than using a no-treatment control group, they are often more acceptable to participants. It should be noted, however, that such randomized experiments will require investments of expertise, financial support, and time that will be at least as large as those required by experiments that have no-treatment control groups.

Oversight and monitoring of all phases of evaluation are necessary to provide quality control and to safeguard the integrity of the research. Evaluation is often a sensitive issue for both project and evaluation staff because of the possibility that it will show that projects are not as effective as they believed. The panel believes that independent oversight of an evaluation can help curb the pressures to show artificially positive effects, and it also can provide additional expertise for solving difficult technical issues.

OUTCOMES

The panel's final conclusion concerns program objectives and outcome measures. Carefully defined program goals and objectives are needed to select appropriate outcome measures to test the effectiveness of a program. Evaluations of past intervention efforts have been hampered by poorly defined program objectives, which do not reflect desired proximate outcomes. Therefore the panel recommends that all intervention programs, in addition to the general goal of reducing HIV transmission, should have explicit objectives framed in terms of measurable biological, behavioral, or psychological outcomes.

In Chapter 2, the panel concludes that behavioral measures should be the primary outcome variables for most AIDS intervention programs. The panel considered the usefulness of biological indicators, including HIV incidence data, rates of sexually transmitted diseases, and fertility rates (for HIV positive women). For most interventions, the panel concludes that these biological measures would be of secondary importance. The proximate outcome most relevant to reducing HIV transmission in most situations will be the adoption and maintenance of behaviors that protect uninfected individuals from contracting HIV and protect infected individuals from transmitting HIV. Appropriate changes in "risky" behavior, other things being equal, will reduce HIV transmission in populations in which the virus is heavily seeded, and it will protect populations in which HIV is yet not well established. Thus, accurate measurements of these behaviors will often be the most relevant indicators of the success of a program in retarding HIV transmission.

The panel also considered using direct measurements of the incidence of new HIV infections as a primary outcome variable. The panel concludes that–although they may be appropriate in some circumstances[1] –HIV incidence data would not be a sensitive indicator for populations in which HIV infection was rare (e.g., heterosexual adolescents in most parts of the country), and they would provide no information about relevant outcomes in seropositive persons. Furthermore, HIV incidence data are not only difficult to obtain, but they are also difficult to interpret. HIV incidence rates require extremely large samples and protracted testing to determine a program's effectiveness. Moreover, the rates can reflect other conditions unrelated to the effects of the program, such as the absence of or saturation of the infection in a given locale.

THE MEDIA CAMPAIGN

In Chapter 3, the panel's discussion of evaluating the media campaign contains two elements that are unique to this program. Specifically,

---

[1] Newborn HIV incidence rates, for example, are discussed in Chapter 6 as potential indicators of project effects.

the panel adds a question–"*Can* the campaign make a difference?"– to evaluate campaign efficacy (i.e., the campaign's likely effects if it were implemented optimally), and it also discusses the use of formative evaluation during program development to determine the effectiveness of a campaign message prior to large-scale dissemination.

The panel strongly believes that the efficacy of a *proposed* media campaign or campaign phase should be carefully evaluated in a number of randomly selected test market areas and that the results from these areas should be compared with the results from a number of other randomly selected test areas in which the campaign is not presented. It is often impossible to predict the effects of a given strategy. In order for future efforts to build on past knowledge, negative outcomes are potentially as important as positive ones.

Process evaluation of the multiphase national AIDS media campaign and its program of public service announcements (PSAs) requires knowledge of whether the campaign was aired, how often it was shown, and who saw or heard it. In its review of the process evaluation of media programs, the panel finds the data to be less than complete and urges that program presentation, including PSAs, be measured more conscientiously. In particular, the committee recommends that more attention be given to the following data collection efforts: population surveys to gauge the public's general awareness of the campaign; telephone surveys directed toward particular market areas after PSA broadcasts; and coincidental surveys following PSA presentation to help chart the extent of viewing and message recall. The panel also recommends augmentation of the data collection capabilities of the national AIDS hotline.

To assess the relative effects of different media campaigns or different program components, the panel recommends randomized experiments of alternative approaches. The panel recommends that experimental trials of alternative messages in the media campaign be undertaken during the development of the campaign rather than after its full implementation. To determine whether a campaign is effective, the panel presents a number of approaches that use randomized and quasi-experimental effectiveness trials in various designs (e.g., lagged implementation, switching replication).

COMMUNITY-BASED ORGANIZATIONS

CBO projects vary considerably, reflecting the diversity of the organizations through which they are delivered and the communities they serve. The panel believes it is important to recognize and describe this diversity, and in Chapter 4 we suggest case studies of selected projects and an administrative reporting system for the CBOs. Administrative reports can document the scope of CBOs' efforts, and case studies can provide detailed, in-depth descriptions as well as a context in which to explore intervention and evaluation questions.

The panel urges the use of randomized experiments to test the effects of the different CBO projects and to compare the relative effectiveness of different approaches. For new CBO projects, the panel believes that individuals seeking services might be assigned either to participate in the CBO project or to be part of a control condition in which they avail themselves of other options in the community. After experience is gained with such experiments, the panel proposes that a subset of capably staffed CBOs participate in comparative evaluations of alternative treatments in which the effects of their projects will be estimated.

The selection of CBO projects for outcome evaluation should be based on the organizations' capacity and willingness to engage in randomized tests. Both willingness and capacity can be enhanced by CDC's investment in a contractual process that encourages CBOs to collaborate with experts in randomized experimentation (and vice versa), and by commitment to an oversight mechanism for research administration that goes well beyond the usual advisory committee duties.

Furthermore, the panel suggests that CDC invest its resources in carefully evaluating a selected sample of projects rather than superficially evaluating all of them. This fewer-but-better approach is justified not only by financial limitations but also on practical grounds: despite their willingness, many projects will not have the case flow, resources, or capacity to participate in a long-term program of experiments.

The panel believes that nonexperimental before-and-after evaluation designs can be useful for looking at a project's proficiency in delivering services to its participants but that it is a weak design for measuring program effectiveness. The inference of cause and effect from such designs is highly problematic because competing explanations for across-time changes in attitudes and behaviors cannot be ruled out.

HIV TESTING AND COUNSELING

The panel concludes in Chapter 5 that it is neither practical nor ethical to conduct experiments with no-treatment control groups to determine the effects of HIV testing and counseling projects. The assignment of individuals to a control group that does not allow them to learn if they are infected or does not offer counseling has serious consequences for personal planning and medical management of HIV disease and AIDS.

While no-treatment control groups are inappropriate to determine if counseling and testing makes a difference, there remains a need to understand what is being delivered in the counseling and testing projects and to determine if there are better strategies for facilitating behavioral change. Determining what services are provided includes how well they are provided, whether they are accessible and attractive, and whether they satisfy *a priori* standards of quality. The panel recommends that data be gathered from multiple sources–including testing sites, clients, independent observers, and groups at increased risk for HIV infection–to evaluate five aspects of service delivery: the adequacy of the testing and counseling protocol, the adequacy of the counseling that is actually provided, the proportion of clients who complete the full protocol, the accessibility of services, and the barriers faced by potential clients in seeking and completing a testing and counseling protocol.

The panel recommends using randomized experiments with alternative-treatment controls to determine if some forms of counseling and testing work better than the standard approach. Alternative treatments can test the effects of different settings and different counseling protocols and services on such outcomes as clients' willingness to return to a site for test results, knowledge of risks, reduction of risk-associated behavior, and the minimizing of negative side effects (e.g., psychological distress) of HIV testing.

RANDOMIZED AND OBSERVATIONAL APPROACHES TO EVALUATION

In Chapter 6, as in earlier chapters, the panel recommends that randomized controlled experiments be used in outcome evaluations of a small number of important and carefully selected AIDS prevention programs. It is the panel's judgment that well-executed randomized experiments provide the most certainty concerning the effects of these programs. This is so because random assignment of individuals or groups to intervention or control conditions creates subgroups that are not expected (on average) to differ on factors that affect the intervention's outcomes.

The panel devotes one section of this chapter to an in depth examination of randomized experiments and their pitfalls. Because we believe that randomized trials have the best chance of avoiding selection bias, and thus provide the most trustworthy estimates of effects, we recommend that they constitute the backbone of an evaluation strategy for new AIDS prevention services. The panel notes, however, that such experiments can be compromised, and we recommend studies of ways to reduce such threats to executing experiments as attrition and noncompliance. The panel also specifies a number of conditions under which randomization may not be feasible or appropriate.

In situations where randomization is not appropriate or feasible, the panel invites serious consideration of nonrandomized studies to evaluate AIDS interventions. The panel categorizes nonexperimental studies according to the two general approaches they take to control for selection bias and yield fair comparisons. The first approach is the *design of comparability* through the creation of nonrandomized comparison groups–i.e., through quasi-experiments, natural experiments, and matching. The second approach involves *post hoc statistical adjustments* for selection bias through model-based data analyses–i.e., through analysis of covariance, structural equation modeling, and selection modeling.

An example of *a priori* design is the quasi-experiment. In this type of evaluation, some individuals are assigned to receive an intervention, and a comparison group is devised of individuals who will not be assigned to receive it, for reasons theoretically unrelated to the outcome variable. Two quasi-experimental designs that the panel believes are promising are the interrupted time series and the regression displacement/regression discontinuity designs. The panel discusses some data sources that can be tapped for evaluating future activities with quasi-experiments (the CDC/NIH neonatal screening survey and the National Health Interview Survey).

A design variation is the natural experiment, a situation in which investigators attempt to assess the effects of an exogenously introduced intervention by comparing treated and untreated groups. The assumption of natural experiments is that the comparison group is identical to the treatment group except for the lack of the intervention. Weakening that assumption, however, is the fact that the investigator typically has no control over selecting and implementing these treatments. In cases in which the investigator can foresee a natural experiment in the making (e.g., AIDS-related legislation that will affect some but not all locales), pre-test measures can be collected, which will enhance the credibility of an evaluation of project effects.

The third kind of *a priori* method discussed is matching, which involves selecting a comparison that "looks like" a project participant with respect to variables that are believed affect project participation (such as age). Although matching can control *known* sources of bias, the panel believes that the resulting comparisons may often be misleading because unknown and uncontrolled confounding variables can influence the outcome.

The credibility of *a posteriori* data analysis (e.g., analysis of covariance and modeling approaches) to evaluate AIDS prevention programs rests on the credibility of its underlying theory and the quality of data available to use with these procedures.

The panel is concerned about efforts to establish comparability using statistical adjustment and modeling procedures in the AIDS arena because they may fail (without detection) because of either flaws in data quality or errors in the assumptions that are made about the relationship of variables that affect selection and outcome. First, although it may seem obvious, the panel wishes to emphasize that the knowledge base is woefully inadequate about the behavioral and other characteristics that are important in changing behaviors that transmit HIV. The absence of a wealth of tested theory or empirical evidence shrinks the basis for the assumptions required by these models.

Although the panel is not optimistic about our present ability to use structural equation or selection models and data from nonrandomized studies as the primary strategy for evaluating the effectiveness of AIDS prevention programs, we do believe that such models will have a role to play and we suspect that this role may grow in the future. In particular, the panel believes that much might be gained by the judicious use of such models as an adjunct to randomized experiments. Structural equation modeling might be used, for example, to improve our understanding of the individual and contextual factors that mediate between a treatment and an outcome. Furthermore, the panel would observe that as experience accrues in situations where modeling is done *in tandem with experiments,* we anticipate the development of theory and data that may allow modeling approaches to substitute for some experiments in the future.

Finally, the panel notes that trustworthy evaluation requires a reservoir of evidence whether it comes from randomized or nonrandomized studies. A difficulty in comparing data drawn from several studies, however, arises when studies use different definitions of target audiences, different specification of causal variables, different outcome measures, different wordings in survey instruments, and so on. Not only do these differences make it hard to compare studies and projects, they make results difficult to generalize. Thus, we recommend that subsets of common data elements be repeated across studies as a way to ensure comparability and improve data reliability.

SPECIFIC RECOMMENDATIONS

The formal recommendations of the Panel on the Evaluation of AIDS Interventions are listed below. The first group of recommendations covers all of the separate programs, with one exception: recommendation

2 does not apply to the counseling and testing program. Additional recommendations that are specific to each program are listed separately.

All AIDS Intervention Programs

1. To improve interventions that are already broadly implemented, the panel recommends the use of randomized field experiments of alternative or enhanced interventions.

2. Before a new intervention is broadly implemented, the panel recommends that it be pilot tested in a randomized field experiment. (This recommendation applies to the media campaign and CBO projects but not to the HIV testing and counseling program.)

3. The panel recommends that any intensive evaluation of an intervention be conducted on a subset of projects selected according to explicit criteria. These criteria should include the replicability of the project, the feasibility of evaluation, and the project's potential effectiveness for prevention of HIV transmission.

4. The panel recommends that evaluation be conducted and replicated across major types of subgroups, programs, and settings. Attention should be paid to geographic areas with low and high AIDS prevalence, as well as to subpopulations at low and high risk for AIDS.

5. When evaluation is to be conducted by a number of different evaluation teams, the panel recommends establishing an independent scientific committee to oversee project selection and research efforts, corroborate the impartiality and validity of results, conduct cross-site analyses, and prepare reports on the progress of the evaluations.

6. The panel recommends that CDC recruit and retain behavioral, social, and statistical scientists trained in evaluation methodology to facilitate the implementation of the evaluation research recommended in this report.

7. In addition to the overarching goal of eliminating HIV transmission, the panel recommends that explicit objectives be written for each of the major intervention programs and that these objectives be framed as measurable biological, psychological, and behavioral outcomes.

8. The panel recommends that all evaluation protocols provide for the assessment of potential harmful effects, as well as the assessment of desired effects.

9. The panel recommends that once goals are met, projects be reevaluated periodically to monitor their continued effectiveness.

10. The panel recommends that the Office of the Assistant Secretary for Health allocate sufficient funds in the budget of each major AIDS prevention program, including future wide-scale programs, to implement the evaluation strategies recommended herein.

11. The panel recommends that studies be conducted on ways to systematically increase participant involvement in projects and to reduce attrition through outreach to project dropouts. All trials should assess levels of participation and variability in the strength of the treatment provided.

12. The panel recommends that new or improved AIDS prevention services be implemented as part of coordinated collaborative research and demonstration grants requiring controlled randomized trials of the effects of the services.

13. The panel recommends that the National Science Foundation sponsor research into the empirical accuracy of estimates of program effects derived from selection model methods.

14. The panel recommends that the Public Health Service and other agencies that sponsor the evaluation of AIDS prevention research require the collection of selected subsets of common data elements across evaluation studies to ensure comparability across sites and to establish and improve data validity and reliability.

National AIDS Media Campaign

15. The panel recommends the expanded use of formative evaluation or developmental research in designing media projects.

16. The panel recommends systematic comparative tests of paid advertising versus public service announcement campaigns.

17. The panel recommends that items be added to the National Health Interview Survey to evaluate exposure to, recall of, responses to, and changes resulting from new phases of the media campaign.

18. The panel recommends that CDC increase the usefulness of hotline data for media campaign assessments by collecting evaluation-related data such as the caller's geographic location, selected caller characteristics, issue(s) of concern, and counselor responses.

19. The panel recommends that CDC initiate changes in its time schedules for the dissemination of public service announcements to facilitate the evaluation of the media campaign. To enable the staggered implementation of television broadcasts, changes are needed in (1) the distribution schedule of public service announcements within the National AIDS Information and Education Program's consortium of

media distributors and (2) the period of time between Public Health Service approval and release of new phases of the campaign.

20. The panel recommends that CDC initiate changes in its data collection and data sharing activities to facilitate the evaluation of the media campaign. To generate needed data, changes are needed in (1) the period of time for internal approval of data items for the National Health Interview Survey, and (2) expeditious data sharing between the National Center for Health Statistics and other divisions of CDC.

Community-Based Organizations

21. The panel recommends that a simple standardized reporting system for health education/risk reduction projects be developed and used to address the question of what activities are planned and under way.

22. The panel also recommends the expanded use of case studies.

Testing and Counseling

23. The panel recommends that data be gathered from multiple sources–including testing sites, clients, groups at increased risk of HIV infection, and independent observers–to evaluate five aspects of service delivery: the adequacy of the counseling and testing protocol, the adequacy of the counseling that is actually provided, the proportion of clients that complete the full protocol, the accessibility of services, and the nature of the barriers, if any, to clients seeking and completing counseling and testing.

24. The panel recommends that evaluations of "What works better?" focus on the comparative effectiveness of testing and counseling services that (1) are delivered in different settings, (2) have different content, duration, and intensity, and (3) are accompanied by different types of supportive services.

25. The panel recommends that the National Health Interview Survey (NHIS) be periodically augmented with several questions about accessibility and barriers to HIV testing and counseling services.

1

Design and Implementation
of Evaluation Research

Evaluation has its roots in the social, behavioral, and statistical sciences, and it relies on their principles and methodologies of research, including experimental design, measurement, statistical tests, and direct observation. What distinguishes evaluation research from other social science is that its subjects are ongoing social action programs that are intended to produce individual or collective change. This setting usually engenders a great need for cooperation between those who conduct the program and those who evaluate it. This need for cooperation can be particularly acute in the case of AIDS prevention programs because those programs have been developed rapidly to meet the urgent demands of a changing and deadly epidemic.

Although the characteristics of AIDS intervention programs place some unique demands on evaluation, the techniques for conducting good program evaluation do not need to be invented. Two decades of evaluation research have provided a basic conceptual framework for undertaking such efforts (see, e.g., Campbell and Stanley [1966] and Cook and Campbell [1979] for discussions of outcome evaluation; see Weiss [1972] and Rossi and Freeman [1982] for process and outcome evaluations); in addition, similar programs, such as the antismoking campaigns, have been subject to evaluation, and they offer examples of the problems that have been encountered.

In this chapter the panel provides an overview of the terminology, types, designs, and management of research evaluation. The following chapter provides an overview of program objectives and the selection and measurement of appropriate outcome variables for judging the effectiveness of AIDS intervention programs. These issues are discussed in detail in the subsequent, program-specific Chapters 3-5.

TYPES OF EVALUATION

The term evaluation implies a variety of different things to different people. The recent report of the Committee on AIDS Research and the Behavioral, Social, and Statistical Sciences defines the area through a series of questions (Turner, Miller, and Moses, 1989:317-318):

> Evaluation is a systematic process that produces a trustworthy account of what was attempted and why; through the examination of results—the outcomes of intervention programs—it answers the questions, "What was done?" "To whom, and how?" and "What outcomes were observed?" Well-designed evaluation permits us to draw inferences from the data and addresses the difficult question: "What do the outcomes mean?"

These questions differ in the degree of difficulty of answering them. An evaluation that tries to determine the outcomes of an intervention and what those outcomes mean is a more complicated endeavor than an evaluation that assesses the process by which the intervention was delivered. Both kinds of evaluation are necessary because they are intimately connected: to establish a project's success, an evaluator must first ask whether the project was implemented as planned and then whether its objective was achieved. Questions about a project's implementation usually fall under the rubric of *process evaluation.* If the investigation involves rapid feedback to the project staff or sponsors, particularly at the earliest stages of program implementation, the work is called *formative evaluation.* Questions about effects or effectiveness are often variously called summative evaluation, impact assessment, or *outcome evaluation,* the term the panel uses.

Formative evaluation is a special type of early evaluation that occurs during and after a program has been designed but before it is broadly implemented. Formative evaluation is used to understand the need for the intervention and to make tentative decisions about how to implement or improve it. During formative evaluation, information is collected and then fed back to program designers and administrators to enhance program development and maximize the success of the intervention. For example, formative evaluation may be carried out through a pilot project before a program is implemented at several sites. A pilot study of a community-based organization (CBO), for example, might be used to gather data on problems involving access to and recruitment of targeted populations and the utilization and implementation of services; the findings of such a study would then be used to modify (if needed) the planned program.

Another example of formative evaluation is the use of a "story board" design of a TV message that has yet to be produced. A story board is a series of text and sketches of camera shots that are to be produced in a commercial. To evaluate the effectiveness of the message and forecast some of the consequences of actually broadcasting it to the general public, an advertising agency convenes small groups of people to react to and comment on the proposed design.

Once an intervention has been implemented, the next stage of evaluation is *process evaluation,* which addresses two broad questions: "What was done?" and "To whom, and how?" Ordinarily, process evaluation is carried out at some point in the life of a project to determine how and how well the delivery goals of the program are being met. When intervention programs continue over a long period of time (as is the case for some of the major AIDS prevention programs), measurements at several times are warranted to ensure that the components of the intervention continue to be delivered by the right people, to the right people, in the right manner, and at the right time. Process evaluation can also play a role in improving interventions by providing the information necessary to change delivery strategies or program objectives in a changing epidemic.

Research designs for process evaluation include direct observation of projects, surveys of service providers and clients, and the monitoring of administrative records. The panel notes that the Centers for Disease Control (CDC) is already collecting some administrative records on its counseling and testing program and community-based projects. The panel believes that this type of evaluation should be a continuing and expanded component of intervention projects to guarantee the maintenance of the projects' integrity and responsiveness to their constituencies.

The purpose of *outcome evaluation* is to identify consequences and to establish that consequences are, indeed, attributable to a project. This type of evaluation answers the questions, "What outcomes were observed?" and, perhaps more importantly, "What do the outcomes mean?" Like process evaluation, outcome evaluation can also be conducted at intervals during an ongoing program, and the panel believes that such periodic evaluation should be done to monitor goal achievement.

The panel believes that these stages of evaluation (i.e., formative, process, and outcome) are essential to learning how AIDS prevention programs contribute to containing the epidemic. After a body of findings has been accumulated from such evaluations, it may be fruitful to launch another stage of evaluation: *cost-effectiveness analysis* (see Weinstein et al., 1989). Like outcome evaluation, cost-effectiveness analysis also measures program effectiveness, but it extends the analysis by adding a measure of program cost. The panel believes that consideration of cost-effective analysis should be postponed until more experience is gained with formative, process, and outcome evaluation of the CDC AIDS prevention programs.

EVALUATION RESEARCH DESIGN

Process and outcome evaluations require different types of research designs, as discussed below. Formative evaluations, which are intended to both assess implementation and forecast effects, use a mix of these designs.

Process Evaluation Designs

To conduct process evaluations on how well services are delivered, data need to be gathered on the content of interventions and on their delivery systems. Suggested methodologies include direct observation, surveys, and record keeping.

Direct observation designs include case studies, in which participant-observers unobtrusively and systematically record encounters within a program setting, and nonparticipant observation, in which long, open-ended (or "focused") interviews are conducted with program participants.[1] For example, "professional customers" at counseling and testing sites can act as project clients to monitor activities unobtrusively;[2] alternatively, nonparticipant observers can interview both staff and clients. *Surveys*—either censuses (of the whole population of interest) or samples—elicit information through interviews or questionnaires completed by project participants or potential users of a project. For example, surveys within community-based projects can collect basic statistical information on project objectives, what services are provided, to whom, when, how often, for how long, and in what context.

Record keeping consists of administrative or other reporting systems that monitor use of services. Standardized reporting ensures consistency in the scope and depth of data collected. To use the media campaign as an example, the panel suggests using standardized data on the use of the AIDS hotline to monitor public attentiveness to the advertisements broadcast by the media campaign.

---

[1] On occasion, nonparticipants observe behavior during or after an intervention. Chapter 3 introduces this option in the context of formative evaluation.

[2] The use of professional customers can raise serious concerns in the eyes of project administrators at counseling and testing sites. The panel believes that site administrators should receive advance notification that professional customers may visit their sites for testing and counseling services and provide their consent before this method of data collection is used.

These designs are simple to understand, but they require expertise to implement. For example, observational studies must be conducted by people who are well trained in how to carry out on-site tasks sensitively and to record their findings uniformly. Observers can either complete narrative accounts of what occurred in a service setting or they can complete some sort of data inventory to ensure that multiple aspects of service delivery are covered. These types of studies are time consuming and benefit from corroboration among several observers. The use of surveys in research is well-understood, although they, too, require expertise to be well implemented. As the program chapters reflect, survey data collection must be carefully designed to reduce problems of validity and reliability and, if samples are used, to design an appropriate sampling scheme. Record keeping or service inventories are probably the easiest research designs to implement, although preparing standardized internal forms requires attention to detail about salient aspects of service delivery.

Outcome Evaluation Designs

Research designs for outcome evaluations are meant to assess principal and relative effects. Ideally, to assess the effect of an intervention on program participants, one would like to know what would have happened to the same participants in the absence of the program. Because it is not possible to make this comparison directly, inference strategies that rely on proxies have to be used. Scientists use three general approaches to construct proxies for use in the comparisons required to evaluate the effects of interventions: (1) nonexperimental methods, (2) quasi-experiments, and (3) randomized experiments. The first two are discussed below, and randomized experiments are discussed in the subsequent section.

Nonexperimental and Quasi-Experimental Designs[3]

The most common form of nonexperimental design is a before-and-after study. In this design, pre-intervention measurements are compared with equivalent measurements made after the intervention to detect change in the outcome variables that the intervention was designed to influence.

Although the panel finds that before-and-after studies frequently provide helpful insights, the panel believes that these studies do not provide sufficiently reliable information to be the cornerstone for evaluation research on the effectiveness of AIDS prevention programs. The panel's

---

[3]Parts of this section are adopted from Turner, Miller, and Moses, (1989:324-326).

conclusion follows from the fact that the postintervention changes cannot usually be attributed unambiguously to the intervention.[4] Plausible competing explanations for differences between pre- and postintervention measurements will often be numerous, including not only the possible effects of other AIDS intervention programs, news stories, and local events, but also the effects that may result from the maturation of the participants and the educational or sensitizing effects of repeated measurements, among others.

Quasi-experimental and matched control designs provide a separate comparison group. In these designs, the control group may be selected by matching nonparticipants to participants in the treatment group on the basis of selected characteristics. It is difficult to ensure the comparability of the two groups even when they are matched on many characteristics because other relevant factors may have been overlooked or mismatched or they may be difficult to measure (e.g., the motivation to change behavior). In some situations, it may simply be impossible to measure all of the characteristics of the units (e.g., communities) that may affect outcomes, much less demonstrate their comparability.

Matched control designs require extraordinarily comprehensive scientific knowledge about the phenomenon under investigation in order for evaluators to be confident that all of the relevant determinants of outcomes have been properly accounted for in the matching. Three types of information or knowledge are required: (1) knowledge of intervening variables that also affect the outcome of the intervention and, consequently, need adjustment to make the groups comparable; (2) measurements on all intervening variables for all subjects; and (3) knowledge of how to make the adjustments properly, which in turn requires an understanding of the functional relationship between the intervening variables and the outcome variables. Satisfying each of these information requirements is likely to be more difficult than answering the primary evaluation question, "Does this intervention produce beneficial effects?"

Given the size and the national importance of AIDS intervention programs and given the state of current knowledge about behavior change in general and AIDS prevention, in particular, the panel believes that it would be unwise to rely on matching and adjustment strategies as the primary design for evaluating AIDS intervention programs. With differently constituted groups, inferences about results are hostage to uncertainty about the extent to which the observed outcome actually

---

[4]This weakness has been noted by CDC in a sourcebook provided to its HIV intervention project grantees (CDC, 1988:F-14).

results from the intervention and is not an artifact of intergroup differences that may not have been removed by matching or adjustment.

Randomized Experiments

A remedy to the inferential uncertainties that afflict nonexperimental designs is provided by *randomized experiments*. In such experiments, one singly constituted group is established for study. A subset of the group is then randomly chosen to receive the intervention, with the other subset becoming the control. The two groups are not identical, but they are comparable. Because they are two *random* samples drawn from the same population, they are not systematically different in any respect, which is important for all variables—both known and unknown—that can influence the outcome. Dividing a singly constituted group into two random and therefore comparable subgroups cuts through the tangle of causation and establishes a basis for the valid comparison of respondents who do and do not receive the intervention. Randomized experiments provide for clear causal inference by solving the problem of group comparability, and may be used to answer the evaluation questions "Does the intervention work?" and "What works better?"

Which question is answered depends on whether the controls receive an intervention or not. When the object is to estimate whether a given intervention has any effects, individuals are randomly assigned to the project or to a zero-treatment control group. The control group may be put on a waiting list or simply not get the treatment. This design addresses the question, "Does it work?"

When the object is to compare variations on a project—e.g., individual counseling sessions versus group counseling—then individuals are randomly assigned to these two regimens, and there is no zero-treatment control group. This design addresses the question, "What works better?" In either case, the control groups must be followed up as rigorously as the experimental groups.

Rationale. A randomized experiment requires that individuals, organizations, or other treatment units be randomly assigned to one of two or more treatments or program variations. Random assignment ensures that the estimated differences between the groups so constituted are statistically unbiased; that is, that any differences in effects measured between them are a result of treatment. The absence of statistical bias in groups constituted in this fashion stems from the fact that random assignment ensures that there are no systematic differences between them, differences that can and usually do affect groups composed in ways that are not random.[5] The panel believes this approach is far superior for outcome evaluations of AIDS interventions than the nonrandom and quasi-experimental approaches. Therefore,

To improve interventions that are already broadly implemented, the panel recommends the use of randomized field experiments of alternative or enhanced interventions.

Under certain conditions, the panel also endorses randomized field experiments with a nontreatment control group to evaluate new interventions. In the context of a deadly epidemic, ethics dictate that treatment not be withheld simply for the purpose of conducting an experiment. Nevertheless, there may be times when a randomized field test of a new treatment with a no-treatment control group is worthwhile. One such time is during the design phase of a major or national intervention.

Before a new intervention is broadly implemented, the panel recommends that it be pilot tested in a randomized field experiment.

The panel considered the use of experiments with delayed rather than no treatment. A delayed-treatment control group strategy might be pursued when resources are too scarce for an intervention to be widely distributed at one time. For example, a project site that is waiting to receive funding for an intervention would be designated as the control group. If it is possible to randomize which projects in the queue receive the intervention, an evaluator could measure and compare outcomes after the experimental group had received the new treatment but before the control group received it. The panel believes that such a design can be applied only in limited circumstances, such as when groups would have access to related services in their communities and that conducting the study was likely to lead to greater access or better services. For example, a study cited in Chapter 4 used a randomized delayed-treatment experiment to measure the effects of a community-based risk reduction program. However, such a strategy may be impractical for several reasons, including:

- sites waiting for funding for an intervention might seek resources from another source;
- it might be difficult to enlist the nonfunded site and its clients to participate in the study;

---

[5]The significance tests applied to experimental outcomes calculate the probability that any observed differences between the sample estimates might result from random variations between the groups.

- there could be an appearance of favoritism toward projects whose funding was not delayed.

Pitfalls. Although randomized experiments have many benefits, the approach is not without pitfalls. In the planning stages of evaluation, it is necessary to contemplate certain hazards, such as the Hawthorne effect[6] and differential project dropout rates. Precautions must be taken either to prevent these problems or to measure their effects. Fortunately, there is some evidence suggesting that the Hawthorne effect is usually not very large (Rossi and Freeman, 1982:175-176).

Attrition is potentially more damaging to an evaluation, and it must be limited if the experimental design is to be preserved. If sample attrition is not limited in an experimental design, it becomes necessary to account for the potentially biasing impact of the loss of subjects in the treatment and control conditions of the experiment. The statistical adjustments required to make inferences about treatment effectiveness in such circumstances can introduce uncertainties that are as worrisome as those afflicting nonexperimental and quasi-experimental designs. Thus, the panel's recommendation of the selective use of randomized design carries an implicit caveat: To realize the theoretical advantages offered by randomized experimental designs, substantial efforts will be required to ensure that the designs are not compromised by flawed execution.

Another pitfall to randomization is its appearance of unfairness or unattractiveness to participants and the controversial legal and ethical issues it sometimes raises. Often, what is being criticized is the control of project assignment of participants rather than the use of randomization itself. In deciding whether random assignment is appropriate, it is important to consider the specific context of the evaluation and how participants would be assigned to projects in the absence of randomization. The Federal Judicial Center (1981) offers five threshold conditions for the use of random assignment.

- Does present practice or policy need improvement?
- Is there significant uncertainty about the value of the proposed regimen?
- Are there acceptable alternatives to randomized experiments?
- Will the results of the experiment be used to improve practice or policy?

---

[6]Research participants' knowledge that they were being observed had a positive effect on their responses in a series of famous studies made at General Electric's Hawthorne Works in Chicago (Roethlisberger and Dickson, 1939); the phenomenon is referred to as the Hawthorne effect.

- Is there a reasonable protection against risk for vulnerable groups (i.e., individuals within the justice system)?

The parent committee has argued that these threshold conditions apply in the case of AIDS prevention programs (see Turner, Miller, and Moses, 1989:331-333).

Although randomization may be desirable from an evaluation and ethical standpoint, and acceptable from a legal standpoint, it may be difficult to implement from a practical or political standpoint. Again, the panel emphasizes that questions about the practical or political feasibility of the use of randomization may in fact refer to the control of program allocation rather than to the issues of randomization itself. In fact, when resources are scarce, it is often more ethical and politically palatable to randomize allocation rather than to allocate on grounds that may appear biased.

It is usually easier to defend the use of randomization when the choice has to do with assignment to groups receiving *alternative* services than when the choice involves assignment to groups receiving no treatment. For example, in comparing a testing and counseling intervention that offered a special "skills training" session in addition to its regular services with a counseling and testing intervention that offered no additional component, random assignment of participants to one group rather than another may be acceptable to program staff and participants because the relative values of the alternative interventions are unknown.

The more difficult issue is the introduction of new interventions that are perceived to be needed and effective in a situation in which there are no services. An argument that is sometimes offered against the use of randomization in this instance is that interventions should be assigned on the basis of need (perhaps as measured by rates of HIV incidence or of high-risk behaviors). But this argument presumes that the intervention will have a positive effect—which is unknown before evaluation—and that relative need can be established, which is a difficult task in itself.

The panel recognizes that community and political opposition to randomization to zero treatments may be strong and that enlisting participation in such experiments may be difficult. This opposition and reluctance could seriously jeopardize the production of reliable results if it is translated into noncompliance with a research design. The feasibility of randomized experiments for AIDS prevention programs has already been demonstrated, however (see the review of selected experiments in Turner, Miller, and Moses, 1989:327-329). The substantial effort involved in mounting randomized field experiments is repaid by the fact that they can provide unbiased evidence of the effects of a program.

Unit of Assignment. The unit of assignment of an experiment may be an individual person, a clinic (i.e., the clientele of the clinic), or another organizational unit (e.g., the community or city). The treatment unit is selected at the earliest stage of design. Variations of units are illustrated in the following four examples of intervention programs.

1. Two different pamphlets (A and B) on the same subject (e.g., testing) are distributed in an alternating sequence to individuals calling an AIDS hotline. The outcome to be measured is whether the recipient returns a card asking for more information.

2. Two instruction curricula (A and B) about AIDS and HIV infections are prepared for use in high school driver education classes. The outcome to be measured is a score on a knowledge test.

3. Of all clinics for sexually transmitted diseases (STDs) in a large metropolitan area, some are randomly chosen to introduce a change in the fee schedule. The outcome to be measured is the change in patient load.

4. A coordinated set of community-wide interventions—involving community leaders, social service agencies, the media, community associations and other groups—is implemented in one area of a city. Outcomes are knowledge as assessed by testing at drug treatment centers and STD clinics and condom sales in the community's retail outlets.

In example (1), the treatment unit is an individual *person* who receives pamphlet A or pamphlet B. If either "treatment" is applied again, it would be applied to a person. In example (2), the high school *class* is the treatment unit; everyone in a given class experiences either curriculum A or curriculum B. If either treatment is applied again, it would be applied to a class. The treatment unit is the *clinic* in example (3), and in example (4), the treatment unit is a *community.*

The consistency of the effects of a particular intervention across repetitions justly carries a heavy weight in appraising the intervention. It is important to remember that repetitions of a treatment or intervention are the number of treatment units to which the intervention is applied. This is a salient principle in the design and execution of intervention programs as well as in the assessment of their results.

The adequacy of the proposed sample size (number of treatment units) has to be considered in advance. Adequacy depends mainly on two factors:

- How much variation occurs from unit to unit among units receiving a common treatment? If that variation is large, then the number of units needs to be large.

- What is the minimum size of a possible treatment difference that, if present, would be practically important? That is, how small a treatment difference is it essential to detect if it is present? The smaller this quantity, the larger the number of units that are necessary.

Many formal methods for considering and choosing sample size exist (see, e.g., Cohen, 1988). Practical circumstances occasionally allow choosing between designs that involve units at different levels; thus, a classroom might be the unit if the treatment is applied in one way, but an entire school might be the unit if the treatment is applied in another. When both approaches are feasible, the use of a power analysis for each approach may lead to a reasoned choice.

Choice of Methods

There is some controversy about the advantages of randomized experiments in comparison with other evaluative approaches. It is the panel's belief that when a (well executed) randomized study is feasible, it is superior to alternative kinds of studies in the strength and clarity of whatever conclusions emerge, primarily because the experimental approach avoids selection biases.[7] Other evaluation approaches are sometimes unavoidable, but ordinarily the accumulation of valid information will go more slowly and less securely than in randomized approaches.

Experiments in medical research shed light on the advantages of carefully conducted randomized experiments. The Salk vaccine trials are a successful example of a large, randomized study. In a double-blind test of the polio vaccine,[8] children in various communities were randomly assigned to two treatments, either the vaccine or a placebo. By this method, the effectiveness of Salk vaccine was demonstrated in one summer of research (Meier, 1957).

A sufficient accumulation of relevant, observational information, especially when collected in studies using different procedures and sample populations, may also clearly demonstrate the effectiveness of a treatment or intervention. The process of accumulating such information can

---

[7]Participants who self-select into a program are likely to be different from non-random comparison groups in terms of interests, motivations, values, abilities, and other attributes that can bias the outcomes.

[8]A double-blind test is one in which neither the person receiving the treatment nor the person administering it knows which treatment (or when no treatment) is being given.

be a long one, however. When a (well-executed) randomized study is feasible, it can provide evidence that is subject to less uncertainty in its interpretation, and it can often do so in a more timely fashion. In the midst of an epidemic, the panel believes it proper that randomized experiments be one of the primary strategies for evaluating the effectiveness of AIDS prevention efforts. In making this recommendation, however, the panel also wishes to emphasize that the advantages of the randomized experimental design can be squandered by poor execution (e.g., by compromised assignment of subjects, significant subject attrition rates, etc.). To achieve the advantages of the experimental design, care must be taken to ensure that the integrity of the design is not compromised by poor execution.

In proposing that randomized experiments be one of the primary strategies for evaluating the effectiveness of AIDS prevention programs, the panel also recognizes that there are situations in which randomization will be impossible or, for other reasons, cannot be used. In its next report the panel will describe at length appropriate nonexperimental strategies to be considered in situations in which an experiment is not a practical or desirable alternative.

THE MANAGEMENT OF EVALUATION

Conscientious evaluation requires a considerable investment of funds, time, and personnel. Because the panel recognizes that resources are not unlimited, it suggests that they be concentrated on the evaluation of a subset of projects to maximize the return on investment and to enhance the likelihood of high-quality results.

Project Selection

Deciding which programs or sites to evaluate is by no means a trivial matter. Selection should be carefully weighed so that projects that are not replicable or that have little chance for success are not subjected to rigorous evaluations.

The panel recommends that any intensive evaluation of an intervention be conducted on a subset of projects selected according to explicit criteria. These criteria should include the replicability of the project, the feasibility of evaluation, and the project's potential effectiveness for prevention of HIV transmission.

If a project is replicable, it means that the particular circumstances of service delivery in that project can be duplicated. In other words, for

CBOs and counseling and testing projects, the content and setting of an intervention can be duplicated across sites. Feasibility of evaluation means that, as a practical matter, the research can be done: that is, the research design is adequate to control for rival hypotheses, it is not excessively costly, and the project is acceptable to the community and the sponsor. Potential effectiveness for HIV prevention means that the intervention is at least based on a reasonable theory (or mix of theories) about behavioral change (e.g., social learning theory [Bandura, 1977], the health belief model [Janz and Becker, 1984], etc.), if it has not already been found to be effective in related circumstances.

In addition, since it is important to ensure that the results of evaluations will be broadly applicable,

The panel recommends that evaluation be conducted and replicated across major types of subgroups, programs, and settings. Attention should be paid to geographic areas with low and high AIDS prevalence, as well as to subpopulations at low and high risk for AIDS.

Research Administration

The sponsoring agency interested in evaluating an AIDS intervention should consider the mechanisms through which the research will be carried out as well as the desirability of both independent oversight and agency in-house conduct and monitoring of the research. The appropriate entities and mechanisms for conducting evaluations depend to some extent on the kinds of data being gathered and the evaluation questions being asked.

Oversight and monitoring are important to keep projects fully informed about the other evaluations relevant to their own and to render assistance when needed. Oversight and monitoring are also important because evaluation is often a sensitive issue for project and evaluation staff alike. The panel is aware that evaluation may appear threatening to practitioners and researchers because of the possibility that evaluation research will show that their projects are not as effective as they believe them to be. These needs and vulnerabilities should be taken into account as evaluation research management is developed.

Conducting the Research

To conduct some aspects of a project's evaluation, it may be appropriate to involve project administrators, especially when the data will be used to evaluate delivery systems (e.g., to determine when and which services are being delivered). To evaluate outcomes, the services of an outside evaluator[9] or evaluation team are almost always required because few practitioners have the necessary professional experience or the time and resources necessary to do evaluation. The outside evaluator must have relevant expertise in evaluation research methodology and must also be sensitive to the fears, hopes, and constraints of project administrators.

Several evaluation management schemes are possible. For example, a prospective AIDS prevention project group (the contractor) can bid on a contract for project funding that includes an intensive evaluation component. The actual evaluation can be conducted either by the contractor alone or by the contractor working in concert with an outside independent collaborator. This mechanism has the advantage of involving project practitioners in the work of evaluation as well as building separate but mutually informing communities of experts around the country. Alternatively, a contract can be let with a single evaluator or evaluation team that will collaborate with the subset of sites that is chosen for evaluation. This variation would be managerially less burdensome than awarding separate contracts, but it would require greater dependence on the expertise of a single investigator or investigative team. (Appendix A discusses contracting options in greater depth.) Both of these approaches accord with the parent committee's recommendation that collaboration between practitioners and evaluation researchers be ensured. Finally, in the more traditional evaluation approach, independent principal investigators or investigative teams may respond to a request for proposal (RFP) issued to evaluate individual projects. Such investigators are frequently university-based or are members of a professional research organization, and they bring to the task a variety of research experiences and perspectives.

Independent Oversight

The panel believes that coordination and oversight of multisite evaluations is critical because of the variability in investigators' expertise and in the results of the projects being evaluated. Oversight can provide quality control for individual investigators and can be used to review and integrate findings across sites for developing policy. The independence of an oversight body is crucial to ensure that project evaluations do not succumb to the pressures for positive findings of effectiveness.

When evaluation is to be conducted by a number of different evaluation teams, the panel recommends establishing

---

[9] As discussed under "Agency In-House Team," the outside evaluator might be one of CDC's personnel. However, given the large amount of research to be done, it is likely that non-CDC evaluators will also need to be used.

an independent scientific committee to oversee project selection and research efforts, corroborate the impartiality and validity of results, conduct cross-site analyses, and prepare reports on the progress of the evaluations.

The composition of such an independent oversight committee will depend on the research design of a given program. For example, the committee ought to include statisticians and other specialists in randomized field tests when that approach is being taken. Specialists in survey research and case studies should be recruited if either of those approaches is to be used. Appendix B offers a model for an independent oversight group that has been successfully implemented in other settings—a project review team, or advisory board.

Agency In-House Team

As the parent committee noted in its report, evaluations of AIDS interventions require skills that may be in short supply for agencies invested in delivering services (Turner, Miller, and Moses, 1989:349). Although this situation can be partly alleviated by recruiting professional outside evaluators and retaining an independent oversight group, the panel believes that an in-house team of professionals within the sponsoring agency is also critical. The in-house experts will interact with the outside evaluators and provide input into the selection of projects, outcome objectives, and appropriate research designs; they will also monitor the progress and costs of evaluation. These functions require not just bureaucratic oversight but appropriate scientific expertise.

This is not intended to preclude the direct involvement of CDC staff in *conducting* evaluations. However, given the great amount of work to be done, it is likely a considerable portion will have to be contracted out. The quality and usefulness of the evaluations done under contract can be greatly enhanced by ensuring that there are an adequate number of CDC staff trained in evaluation research methods to monitor these contracts.

The panel recommends that CDC recruit and retain behavioral, social, and statistical scientists trained in evaluation methodology to facilitate the implementation of the evaluation research recommended in this report.

Interagency Collaboration

The panel believes that the federal agencies that sponsor the design of basic research, intervention programs, and evaluation strategies would profit from greater interagency collaboration. The evaluation of AIDS intervention programs would benefit from a coherent program of studies that should provide models of efficacious and effective interventions to prevent further HIV transmission, the spread of other STDs, and unwanted pregnancies (especially among adolescents). A marriage could then be made of basic and applied science, from which the best evaluation is born. Exploring the possibility of interagency collaboration and CDC's role in such collaboration is beyond the scope of this panel's task, but it is an important issue that we suggest be addressed in the future.

Costs of Evaluation

In view of the dearth of current evaluation efforts, the panel believes that vigorous evaluation research must be undertaken over the next few years to build up a body of knowledge about what interventions can and cannot do. Dedicating no resources to evaluation will virtually guarantee that high-quality evaluations will be infrequent and the data needed for policy decisions will be sparse or absent. Yet, evaluating every project is not feasible simply because there are not enough resources and, in many cases, evaluating every project is not necessary for good science or good policy.

The panel believes that evaluating only some of a program's sites or projects, selected under the criteria noted in Chapter 4, is a sensible strategy. Although we recommend that intensive evaluation be conducted on only a subset of carefully chosen projects, we believe that high-quality evaluation will require a significant investment of time, planning, personnel, and financial support. The panel's aim is to be realistic—not discouraging—when it notes that the costs of program evaluation should not be underestimated. Many of the research strategies proposed in this report require investments that are perhaps greater than has been previously contemplated. This is particularly the case for outcome evaluations, which are ordinarily more difficult and expensive to conduct than formative or process evaluations. And those costs will be additive with each type of evaluation that is conducted.

Panel members have found that the cost of an outcome evaluation sometimes equals or even exceeds the cost of actual program delivery. For example, it was reported to the panel that randomized studies used to evaluate recent manpower training projects cost as much as the projects themselves (see Cottingham and Rodriguez, 1987). In another case, the principal investigator of an ongoing AIDS prevention project told the panel that the cost of randomized experimentation was approximately three times higher than the cost of delivering the intervention (albeit the study was quite small, involving only 104 participants) (Kelly et al., 1989). Fortunately, only a fraction of a program's projects or sites need to be intensively evaluated to produce high-quality information, and not all will require randomized studies.

Because of the variability in kinds of evaluation that will be done as well as in the costs involved, there is no set standard or rule for judging what fraction of a total program budget should be invested in evaluation. Based upon very limited data[10] and assuming that only a small *sample* of projects would be evaluated, the panel suspects that program managers might reasonably anticipate spending 8 to 12 percent of their intervention budgets to conduct high-quality evaluations (i.e., formative, process, and outcome evaluations).[11] Larger investments seem politically infeasible and unwise in view of the need to put resources into program delivery. Smaller investments in evaluation may risk studying an inadequate sample of program types, and it may also invite compromises in research quality.

The nature of the HIV/AIDS epidemic mandates an unwavering commitment to prevention programs, and the prevention activities require a similar commitment to the evaluation of those programs. The magnitude of what can be learned from doing good evaluations will more than balance the magnitude of the costs required to perform them. Moreover, it should be realized that the costs of shoddy research can be substantial, both in their direct expense and in the lost opportunities to identify effective strategies for AIDS prevention. Once the investment has been made, however, and a reservoir of findings and practical experience has accumulated, subsequent evaluations should be easier and less costly to conduct.

REFERENCES

Bandura, A. (1977) Self-efficacy: Toward a unifying theory of behavioral change. *Psychological Review* 34:191-215.

Campbell, D. T., and Stanley, J. C. (1966) *Experimental and Quasi-Experimental Design and Analysis*. Boston: Houghton-Mifflin.

Centers for Disease Control (CDC) (1988) Sourcebook presented at the National Conference on the Prevention of HIV Infection and AIDS Among Racial and Ethnic Minorities in the United States (August).

---

[10]See, for example, chapter 3 which presents cost estimates for evaluations of media campaigns. Similar estimates are not readily available for other program types.

[11]For example, the U. K. Health Education Authority (that country's primary agency for AIDS education and prevention programs) allocates 10 percent of its AIDS budget for research and evaluation of its AIDS programs (D. McVey, Health Education Authority, personal communication, June 1990). This allocation covers both process and outcome evaluation.

Cohen, J. (1988) *Statistical Power Analysis for the Behavioral Sciences.* 2nd ed. Hillsdale, N.J.: L. Erlbaum Associates.

Cook, T., and Campbell, D. T. (1979) *Quasi-Experimentation: Design and Analysis for Field Settings.* Boston: Houghton-Mifflin.

Federal Judicial Center (1981) *Experimentation in the Law.* Washington, D.C.: Federal Judicial Center.

Janz, N. K., and Becker, M. H. (1984) The health belief model: A decade later. *Health Education Quarterly* 11(1):1-47.

Kelly, J. A., St. Lawrence, J. S., Hood, H. V., and Brasfield, T. L. (1989) Behavioral intervention to reduce AIDS risk activities. *Journal of Consulting and Clinical Psychology* 57:60-67.

Meier, P. (1957) Safety testing of poliomyelitis vaccine. *Science* 125(3257): 1067-1071.

Roethlisberger, F. J. and Dickson, W. J. (1939) *Management and the Worker.* Cambridge, Mass.: Harvard University Press.

Rossi, P. H., and Freeman, H. E. (1982) *Evaluation: A Systematic Approach.* 2nd ed. Beverly Hills, Cal.: Sage Publications.

Turner, C. F., Miller, H. G., and Moses, L. E., eds. (1989) *AIDS, Sexual Behavior, and Intravenous Drug Use.* Report of the NRC Committee on AIDS Research and the Behavioral, Social, and Statistical Sciences. Washington, D.C.: National Academy Press.

Weinstein, M. C., Graham, J. D., Siegel, J. E., and Fineberg, H. V. (1989) Cost-effectiveness analysis of AIDS prevention programs: Concepts, complications, and illustrations. In C.F. Turner, H. G. Miller, and L. E. Moses, eds., *AIDS, Sexual Behavior, and Intravenous Drug Use.* Report of the NRC Committee on AIDS Research and the Behavioral, Social, and Statistical Sciences. Washington, D.C.: National Academy Press.

Weiss, C. H. (1972) *Evaluation Research.* Englewood Cliffs, N.J.: Prentice-Hall, Inc.

2

Measurement of Outcomes

Before an evaluation can be designed, the goals of the intervention program must be set. Indeed, goal setting should precede the design and implementation of a program. This chapter provides an overview of goal setting, the strengths and weaknesses of various outcome objectives, and the measurement of outcomes for AIDS prevention programs.

PROGRAM OBJECTIVES

CDC's overall mission has been "to prevent the spread of HIV infection" (CDC, 1989), an objective shared by the three programs of interest here. For the media program, campaign efforts were to be focused on the general population "for an improved understanding of the risk factors [for HIV diffusion, and] . . . for affecting a change in attitude, understanding and behaviour" to result in "curbing the further spread of AIDS and HIV" (Ogilvy & Mather, 1987). The stated national program goals of the new direct grants program that will fund CBOs and the goals of the testing and counseling project network were: (1) to institute surveillance programs; (2) "to reduce the risk of HIV infection and to effect, maintain, measure, and evaluate the significance of behavioral change" among the general population and high-risk groups; and (3) "to inform and educate the general public in order to gain broad support" for HIV prevention programs (CDC, 1988).

The overall goal of reducing the spread of HIV is appropriate from a "big picture" perspective, but as stated it is inadequate as an evaluation objective. First, it is too general: it does not specify how the spread of HIV will be reduced by specific interventions among specific populations and in specific contexts. Furthermore, it is too distant: reducing the rate of HIV transmission is a long-term goal that will have to be measured and remeasured over a long period of time. Finally, focusing on HIV alone can be misleading in some contexts: for example, in a community that begins with zero HIV prevalence, an outcome of zero prevalence following an intervention cannot be taken as evidence of the intervention's effectiveness.

In addition to the overarching goal of eliminating HIV transmission, the panel recommends that explicit objectives be written for each of the major intervention programs and that these objectives be framed as measurable biological, psychological, and behavioral outcomes.

Objectives should be framed as proximate outcomes of behavior—that is, as near-term or intermediate outcomes that are linked to long-term goals. In fact, when an intermediate goal is known to lead to a long-term outcome, the need to evaluate results beyond the first stage is obviated (Weiss, 1972:38-39). The long-term goal, of course, is the elimination of the transmission of HIV, or at least its reduction to a reproductive rate of less than 1.0.[1] As for proximate outcomes, the panel believes that the appropriate, linked, intermediate objectives include (1) accurate knowledge about HIV risks, (2) the reduction of risk behaviors, and (3) the adoption of protective behaviors. Biological outcomes are not on this list because their interpretation is much more problematic than these three (see discussion below). Of these three intermediate objectives, the panel believes that valid and reliable indicators of the frequency of both risk-associated and protective behaviors (the second and third objectives) are the most appropriate proximate outcomes for AIDS prevention efforts. The hope of an intervention program is that any changes that occur as a result of its efforts will show up rapidly in these indicators and that those changes, if maintained, will lead to the achievement of the program's long-term goal of reducing HIV transmission.

Suchman (1967:39-41) has suggested guidelines for goal setting that the panel believes would be helpful to CDC in specifying outcome objectives, including:

- the content of the objective (e.g., whether a goal is to change or to eliminate behaviors);

---

[1] Studies of the dynamics of epidemics of measles and smallpox have demonstrated that the reproductive rate of an infectious disease must exceed 1.0 to sustain an epidemic. When the rate drops below 1.0, the epidemic will dwindle, although small, infected segments of the population may remain. One implication of this fact is that, as a first step toward eliminating AIDS, it is not necessary to prevent all new HIV infections to halt the epidemic spread of HIV.

- the target audience;
- when the change is to take place (i.e., short-term versus long-term changes);
- whether the objectives are unitary or multiple and whether they have potential side effects;
- the desired magnitude of effect; and
- how the objective is to be attained (i.e., the instrumentation of the program).

One of the guidelines Suchman suggests for setting objectives addresses the side effects or unwanted (and sometimes unanticipated) consequences that may attend efforts to achieve a particular goal. Side effects are not a trivial concern, and the panel believes that the negative effects of AIDS interventions should be assessed along with the positive outcomes. Negative side effects—such as excessive fear or psychological distress—can often be anticipated at the time of program design from data derived from comparable studies or from anecdotal evidence.

A side effect that has received attention recently is the impact of AIDS-related stressors on individuals' mental health. In the case of testing and counseling, in particular, there is increasing evidence that for some individuals, learning about one's seropositivity is associated with certain types of psychological distress symptoms (e.g., anxiety, anger, depression, sexual dysfunction) and other untoward effects (e.g., disruption of one's partner relationship, increased illicit drug use); see, for example, Coates, Morin, and McKusick (1987), Grant and Anns (1988), Ostrow et al. (1988), Martin et al. (1989). It is generally not the test itself that is the source of the distress; rather, it is the message an individual receives that he or she has tested positive for HIV and is susceptible to developing a fatal disease.[2] How to deliver this message and provide the requisite emotional support and medical referral deserve serious attention.

The panel recommends that all evaluation protocols provide for the assessment of potential harmful effects as well as the assessment of desired effects.

In the following section the panel discusses a variety of project objectives that are suitable outcomes for HIV/AIDS prevention programs, along with the strengths and weaknesses of each.

---

[2]The test itself may be a culprit in certain cases in which it is taken involuntarily, such as in a drug treatment center, hospital, or prison. More attention to negative effects is thus warranted in the case of involuntary testing.

OUTCOMES FOR EVALUATIONS OF
HIV PREVENTION PROGRAMS

There are a wide range of possible evaluation outcome variables, the choice of which will vary among projects. For example, the cognitive or behavioral outcomes that are appropriate to a counseling and testing session at a gay men's health clinic will be different from those associated with an information program offered in a drug treatment center. The objective for the former project may be abstinence from anal intercourse; for the latter project, it may be the adoption of using bleach with drug paraphernalia. The specific objective or objectives selected by a community-based organization or a testing and counseling center should be consonant with the overarching goal of reduced HIV transmission, but this does not mean that they must or should be identical from project to project. Indeed, the panel believes that CDC should seek advice from project staffs and communities concerning potential outcome variables.

We discuss potential outcome variables in three categories: biological, behavioral, and psychological. Before discussing the strengths and weaknesses of each type of outcome, the variables in each category are described below. Table 2-1 summarizes the evaluation outcome measures discussed in the following pages.

Biological Outcomes

New HIV infection (in the form of seroconversion rates in specific populations) is the most informative biological outcome variable to indicate the spread of the disease among adults or adolescents. This variable is quite appealing as an outcome measure because it relates directly to the overarching goal of CDC's prevention programs. If reliable data from representative samples of the target populations could be collected, HIV incidence rates might prove to be useful indicators of program effectiveness. However, incidence data on HIV infection must be used with caution because so many factors other than risk reduction efforts—such as the saturation of the virus in a given population—influence these rates.

While incidence rates for AIDS might also be used, they could lead to faulty inferences because they reflect HIV infections contracted several years prior to the onset of the disease. The most recent estimated mean incubation period for AIDS is 9.8 years (Longini et al., 1989), and even this estimate may be revised upward as new cases and longer latencies are recorded. Rates of sexually transmitted diseases (STDs) may also be useful, as they should respond (other things being equal) to changes in sexual behaviors that risk HIV transmission. Moreover, data on STD rates may be useful for validating self-reported behavior changes. Like

TABLE 2-1   Summary of Possible Evaluation Outcome Measures

I. Biological Outcomes

A. Incidence of HIV infection

B. Fertility rate

C. Incidence of sexually transmitted diseases

II. Behavioral Outcomes

A. Primary prevention behaviors
1. Elimination of risk behaviors
   a. Abstinence from all sexual contact
   b. Abstinence from all IV drug use
   c. Avoidance of anal and vaginal intercourse
   d. Avoidance of unsterilized IV drug injection equipment
   e. Avoidance of pregnancy by HIV-positive women
2. Reduction of risk behaviors
   a. Monogamy
   b. Avoidance of anonymous and extradomestic sex
   c. Avoidance of "shooting galleries"
3. Protective behaviors
   a. Use of condoms
   b. Use of anti-HIV spermicides
   c. Use of bleach for cleaning IV drug paraphernalia
   d. Participation in needle exchange program

B. Complementary prevention behaviors
1. HIV antibody counseling
2. HIV antibody testing
3. Enrolling in drug treatment programs
4. Determining HIV status of sexual or drug partners
5. Providing names of contacts to public health agents
6. Using family planning services
7. Personal involvement in HIV prevention program

III. Psychological outcomes

A. Awareness of AIDS and HIV

B. Knowledge of AIDS and HIV transmission modes

C. Stigmatization of persons with AIDS and HIV infection

seroconversion data, however, STD rates must be viewed with some caution, since many other factors influence these rates.

Fertility rates may also be reasonable biological measures for evaluating AIDS prevention efforts aimed at certain samples of women, e.g. those who are seropositive or at high risk of infection such as intravenous drug users or the sexual partners of intravenous drug users.

Strengths and Weaknesses of Biological Outcomes

Using serological data on HIV infection as the primary outcome of an evaluation effort seems intuitively appealing. After all, HIV infection is exactly what one wants to prevent. In addition, the approach to evaluation using HIV infections as the outcome variable of interest seems straightforward: to the extent that there are fewer new cases of infection among people involved in an intervention program, compared with an equivalent group of people who were not involved, one would conclude that the prevention campaign was effective; to the extent that the incidence rates of HIV infection were similar in both groups, one would conclude that the interventions had no effect.

But the use of these data is often problematic. There must be a certain level of occurrence of a particular event (i.e., seroconversions, or the change from HIV negative to HIV positive) before statistical tests can determine whether a particular program is effective. HIV seroconversion is a relatively rare event, even in the highest risk populations in the United States. Seroconversion among urban gay men was in the range of 0.5-2.0 percent per year as of 1987. Among East Coast IV drug users, the rate was probably as high as 3.0-7.0 percent per year, as of 1987.[3] With such low rates of occurrence, evaluation requires extremely large samples and long intervals of time before there are enough occurrences of the event to conduct statistical tests of program effectiveness. Such evaluation studies must use a longitudinal cohort study design to establish a fixed denominator of susceptible individuals for all treatment and control groups. This type of design may require the screening of thousands of individuals to assemble a sufficiently large HIV-negative cohort, a process that requires great time and expense. In addition, once screening and study enrollment have been accomplished, reevaluation and tracing procedures must be implemented. Like screening, these tasks are highly labor intensive, and they will be very expensive and time-consuming if sample sizes must be very large.

---

[3]These rates contrast sharply with those in other countries such as Thailand, where seroconversion rates of more than 2 percent *per month* have been observed recently among IV drug users.

Another factor that argues for limiting the number of evaluation studies that rely on HIV seroconversion as an outcome is that such studies tend to focus primarily on those who are uninfected. Although the goal of HIV prevention efforts is to keep people uninfected, a significant determinant of a person's remaining HIV negative involves the behavior of those who are infected—that is, HIV-positive individuals. To maximize prevention of HIV infection, intervention efforts should not be limited only to the uninfected but should include all members of a population. Hence, the use of seroconversion as an outcome measure excludes a part of the population that should be included in prevention programs.

Despite these substantial reservations, however, there may be instances in which HIV seroconversion is a major variable of interest in an evaluation.[4] One example would be a study of transmission rates among couples in which one partner was seropositive. In those cases, it is advisable to include a range of sound behavioral measures in the study protocols. This approach will not only allow the detection of biological program effects but will also help in interpreting and understanding the reasons for the presence or absence of such effects.

Sexually transmitted and blood-borne diseases that occur with higher incidence rates than HIV can sometimes provide a biological outcome of practical value in the evaluation of AIDS prevention programs. The logic for the use of other STDs as outcome measures is that the behavioral changes that protect individuals against HIV will also protect against gonorrhea, syphilis, chlamydia, hepatitis, and similar diseases. But for these outcomes, too, low incidence rates may require use of relatively large samples or long periods of follow-up. However, the incidence rates for these diseases are generally much higher than for HIV, and in some populations the frequency of such infection can be quite high; see, for example, Strobino's (1987:94-105) review of STD infections among adolescents.

In considering the use of other STDs and blood-borne infections as outcomes, two considerations are important. First, evaluations using such outcome measures will ordinarily require scheduling clinical examinations or serological testing of the individuals taking part in the study.

---

[4] The panel notes a number of large cohort studies are currently monitoring HIV seroconversion rates among high-risk groups in the United States. Many of these studies include components that assess knowledge, beliefs, coping, social skills, psychological factors, and social supports, as well as other variables of interest. However, most of these studies are funded as scientific projects by specific biomedical agencies (such as the National Institute of Allergy and Infectious Diseases) rather than as efforts to protect the public health. Thus, seroconversion rates are being carefully monitored, as are their potential determinants. These studies are valuable, and the panel notes that the aging cohorts might well be supplemented with new recruits to enhance the usefulness of their data.

Official STD statistics are not appropriate for use in program evaluations since they do not identify the individuals who have been exposed to particular AIDS prevention programs. (These statistics also vary in quality from locale to locale.) Second, interpreting changes in STD rates can be difficult without reliable data on the behaviors that place individuals at risk of infection and data on trends over time in the prevalence of infection in the local community. It is possible, for example, for an increase in STD rates to occur in a group under study despite declines in their frequency of risky behavior. This seemingly paradoxical outcome can result from rising STD rates in the population at large, which masks the protective effect of behavioral change in a target group. In this situation, fewer episodes of risky behavior enacted with partners who are more likely to be infected may result in an increased overall risk of infection.

Behavioral Outcomes

The list of possible behavioral outcomes for evaluating HIV prevention programs is quite extensive and can be subdivided in a number of ways. The first main distinction is between those behaviors that have a direct influence on the risk of acquiring HIV infection and those that have an indirect influence. The former can be called primary prevention behaviors because adopting or not adopting them has a direct bearing on an individual's chances of infection. The latter can be called complementary prevention behaviors because they increase the likelihood of engaging in primary prevention behaviors but do not themselves alter the risk of infection.

A further useful distinction can be made among primary prevention behaviors between those behaviors that eliminate or reduce the risk of infection and those that increase the ability to protect against infection. Eliminating or reducing risk generally involves the elimination of a behavior from the behavioral repertoire; increasing protection involves adding a new behavior. Each of these processes is psychologically distinct in terms of the skills required, and each of them may require different types of intervention or prevention programs. Even if both the acquisition and elimination of behaviors are included in a prevention program, the standards used to evaluate the effectiveness of the program (e.g., what size of effect will be considered important) may vary, depending on whether the focus is on risk reduction or increased protection.

Primary Prevention Behaviors

Risk Reduction. The first group of behaviors that have a direct influence on HIV transmission includes anal and vaginal intercourse; the use of le drug injection equipment; and pregnancy for women who are ͻpositive.[5] These behaviors account for more than 96 percent of ... new cases of HIV infection occurring worldwide, and they are the central means by which the infection is passed from person to person. Any infected individual who avoids these three behaviors virtually eliminates the possibility that he or she will transmit HIV to an uninfected person; any uninfected individual who avoids these behaviors virtually eliminates the possibility that he or she will acquire HIV from an infected person.

A second group of direct behaviors that may be of interest in evaluation research on HIV prevention programs involve the partial elimination of risk. These behaviors include monogamy; avoidance of extradomestic sexual activity (e.g., sex in bathhouses, backroom bars, and so on); and avoidance of drug "shooting galleries." However, these behavioral outcomes are not as useful or informative as those involving intercourse, shared drug injection equipment, and pregnancy because the extent to which they actually contribute to a person's risk reduction depends on the characteristics of his or her sexual or drug shooting partners and on the particular behaviors in which all of these individuals engage.

Protective Behaviors. A third set of behaviors that bear directly on HIV transmission emphasizes increased protection against risk rather than the elimination or reduction of risk-taking activity. These behaviors include the use of barrier contraception (condoms) during anal or vaginal intercourse; the use of anti-HIV agents (contained in some spermicides); the cleaning of injection equipment with bleach and water prior to use; and participation in a needle exchange program. The adoption of these behaviors are only important among those individuals who continue to engage in the primary HIV risk behaviors— anal or vaginal intercourse or drug injection.

Complementary Prevention Behaviors

As defined above, complementary prevention behaviors have an indirect bearing on HIV transmission risk. By increasing an individual's chances of either practicing risk elimination or risk reduction behavior or of engaging in protective behavior; they do not in themselves reduce an individual's risk of acquiring or transmitting the virus. Nevertheless, these behaviors may be important as evaluation outcomes of HIV prevention programs. Complementary prevention behaviors include HIV antibody counseling; HIV antibody testing; enrollment in a drug treatment program; informing sexual and drug partners of one's HIV status; providing

---

[5]Pregnancy, of course, is a condition, not a behavior. It is used here as shorthand for the behaviors that constitute the risk of transmission of HIV from an infected mother to an unborn child.

names of drug and sexual contacts to public health officials; the use of family planning services; and personal involvement in or establishment of an HIV prevention program.

Some of these complementary prevention behaviors are themselves part of a prevention or intervention program that is in need of evaluation. For example, there is currently great interest in evaluating whether HIV counseling and testing programs help people to reduce risk or to practice protection. There have been similar calls for assessing whether partner notification (of sexual or drug partners) helps to prevent HIV infection. Despite the lack of empirical data on the effectiveness of these complementary behaviors in preventing HIV infection, they remain defensible evaluation outcomes if one is willing to assume that they promote risk reduction or protection.

Strengths and Weaknesses of Behavioral Outcomes
The past eight years of research on AIDS and HIV transmission have confirmed the specific behaviors that are overwhelmingly responsible for HIV infection. Consequently, it is not necessary to rely on HIV seroconversion as the primary outcome of evaluation studies of HIV prevention programs because those specific behaviors can be targeted for assessment.

In contrast to studies that rely on seroconversion as the primary outcome, studies that rely on behavioral outcomes can be conducted more quickly and less expensively because they need not carry out the extensive screening required in seroconversion studies. (This is not to say, however, that behavioral studies are inexpensive.) Because both primary and complementary risk behaviors occur at rates that far exceed the rate of seroconversions, it is possible to make reliable estimates of specific behaviors using smaller samples—thereby making the research less costly—than for seroconversion studies.

In addition, a reliance on behavioral outcomes rather than seroconversion circumvents the problem of the reluctance of some people to be tested. HIV antibody testing is not routine among the general population, although the picture is mixed among high-risk individuals. There is evidence from a number of cohort studies of the willingness of gay men to be tested, although what proportion of people in those communities is willing to be tested is unknown. But there is evidence that many individuals in drug treatment programs or STD clinics are not willing to be tested (see, e.g., Hull et al., 1988; Fleming et al., 1989). Thus, if AIDS prevention programs and their companion evaluation studies can avoid the need to conduct HIV testing, they may be likely to reach a wider and more representative portion of their target populations.

For those evaluation protocols that must include HIV testing, the use of behavioral outcomes is nonetheless important for adequate evaluation. For an individual who is HIV positive, the primary behaviors of interest involve behaviors that impose risk on others; e.g., allowing another person to use his or her unsterilized IV drug injection equipment, becoming pregnant. For those who are HIV negative, the primary behaviors of interest involve risk taking; e.g., using unsterilized drug injection equipment.

The main weaknesses of behavioral data involve problems of validity and reliability (see Appendix C). Problems also arise in interpreting data about similar outcomes when wordings of questions differ among studies. Moreover, even the interpretation of the same question may be problematic over time because respondents' willingness to report behaviors may change.

Another problem in research based on self-reports involves respondents' ability to remember and accurately report specific events and behaviors (there is a fairly large literature on this topic). The problem of recall often may be decreased by shortening the time frame over which respondents must recall the occurrence and frequency of behaviors. However, a shorter time frame may change the meaning of a particular outcome: celibacy or monogamy for a week, for example, is quite different from celibacy or monogamy for a year.

Another major issue surrounding behavioral outcomes involves which outcomes to emphasize in prevention programs and which to focus on in evaluation studies. While risk reduction and risk elimination are most desirable outcomes from the standpoint of halting the spread of HIV, protective behaviors may be more practical to teach and maintain.

Psychological Outcomes

There are a handful of psychological outcomes that are also of interest from the standpoint of AIDS prevention. These include an awareness of AIDS and HIV and of the gravity of the problems they pose; knowledge of AIDS and HIV transmission; and stigmatization of individuals who have AIDS or who are infected with HIV. These psychological outcomes do not have a direct bearing on HIV infection in the way that intercourse, drug injection, and pregnancy (for seropositive women) do. Nevertheless, differences in the degree to which individuals are aware of AIDS, understand which behaviors transmit HIV, and disparage or devalue those who are ill or infected may be important determinants of whether they adopt risk reduction or protective behaviors.

Of all the possible goals for the educational campaigns that have been mounted in this country, the greatest progress has been made in the area of increased knowledge and awareness of AIDS (Turner, Miller, and Barker, 1988). This must be seen as an important accomplishment because behavioral change is unlikely to occur without knowledge and awareness of the AIDS problem and the means of HIV transmission. How much of the credit for this increased knowledge belongs to Public Health Service efforts, as compared with efforts originating from other educational institutions, personal experience, news stories, and so forth, can probably never be accurately assessed. From a public health standpoint, it is not crucial to make such a determination. Instead, one of the most important public health goals now should be to maintain the current high level of knowledge and awareness that exists in the population about the risk of HIV transmission by sexual contact and the sharing of infected equipment and dispelling misconceptions about the risk of transmission through casual contact.

Strengths and Weaknesses of Psychological Outcomes

Psychological outcomes that involve awareness of AIDS and HIV, knowledge about AIDS and HIV transmission, and attitudes toward those who are infected and ill may be the easiest outcomes to measure and study, in the sense that these measures are easily incorporated in a survey questionnaire. Nonetheless, the development of specific questions must be carefully done. Questions involving knowledge and attitudes must be sensitively crafted as well as clearly worded in the vernacular of the target population to avoid introducing substantial response bias and error. Similarly, there is a need to test the sensitivity of the measurements to alternative question wordings or interview formats (see Turner and Martin, 1984: Volume 1, Ch. 4-5).

EVALUATION MEASURES

There are several methodological issues involved in developing reliable indicators of changes in knowledge, attitudes, and risky behaviors. Two issues in particular challenge the measurement of program effectiveness: (1) determining the appropriate time intervals between program implementation and the measurement of change and (2) assessing the quality of survey instruments (questionnaires) and the resulting data. Some of the issues addressed in the sections below are generic to program evaluation; others are more specifically related to the measurement of unobserved phenomena, such as sexual behavior or attitudes.

Timing of Measurement

People who adopt new behaviors in the face of the epidemic may discontinue the change, relapse from time to time, or, conversely, enhance the change over time. Measurements taken soon after the intervention has been delivered may show substantial change but that change may decay over time. Because immediate postintervention measurements and delayed measurements may yield different results, periodic measurement is desirable.

One other measurement timing issue warrants mention here. The national media campaign (see Chapter 3) changed its goal—and even its target audience—before measuring any outcomes. Thus, four separate phases of the campaign were launched without measuring what occurred during previous phases. Such haste is dysfunctional. It does not permit evidence to be gathered on what it is about the intervention that works or does not work or which elements should be continued or discontinued in subsequent phases. The panel cautions that other CDC programs, such as the forthcoming program of direct grants to community-based organizations (CBOs) (see Chapter 4) and other projects with multiple objectives are vulnerable to shifting program goals.

The consequences of interventions should be measured and assessed before deciding on new or alternative stages of intervention programs, a policy that will require periodic measurement of program outcomes. In addition, even if a well-planned, well-implemented project has been successful in meeting its specified goal or goals, periodic evaluation efforts should not cease. For example, media messages may lose their impact with repeated use, the audience may change as the population ages, individuals may feel secure and become careless in their behaviors, or the program itself may drift in its purposes.

The panel recommends that once goals are met, projects be reevaluated periodically to monitor their continued effectiveness.

Quality of Measures

There are a number of methodological topics that are related to the quality of survey data: sampling hard-to-reach groups, appropriate designs for intervention research and evaluation, the validity of self-reported information, and the construction of reliable questionnaire items. Because of the importance of data quality when trying to determine whether program objectives have been reached, Appendix C includes a chapter from the recent report of the parent committee (Miller, Turner, and Moses,

1990) reviewing methodological research on the accuracy of surveys measurements of sexual and drug using behaviors.

There are two general methodological issues that should be considered in an assessment of evaluation measures: validity and reliability. Valid measures reflect without bias the presence or intensity of the concept that they intend to quantify. (Bias refers to systematic misrepresentation or other systematic error which may be due to faulty measurement, sampling, or other factors.) Reliable measures will yield the same data if applied repeatedly. In considering the difficulties associated with AIDS evaluation measures, the panel believes that *measurement* validity will pose the most serious and difficult problem. With regard to reliability, the panel notes a small but important set of studies that have begun to examine the reliability of sexual behavior data, collected mainly from gay men, and a limited number of small studies that have examined the reliability of measures of behavioral change made in response to the AIDS epidemic: see, for example, Saltzman and colleagues (1987); Catania and colleagues (1990); Martin and colleagues (1989); and Martin and Dean (1989).

Differential validity, that is, nonequivalent measurement biases in treatment and control groups, is a particularly worrisome concern for outcome evaluations. It is understandable that some individuals would be reluctant to report risky sexual or drug use behaviors. In an outcome evaluation experiment that randomly assigns participants to different treatments, this reporting bias can be expected to be equivalent across groups at the beginning of the experiment. However, the social pressures created by an intervention program can differentially affect the reporting bias. Individuals enrolled in intervention programs should feel an increase in psychological and social pressure to refrain from engaging in risk-associated behavior. Consequently, they may also feel pressure to conceal conduct that is at odds with program objectives. In such a circumstance, differential reporting biases may cause the group that receives the intervention to appear to have adopted safer behavioral patterns than the control group, when in fact the observed effect is due to the effect of the intervention on the reporting bias.

The quality of measures will also depend on the level of detail of information elicited by the survey instrument. For example, to evaluate the effectiveness of an intervention program, it is not be sufficient to know whether respondents have ever used condoms or whether they have begun to use them. It is also important to determine the frequency of use, and it will be helpful to ascertain the conditions that foster use.

This last point underscores the need to collect data that are not only valid and reliable but that are also meaningful. Outcome measures should include comprehensive and up-to-date observations of the attainment of a program's explicitly stated objectives as well as anticipated side effects, if any. Careful measurement in the context of good research design and implementation will then allow thoughtful inferences to be made about what the results of evaluation mean.

REFERENCES

Catania, J. A., Gibson, D. R., Marin, B., Coates, T. J., and Greenblatt, R. M. (1990) Response bias in assessing sexual behaviors relevant to HIV transmission. *Evaluation and Program Planning* 13:19-29.

Centers for Disease Control (CDC) (1988) Announcement No. 901. September 20. *Federal Register* 53 (182):36492-36493.

Centers for Disease Control (CDC) (1989) *A Comprehensive Program to Prevent HIV Transmission.* Fiscal Year 1989 Operating Plan. Washington, D.C.: U.S. Department of Health and Human Services.

Coates, T. J., Morin, S.F., and McKusick, L. (1987) Behavioral consequences of AIDS antibody testing among gay men. *Journal of the American Medical Association* 258:1889.

Fleming, D., Bennett, D., Klockner, R., Gould, J., Cassidy, D., and Foster, L. (1989) HIV Infected STD Clients Who Decline HIV Counseling and Testing. Paper presented at the Fifth International AIDS Conference. Montreal, June 4-9.

Grant, D., and Anns, M. (1988) Counseling AIDS antibody-positive clients: Reactions and treatment. *American Psychologist* 43:72-74.

Hull, H. F., Bettinger, C. J., Gallaher, M. M., Keller, N. M., Wilson, J., and Mertz, G. J. (1988) Comparison of HIV-antibody prevalence in patients consenting to and declining HIV-antibody testing in an STD clinic. *Journal of the American Medical Association* 260:935-938.

Longini, I. M., Jr., Clark, W. S., Horsburgh, C. R., Lemp, G. F., Byers, R. H., Darrow, W. W., and others (1989) Statistical analysis of the stages of HIV infection using a Markov model. Paper presented at the Fifth International AIDS Conference. Montreal, June 4-9.

Martin, J. L., and Dean, L. (1989) Risk factors for AIDS-related bereavement in a cohort of homosexual men in New York City. In B. Cooper and T. Helgason, eds., *Epidemiology and the Prevention of Mental Disorders.* United Kingdom: Routledge.

Martin, J. L., Dean, L., Garcia, M., and Hall, W. (1989) The impact of AIDS on a gay community: Changes in sexual behavior, substance use, and mental health. *American Journal of Community Psychology.* 17(3):269-293

Miller, H. G., Turner, C. F., and Moses, L. E., eds. (1990) *AIDS: The Second Decade.* Report of the NRC Committee on AIDS Research and the Behavioral, Social and Statistical Sciences. Washington, D.C.: National Academy Press.

Ogilvy & Mather (1987) Contract for RFP No. 200-87-0525. Section III (Methodology and Approach). June.

Ostrow, D. G., Joseph, J., Soucey, J., Eller, M., Kessler, R., Phair, J., and Chmiel, J. (1988) Mental health and behavioral correlates of HIV antibody testing in a cohort of gay men. Paper presented at the Fourth International AIDS Conference. Stockholm, June 12-16.

Saltzman, S. P., Stoddard, A. M., McCusher, J., Moon, M. W., and Mayer, K. H. (1987) Reliability of self-reported sexual behavior risk factors for HIV infection in homosexual men. *Public Health Reports* 102:692-697.

Strobino, D. M. (1987) The health and medical consequences of adolescent sexuality and pregnancy: A review of the literature. In S. Hofferth and C. Hayes, eds., *Risking the Future: Adolescent Sexuality, Pregnancy, and Childbearing.* Volume 2, Working Papers and Statistical Appendixes. Report of the NRC Panel on Adolescent Pregnancy and Childbearing. Washington D.C.: National Academy Press.

Suchman, E. A. (1967) *Evaluative Research.* New York: Russell Sage Foundation.

Turner, C. F., and Martin E., eds. (1984) *Surveying Subjective Phenomena*, 2 vols. New York: Russell Sage.

Turner, C. F., Miller, H. G., and Barker, L. (1988) AIDS research and the behavioral and social sciences. In R. Kulstad, ed., *AIDS, 1988*. Washington, D.C.: American Association for the Advancement of Science.

Turner, C. F., Miller, H. G., and Moses, L. E., eds. (1989) *AIDS, Sexual Behavior, and Intravenous Drug Use.* Report of the NRC Committee on AIDS Research and the Behavioral, Social, and Statistical Sciences. Washington, D.C.: National Academy Press.

Weiss, C. H. (1972) *Evaluation Research.* Englewood Cliffs, N.J.: Prentice-Hall, Inc.

3

Evaluating Media Campaigns

This chapter focuses on current and future mass media campaigns centered on the prevention of AIDS. The most visible current effort is the national, multiphase *America Responds to AIDS* campaign of public service announcements and a mass mailing that has been developed through CDC's National AIDS Information and Education Program (NAIEP). However, numerous other campaigns that are usually more local in scope have also been and will be conducted. The panel's suggestions for the evaluation of such media campaigns are relevant for all types, national and local.

The panel focuses on the special problems of evaluating a national mass media effort in the context of an epidemic that will affect the nation for years to come. The assumption that HIV and AIDS will beset U.S. society for the next 20 or 30 years underlies the panel's position that allocating substantial resources to rigorous evaluations at an early stage of program development makes for a wise investment in the long run. In fact, we advocate intensive evaluation at all phases of campaign development precisely to increase the chances of meaningful effects. Evaluation may also help reduce the wasting of resources on ineffective campaign activities; if a campaign phase does not produce effects it can be withdrawn or replaced with more effective material.

In discussing the need for rigorous evaluations, the panel concluded that randomized experiments would produce the most valid account of program effects. We are well aware that this type of evaluation entails high initial costs; nonetheless, we believe that the benefits that may be derived from conducting such experiments will pay off handsomely in the long run. In addition, from a "dollars-and-sense" perspective, we think it is reasonable for CDC to want to know whether its expenditure of millions of dollars on the campaign for the public's education is having the desired effect.

Because the evaluation of mass media campaigns presents special difficulties (see Flay and Cook, 1981), this chapter adds a fourth line of inquiry to the three fundamental questions, "What is delivered?," "Does it make a difference?" and "What works better?"—namely, "*Can* the campaign make a difference?" Another unique feature for the media campaign is that the panel recommends that the latter two questions be answered in controlled settings rather than the real world. The chapter includes discussions of methodological problems and issues related to resources and aspirations under each question. The chapter thus has five major sections:

- Background and objectives
- Formative evaluation: What works better?
- Efficacy trials: Can the campaign make a difference?
- Process evaluation: What is actually delivered?
- Outcome evaluation: Does the campaign make a difference?

BACKGROUND AND OBJECTIVES

Four phases of a national AIDS media campaign have already been launched. Three phases have channeled messages nationwide through a series of public service announcements (PSAs); a fourth phase provided a mass mailing of an informational brochure to all U.S. households. From discussions with CDC staff, it appears that future campaign phases will be focused largely on PSAs. The campaign, *America Responds to AIDS*, has thus far been conducted in a series of six-month phases, although the current (Phase IV) will probably be extended to eight months. For each of the phases, target audiences have been identified and general frameworks provided for the aims of the campaign. These objectives are stated below, as the panel understands them on the basis of extensive discussions with CDC staff.

The general objective of Phase I (October 1987 to March 1988) was to increase the general population's awareness of AIDS and to correct misperceptions about how it is and is not acquired. This phase aimed to "humanize" AIDS and reduce needless fear. The campaign consisted of PSAs aired by television and radio stations throughout the country. CDC and contract staff (the advertising firm of Ogilvy & Mather) conducted a media marketing outreach program to obtain airtime more favorable than PSAs typically receive. Auditing of these PSAs, to the extent that it has been possible, showed that in many "markets" around the country, the PSAs for Phase I were frequently aired, although nearly 90 percent were aired in nonprime time.[1] (It should be noted, however, that over 50 percent of the dollar value of donated air time was in prime time.)

The general objectives of Phase II of the campaign (April to September 1988) were similar to those of Phase I, but this phase used a mass mailing rather than PSAs as the central channel of information. A mass mailing is expected to reach a higher proportion of the national population with more consistent and more detailed information than a PSA campaign. An eight-page brochure, *Understanding AIDS,* was mailed to all households in the United States during the last week of May and first two weeks of June 1988. Under a contract with CDC, Ogilvy & Mather coordinated press releases, a press conference with Surgeon General C. Everett Koop and CDC Director (now Assistant Secretary for Health) James O. Mason, and national marketing of a video news release followed by satellite news interviews and PSAs to promote the mailing.

Phase III of the campaign (October 1988 to March 1989) was directed specifically toward women at risk and sexually active adults with multiple partners. In addition, because a disproportionate number of AIDS cases have been reported among blacks and Hispanics, this phase of the campaign included a number of program elements aimed specifically at these audiences.

Phase IV (April to November 1989) emphasizes families and children. According to an oral presentation in March by NAIEP staff to the panel, this phase has four objectives: (1) to improve parent-child communication about sexual behaviors; (2) to increase the acceptability of abstinence to parents and adolescents (and also to the general population); (3) to increase the acceptability of condom use if abstinence is not practiced; and (4) to increase the availability and adoption of comprehensive school health curricula.[2] Aim (1) concerns the specific target audiences only: changes should be observed only among parents of appropriately aged adolescents and the adolescents themselves and not necessarily in the rest of the population. To be useful in the long term, however, aims (2) and (3) should also influence the general population, eventually affecting social norms regarding the acceptability of abstinence; premarital,

---

[1] The Government Accounting Office (GAO) audited the airing of CDC's PSAs on network TV from December 1987 through February 1988 (GAO, 1988).

[2] A press release (n.d.) on Phase IV casts these objectives in a slightly different voice. The first objective is said to encourage adult-child communication about HIV and AIDS; next, rather than specifying abstinence and condom use, the ensuing objectives are expressed as encouraging youth "to adopt and maintain behaviors that eliminate or reduce their risk of infection;" the final objective is to "raise public awareness of young people's vulnerability to HIV."

extramarital, and casual sex; condom use; etc. Aim (4) appears to be directed toward schools as much as toward parents and children: the aim is to increase the acceptability of comprehensive school health education provided by school personnel and the rate of adoption of such curricula by the nation's schools.

As discussed in the last chapter, the objectives of a campaign, or of any defined component or phase of a campaign, are not useful to an evaluation if they are stated generally. Objectives must be specific before useful evaluations can be conducted and outcomes can be measured. Several possible outcomes of the national AIDS campaign are of interest: knowledge and beliefs about AIDS and its causes, particularly, the clarification of myths; beliefs about susceptibility and the severity of consequences; attitudes toward people with AIDS and toward high-risk situations and protection; intentions regarding personal protection; actual high-risk and protective behaviors; and seroprevalence. (See Chapter 2 for a discussion of these outcomes.)

Consistent with its overall recommendations, the panel urges that the desired outcomes of each future phase of the campaign (1) be made explicit, (2) be measured repeatedly, (3) be reached (or retargeted) prior to developing future phases, and (4) be monitored periodically to ensure that they are maintained once they have been achieved. Maintenance can be ensured either by rerunning some campaign phases or by introducing reinforcing messages in later phases. The panel further suggests that evaluative data from earlier phases drive the choice of target issues and audiences for future phases.

FORMATIVE EVALUATION: WHAT WORKS BETTER?

Formative evaluations of media campaigns are especially useful for obtaining detailed, documented evidence of effectiveness prior to wide or further deployment. During a formative evaluation, alternative campaigns or campaign messages can be tested on a small scale, which will help contain the costs of doing randomized experiments. This type of research partially answers the question "What works better?" (Efficacy trials provide further information on what works in an optimal situation; see the next section).

It is an unfortunate fact that the budgets of most PSA campaigns do not allow the kind of thoughtful formative evaluation that is common in the development of commercial advertisements. Indeed, in many cases, PSA formative evaluation involves nothing more than a review of creative ideas by the officials funding the campaign—perhaps the selection of one campaign from a set of two or three that have been developed to the idea stage—and a selection of the campaign design based on simple intuition. The absence of serious research at this stage of program development can be fatal, and it is always a great disadvantage, since the track records of even the most successful advertising agencies show that changing audience behavior is a difficult enterprise.

A campaign as large and as important as the National AIDS Information and Education Program does not suffer from the same resource deficits that hamper developmental efforts in more typical PSA campaigns. It is possible to do much better than the standard approach in PSA campaign development and to adopt the kinds of research strategies that are more typical of formative evaluations for commercial advertisements. The result is a much stronger campaign and a campaign whose effects can be more easily assessed. Our whole approach to evaluation is designed to lead to the development of effective campaigns. While others have advocated extensive formative evaluation (e.g., the Office of Cancer Communications within the National Cancer Institute) hardly any campaign developers have conducted such careful developmental and evaluation research. A campaign as long as this one deserves such careful attention if we are not to waste millions of dollars.

The panel recommends the expanded use of formative evaluation or developmental research in designing media projects.

There are several standard strategies that are used in formative evaluations of mass media campaigns, and they should be part of a major national campaign such as this one. The panel details one of these approaches here; alternative strategies are provided by Flay (1986), the Office of Cancer Communications (1983, 1984), Palmer (1981), and others. The approach we propose has five basic steps: (1) idea generation, (2) concept testing, (3) the positioning statement, (4) copy testing, and (5) test marketing. The first four of these steps are described below; the fifth is discussed in the next section on efficacy trials. Some of these steps have already been taken by CDC and its contractor; however, we endorse the adoption of all five and hereby underscore their importance.

Step 1: Idea Generation

A media campaign begins with an idea about a message that is thought to have motivational power. There is now a fairly substantial body of research on the cognitive and motivational determinants of and the barriers to behavioral change: see, for example, McKusick, Horstman, and Coates (1987); Joseph and colleagues (1987); McCusker and colleagues

(1988); and Valdiserri and colleagues (1988). This literature is being applied to studies of risk reduction to prevent AIDS, and it can be used to help stimulate the ideas needed to develop campaign messages.

Yet even when ideas are solidly grounded in research, the first step in formative evaluation should be to evaluate the power of the idea. This step is particularly important in cases in which the idea is developed outside of the context of the lives of the people to whom the message will be delivered. The literature on behavioral change interventions is full of examples of ideas that seemed to make perfect sense in the abstract but that failed completely because they clashed with fundamental ideas held by the target population or were not stated in ways that were relevant to the lives of those people. Preliminary evaluation must guard against these "fatal" flaws by evaluating the message's ideas in the context of the lives of the people toward whom the message will be directed. This type of evaluation is usually done in a phase of research known as concept testing.

Step 2: Concept Testing

Concept testing is an iterative process that is usually based on focused interviews and other qualitative research techniques. It attempts to determine the meanings of the behavior one wants to change in the context of the lives of the people one wants to reach. This information is used to assess the appeal of the campaign message in relation to this context. For example, if the message is that condom use helps protect against transmission of the AIDS virus, it is necessary to develop some understanding of the meanings currently associated with condom use, the kinds of reactions that occur when it is claimed that condoms are protective, and the persuasive power of the message that there is danger of infection.

A fuller understanding of these issues might very well lead to a revision of the message that will make it more appealing to the selected audience. It might be discovered, for example, that teenagers are not motivated by the fear of infection, but that they can be reached by appealing to their feelings of insecurity. A revised message based on this insight might emphasize the fact that older, more experienced peers use condoms and that it is only inexperienced youngsters who fail to use them.

A word is in order about the methods used to generate insights of this sort. Qualitative approaches are the standard methods used in this phase of formative evaluation. In commercial applications, a focus group is the qualitative technique that is most commonly used. The use of groups is thought to be superior to individual interviews because group processes help stimulate ideas and uncover resistances that may remain hidden in one-on-one sessions (Morgan and Spanish, 1984). Exploratory work early in the AIDS epidemic with focus groups of gay men documented these advantages by showing that a number of important themes were raised in group discussions but were not found in personal interviews (Joseph et al., 1984). This kind of interaction occurs in part because people in groups talk to each other more than to the group moderator, and this talk tends to be insider talk rather than talk aimed at presenting only the public self. Group interviews, then, can be an extremely valuable tool in preliminary research on the contextual validity of a basic idea or message for the campaign.

At the same time, group processes can sometimes create barriers to understanding when insider behavior involves a good deal of posing and protective actions aimed at presenting an appealing view of oneself. Comprehensive concept testing should use both group and individual methods to guard against the limitations of each mode. The goal of concept testing is to develop insights into the meanings of ideas and messages, which can best be achieved by being open to multiple sources of information. Group interviews, unobtrusive observation, key informants, and focused or in-depth interviews with a cross-section of the selected population all have parts to play.

Once an idea has been refined in this kind of research, it is common to carry out some type of representative survey to guarantee that the themes heard in the focused, qualitative part of the study are representative of the total target population. This research is confirmatory rather than exploratory; its goal is to validate the insights obtained from the individual and group processes. In the development of a campaign for a new commercial product, for example, it is not uncommon for formative evaluation to include several hundred group and individual interviews directed toward refining ideas and messages. This exploratory work is often followed by a nationally representative survey of several thousand respondents to assess whether the themes developed in the exploratory research are representative of the entire selected audience. What is uncommon is to repeat this type of evaluation each time a new phase of a campaign occurs. However, a media campaign whose purpose is to prevent the transmission of HIV is far different in importance and in its different target audiences than a campaign for a commercial product. Thus far, the AIDS campaign has chosen different audiences—the general public, women, adults with multiple sexual partners, parents and youth—for each campaign phase. The panel believes that, under these circumstances, themes and messages should continue to be tested for each new phase and each new target group of the media campaign.

Step 3: The Positioning Statement

The product of concept testing is a positioning statement, that is, an outline of the messages one wants to communicate to the target audience. The positioning statement is the starting point for the development of the creative materials in the campaign. The agency that is developing the campaign begins with the positioning statement and attempts to develop commercials that convey the messages in this statement effectively.

It is conventional for the creative teams in charge of commercial design to develop several different formats for conveying these messages. In early stages, the formats may consist of rough text and descriptions of what the visual components of the advertisements would look like. As formats become more firmly established, several more polished texts are developed with sketches of camera shots. A series of these sketches conveys the entire sequence that would be produced in a final commercial. Several of these sequences, known as story boards, are typically presented to clients for preliminary approval before a more refined phase of development takes place.

In PSA advertisement development, it is not uncommon for the story boards to be the only intermediate version of the advertisement to be reviewed prior to final production. In addition, as noted earlier, it often happens that the selection of the final campaign from among several different story boards is made in a single review meeting, based on the intuitions of the public health clients and advertising executives. Cost constraints often make it difficult to carry out systematic evaluations to select the set of story boards that is likely to make the most effective advertisement. Large and important campaigns, however, should continue the process of formative evaluation at this stage to help in the selection process. By so doing, they not only increase the chances of campaign success by selecting the best set of story boards, but they also obtain information that can be used to make final changes to the story boards that are selected. This data collection is carried out in a type of evaluation known as copy testing.

Step 4: Copy Testing

Copy testing is any research that exposes a test audience to some version of an advertisement and evaluates the success of that advertisement in communicating the intended message. The most superficial kinds of copy testing use small samples of people to read and discuss the advertisements as a way of making sure they are comprehensive and adequate. Systematic copy testing, however, also attempts to assess persuasiveness and does so with experiments.

The simplest kinds of experiments randomly assign a sample of respondents to a laboratory exposure of story boards, animatics (a cartoon or animated story board), or other rough production versions of an advertisement and then evaluate the effects of different formats on self-reported knowledge, attitudes, and behavioral intentions. Debriefing is typically a part of the data collection activity because it allows researchers to pinpoint aspects of the various advertisements that lead to confusion, that convey messages other than those that were intended, or that fail to have the intended persuasive impact. This information can then be used to modify the story boards for another iteration of the process, which continues until a format is developed that has the desired characteristics.

If a researcher is creative, it is possible to use this approach to evaluate real behavioral effects. Wright (1979), for example, evaluated the impact of different formats for risk disclosure about over-the-counter drugs by giving participants in his experiment a free coupon to obtain their choice of several different over-the-counter drugs from a pharmacy next to the theater in which the experiment took place. The evaluation consisted of ratings made by unobtrusive observers on the length of time participants spent reading the warning labels on the packages before choosing a product. Wright found that one version of his advertisement was superior to others in promoting careful reviews of warning statements. One could imagine similar evaluation outcomes in copy-testing experiments of proposed AIDS materials.

A somewhat different kind of copy-testing evaluation is also possible in what is known as a recruit-to-view format of rough productions. This approach recruits participants to view a television program in their homes without telling them that a rough version of the PSA being tested will be one of the commercials on the program. A postviewing interview is then conducted to determine the percentage of the audience who recall the PSA and the aspects they recall most vividly.

This kind of real-life exposure allows researchers to study the intrusiveness of the PSA—that is, its ability to catch the attention of the audience. It also allows them to assess comprehension and knowledge retention in a real-life setting rather than in a laboratory. It often happens that comprehension difficulties are detected in this kind of copy testing that were missed in laboratory research where people are artificially placed in a situation that encourages them to pay more attention to the advertisement than they ordinarily would when watching television at home. The confusion only emerges among people who are half listening, the way many people listen to television commercials.

Sometimes, discoveries at this stage of formative evaluation lead to revisions in final production versions of the advertisements that are extremely important. These can be subtle changes—for instance, changing one word that, if misunderstood, would change the meaning of the message in an important way—or they can be dramatic changes. One might discover, for example, that a message that is easily comprehended in a laboratory situation is delivered in such a low-keyed way that audiences at home take little notice of it and, as a result, never really hear the message. This kind of discovery could lead to a total revision of the campaign and a return to another set of story boards with a more intrusive message.

Methodological Issues

The main methodological problem of formative evaluation is its lack of external validity: that is, one cannot generalize from it because the evaluation is made of a limited or pilot program and not of a program deployed under realistic operating conditions. By conducting small-scale experimental or quasi-experimental evaluations of one-time message exposure in laboratories in forms that are not identical to the final advertisements, evaluators are testing an intervention that is quite different from the final product. Nevertheless, formative research is an important component of program development. Although it may not always result in an effective campaign, it will usually identify an unacceptable or ineffective approach.

Resources and Aspirations

Here and elsewhere in the report we discuss the resources needed to conduct the types of evaluation the panel recommends (i.e., costs, time, staffing), as well as the realistic aspirations for what will be gained from doing the evaluations. It is important to note that all of what has been discussed thus far is not a guarantee of the success of a campaign once it has been fully implemented. But carefully carrying out a systematic formative evaluation will provide clear indications of the types of effects to be expected. Following formative evaluation and subsequent program development efforts, a campaign's implementation and outcomes also need to be evaluated (as described below).

The reader should also recognize that the search for a better campaign —the evaluation of what works better—is inherently limited by the fact that the role of evaluation is to assess ideas rather than to generate them. The success of a campaign such as *America Responds to AIDS* hinges on the stimulation of creative ideas for reaching hard-to-reach population groups. The role of evaluation is not to provide this creativity; rather, it is to recognize it and distinguish efforts that are more likely to be effective from those that are not.

Serious attempts should be made to work through more than one creative idea. Typically, the purchaser of a media campaign will describe a product concept to an advertising agency and contract with the agency to prepare up to six campaign options from which to choose. Often, one of these ideas will be more fully developed than the others, indicating the *agency's* judgment about the most potentially effective option. If a client is not satisfied with the agency's work, the client may negotiate a contract with another agency.

A commercial buyer usually has on staff informed advertising consumers, often with ad agency experience, whose expertise prepares them to choose among multiple options and to decide when to bring in another agency. NAIEP in fact has a staff with substantial ad agency experience, which makes it well-positioned to select from among several creative ideas. To inaugurate the *America Responds to AIDS* campaign, NAIEP solicited proposals and presentations from 13 different agencies before choosing Ogilvy & Mather. That contract is due to expire this fall, and to compete for the next contract, ad agencies will be required to present a proposed campaign in story-board form. The panel endorses this plan, while recognizing that because of the expense of story boards, it may not be possible to get 13 agencies to compete again. For this reason, the panel advocates getting a minimum of three different agencies to develop a campaign to this stage. Because some agencies are unlikely to develop story boards unless they have a contract, the development of boards could be purchased on a fixed-fee basis. This purchase of ideas from multiple agencies is unusual, but the panel believes it is warranted in the present circumstances. Increasing the range of ideas that are nurtured increases the chances that an effective and creative campaign will be produced. When faced with such multiple approaches, evaluation can help determine which of them is likely to be the most effective.

In the preceding section, the panel sketched out an ambitious but not unrealistic approach for formative evaluation. Indeed, this series of activities mimics the standard practices of commercial advertisers in the formation of a major national advertising campaign. Formative evaluation budgets for commercial campaigns are often in the range of $200,000-$500,000.

Formative evaluation should not be left in the hands of the advertising agencies that develop the campaigns, because it is at this critical stage in the decision-making process that it is important to make all reasonable efforts to encourage the development of many ideas for the most creative campaign possible. NAIEP should be able to take advantage of the ad agency backgrounds of its professional staff in the formative evaluation of media messages. The investment of staff time and funds in such research at this stage of campaign development will help to ensure implementation of a good program. Before implementation, however, it is also wise to determine whether the campaign can, indeed, make a difference if it were optimally implemented in markets around the country.

EFFICACY TRIALS: CAN THE CAMPAIGN MAKE A DIFFERENCE?

The ultimate effectiveness of a campaign will depend on its efficacy: with optimal implementation, could it have the desired effects? (An example of optimal implementation is the airing of a PSA during a program that is popular with a target audience.) This type of evaluation or market test should be carried out prior to the launching of the campaign and should be based on test campaigns conducted in a small sample of prototypical markets (rather than in the entire country). Given the enormous potential impact of such national campaigns as *America Responds to AIDS*, it is inappropriate to implement the campaign (or any of its main stages) nationally without some evaluation of whether it is likely to be effective, ineffective, or even harmful. Efficacy evaluation should be distinguished from effectiveness evaluation, which is distinguished by the broad, real-world implementation of a program. It is important to remember that, even with adequate evaluation at this stage, there is no guarantee that a campaign will be effective when finally implemented. It may not be implemented adequately enough to be effective.

Ideally, program developers should separate the determination of a campaign's efficacy—that is, whether it *could* work if it were implemented optimally—from the determination of its effectiveness when actually implemented—that is, whether it *does* work as implemented (usually less than optimally).[3] Otherwise, if less than optimal effects are found only after full-scale implementation, one can never be sure of the reason. Was it because the campaign as designed was not efficacious (could not have produced better effects even if implemented optimally)? Or was it because of less than optimal implementation? In this section the panel considers tests of campaign efficacy. The subsequent section considers tests of campaign effectiveness.

Randomized Experiments

In keeping with its recommendations on randomly controlled trials, the panel believes that campaign efficacy should be determined through the

---

[3] See Flay (1986) for discussion of the efficacy-effectiveness distinction.

use of randomized experiments. The proposed media campaign should be implemented with maximum integrity in several carefully selected test markets, and the data gathered there should be compared with data gathered in several other matched control (nontest) markets. The data sources should be specially designed surveys that are used only in the test and control (nontest) markets. Whenever possible, however, the questions that are to be used in subsequent effectiveness trials should also be used in tests of efficacy.

It is important that the test and control markets chosen for efficacy trials be representative of the selected population one wants to reach. Because of the difficulty of reaching a significant proportion of the audience with more than one message exposure, multiple airings are necessary. In standard test-market studies, a campaign is commonly aired from 6 to 12 months to be sure that most viewers will have been exposed to an ad at least three times. Similarly, the test period for the national AIDS media campaign should be at least six months to provide a sound evaluation of the campaign's exposure effectiveness.

Campaign tracking surveys are a common means of monitoring success in test-market studies. Such surveys might include independent monthly interviews of samples of people in the general population to monitor levels of campaign awareness, recall, understanding, persuasion, and self-reported behavioral change. With parallel surveys in nontest markets, researchers can control for the "confounding" influence of broader societal determinants of change that are unrelated to the campaign. The parallel control market survey is a particularly important design component in an evaluation of an AIDS information campaign because there are many other sources of AIDS information that may be determinants of changes in knowledge, attitudes, and behavior. An evaluation of the unique incremental influence of any new campaign requires a comparison of trends in the test markets with trends in the control markets, which are exposed to all of this other AIDS information but not to the new campaign.

In commercial applications, an important part of test-market evaluation is information about sales trends. An advertising campaign for an automobile is not considered successful unless automobile sales increase more (or decrease less) in the test markets than in the control markets. There may be opportunities for using similar outcome measures in the evaluation of public health information programs. Trends in condom sales, visits to birth control clinics, sales of books about safe sex, and phone calls to the AIDS hotline all provide independent estimates of potential outcomes. (However, the reader should note the cautions regarding the use of trend data in outcome evaluation, discussed below.)

Test-market evaluation should also include the monitoring of negative outcomes, especially in the case of a campaign like the phases of *America Responds to AIDS*. In some cases a message that engenders extreme fear without also offering advice on how to reduce the threat may also engender feelings of helplessness or the denial of susceptibility to the threat. In the case of a disease whose consequences are as deadly as those of AIDS, any negative outcomes resulting from an intervention should be carefully monitored and studied.

Media campaign developers should note that test marketing need not be limited to a single campaign that has been selected as the presumed best among alternatives from prior stages of evaluation. If more than one campaign still seems promising after the copy-testing stage, it is both possible and desirable to carry out randomized comparisons of the two (or more) variations across different markets. AIDS campaign sponsors must decide whether there are, indeed, several potentially effective campaign designs when they carry out their own evaluations of story boards for future stages of the campaign. If there are, the sponsors should not hesitate to produce different campaigns aimed at the same selected population groups and then evaluate the campaigns' comparative efficacy in test markets.

Randomized tests of alternatives can also be used to assess the relative impact of different versions or components of a campaign. For example, to test two approaches to altering norms regarding abstinence, a campaign directed toward parents and children might be run in some markets, and a campaign directed toward the general population might be run in others. A similar approach could be taken to establish the relative strength of different components of any one strategy. Let us take Phase IV of *America Responds to AIDS* as an illustration, even though it will ending in a few months. Phase IV consists of different sets of messages for parents and children; one or the other set might be more acceptable to the group selected for the intervention and thus be more effective. The relative strengths of the two could be determined with an experimental test of alternatives, in which some markets received only the parent messages and some only the children messages; other test strategies might include giving the messages in different orders or both at once. Of course, this approach should be reserved only for questions that remain unresolved after formative research.

Methodological Issues

There are several methodological issues that must be addressed when undertaking efficacy trials of the type recommended by the panel. The fact that PSA campaigns must rely on donated air time makes it difficult to conduct an efficacy trial of this approach to AIDS prevention. To determine efficacy, the selected test markets must air the PSAs on an optimal schedule. To expect this kind of cooperation from randomly selected media markets is unrealistic, but it might be achieved by providing desirable incentives—for example, partial or full payment for the PSAs. Efficacy trials would certainly be feasible using paid air time. The fact that incentives or payment would make the test different from what would occur in the full implementation is not a serious concern: the intent at this stage is to determine what effects the campaign *could have* if it were implemented optimally (efficacy) and not to test what would happen during the real implementation (effectiveness).

Whether a paid advertising campaign would be more cost-effective than a PSA campaign is an untested question. A paid campaign might produce exposure and effects that were so much better than those produced by a PSA campaign that it would be worth the increased costs. Perhaps the exposure and effects of a PSA campaign do not justify the high costs of producing efficacious spots (and certainly nothing can justify the lower costs of producing ineffective spots).

The panel recommends systematic comparative tests of paid advertising versus PSA campaigns.

To conduct such tests, air time on desirable shows (those likely to be viewed by the selected audience for the campaign) must be purchased in some random markets and not in others.

A common alternative to the ideal approach of using multiple, randomly selected test and control markets is to use only one or two cooperative test markets and the same or a larger number of well-matched control sites. Trials of a campaign in "lead" or test markets before national implementation are an example of this approach. Any serious campaign that is planned to last at least six months should be launched in test markets. However, this approach is acceptable only if extensive attempts are made to ensure that the selected control markets are comparable. By conducting a test-market evaluation, researchers study only a small number of areas. These areas, however, do not provide a probability sample of the population the campaign is intended to reach.

In such test-market evaluations, it is important to make a substantive investment in the development of formative evaluation materials and interventions that are as close to the finished product as possible. Animatics or video story boards should be chosen rather than the simple story boards used in laboratory experiments. Without efforts to make the tests as realistic as possible, their implications for the full campaign will be lessened.

Experimental tests of alternatives might seem like an expensive approach to determining whether a campaign can make a difference. There will probably be many instances, however, in which one or another approach will be found to be more effective and the other can then be dropped rather than implemented on a wide scale. Without this way to discriminate among approaches, the less effective strategy may be the one to be implemented on a wide scale. Even if one strategy is no better or no worse than another, the existence of the experimental test of alternatives allows for a more solid assessment of project efficacy. The resources required for such assessments, as well as the limitations that must be accepted, are described below.

Resources and Aspirations

Without high-quality efficacy trial data, policy makers, CDC officials, other public health officials, budgeting staff (at CDC, the Office of Management and Budget, and the Government Accounting Office), and the public are left without any reliable indicators of the likely value of their investments. Yet high-quality trials require professional staff with training and experience in experimental field tests of media campaigns, as well as staff to design and oversee all associated data collection and analysis. Industry typically spends as much as $200,000-$300,000 for efficacy trials (market tests) for a $10 million campaign. Using this figure as a benchmark, we estimate that the resources needed for efficacy trials of an AIDS media campaign prior to national implementation will be 2 to 3 percent of the expected total campaign cost (including donated or in-kind costs from all sources).

There may be a concern that the social context of the epidemic is subject to unexpected rapid developments—e.g., publicity surrounding Rock Hudson's death may have precipitated quick changes in the public's knowledge about AIDS. In this context, the length of time required for mounting the recommended activities (almost a year to conduct formative and efficacy research before a campaign can be fielded) may cause concern. However, it is our contention that one year to develop a campaign is not excessive within the 20-30 years presumed necessary for AIDS prevention. Only rarely are changes likely to be so dramatic and so fast that a campaign idea will have to be dropped halfway through development. However, the possibility of fairly rapid changes serves to emphasize the need for continuous formative research and efficacy and effectiveness trials and for continued monitoring of campaign effects.

The panel recognizes that there are limitations to the generalizability of test-market effects in pilot studies such as these. Of course there will be variant contexts in which campaigns are aired, but the panel believes the substance of the effects will be similar in similar groups. Randomized exposure of campaigns among audiences representative of the target populations will go a long way toward factoring out spurious effects. Then, once efficacy has been determined and the campaign has been implemented, process evaluation can begin to assess the delivery of the intervention.

PROCESS EVALUATION:
WHAT IS ACTUALLY DELIVERED?

The questions of concern in this section involve the implementation of the campaign: whether the campaign was aired at all, how often it was aired, and to whom. There are three major approaches to process evaluations of media campaigns: audits of PSA broadcasts through Broadcast Advertisers Reports data; monitoring of AIDS information requests through calls to AIDS telephone hotlines; and general population surveys of campaign awareness.

In the past, CDC's process evaluation efforts for media campaigns have primarily involved auditing PSA broadcasts through Broadcast Advertisers Reports (BAR) data, which provide information on what PSAs were broadcast on particular stations and at what times. By merging BAR data with information on audience characteristics obtained from A.C. Nielsen, it is possible to generate analyses of the types of people who were exposed to the PSAs.

Another way to evaluate PSA delivery is to monitor whether viewers of a PSA make requests for more information, the opportunity for which is provided by the 800-number telephone hotline associated with the PSA campaign. The AIDS hotline has been operated by the American Social Health Association under contract from CDC since February 1987. By September 1987, the hotline had 17 lines in place; one month later, it had increased its capacity fourfold. Figure 3-1 presents data on the frequency of both taped and operator-handled calls to the hotline from February 1987 to February 1989.

As the figure shows, there was an increase from approximately 70,000 calls per month during the summer of 1987 to approximately 200,000 calls per month in the fall of 1987, a trend that continued through June 1988. This increase might be attributable to the PSA campaign and to the publicity associated with it. However, the proportion of media coverage that actually resulted from the PSA campaign compared with the

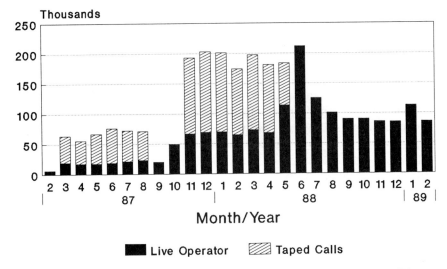

FIGURE 3-1   Calls received by the AIDS hotline by month, from February 1987 to February, 1989. (Note: Hotline calls are reported starting February 16, 1987; there were technical problems with taped responses in September-October, 1987). Source: National AIDS Hotline.

proportion that resulted from other publicity and campaigns is unknown and difficult to estimate accurately.[4] The further increase that occurred in operator-handled calls in May-June 1988 may be attributable to the national mailing and the associated media coverage; the elimination of taped calls in June 1988, however, makes this result less interpretable. Following the May-June increase, the number of hotline calls per month dropped by half from June to August 1988 and remained at that level during subsequent months except for a small increase in January 1989, the cause of which has not been determined.

A more expensive but considerably more effective method for assessing exposure to a media campaign is to take general population surveys of campaign awareness. A special version of this approach is to conduct a telephone survey of a random sample of television households that limits contact to the few minutes directly following the broadcast of a PSA in a particular market. Coincidental surveys of this type are a unique way of determining how many people actually sit through a PSA when

---

[4] Although *America Responds to AIDS* is the only campaign to have aired the hotline telephone number, the number is readily available through directory assistance and AIDS support groups.

it is broadcast (rather than leaving the room or shifting their attention elsewhere).

Methodological Issues

All of the above strategies can provide information for process evaluation, but each has methodological problems that act as counterweights to potential benefits. Some of the problems can be corrected when, as in this instance, the approaches are used for process evaluation. However, when these approaches are used to assess effectiveness (discussed in the next section), the problems often are much harder to resolve.

The Broadcast Advertisers Reports (BAR) data are limited in their ability to provide complete and accurate information on how often PSA messages are broadcast. Information on PSAs is not routinely collected at the same level of detail as information on commercial advertisements. PSA data are limited to major television markets and are reported only once every four weeks. Although this limitation is not a major problem for monitoring general trends (because most television stations use a standard PSA rotation scheme that is fairly constant from one week to the next over short periods of time), the limitation of BAR data to major markets is a serious constraint on the ability to gauge where and how often PSAs appear.

Several methods are available to remedy this situation. One common approach used by agencies that manage PSAs is to send a mail questionnaire (or "bounce-back" postcard) on PSA airing and rotation schedules to station managers responsible for PSA scheduling. This method is not particularly accurate, however, because only a small percentage of the questionnaires or cards are returned. A better method is to conduct a systematic telephone survey with the managers. A probability sample could be selected in a rolling panel design[5] that would minimize the cost of the survey and the burden borne by respondents and yet still yield unbiased and efficient estimates of how often the campaign PSAs are being broadcast throughout the country.

An evaluation of campaign exposure in all markets throughout the country might produce more accurate information by making use of the AIDS hotline callers as respondents. It is known that hotline calls increase for a short period of time after the broadcast of a PSA. The monitoring system for hotline calls could easily be enhanced to record the telephone exchange numbers or area codes of all callers and the time

---

[5] A rolling panel design is one in which a portion of the panel is dropped at every wave and a new representative sample added.

of their calls; alternatively, callers could be asked to provide their zip codes. These data could be used to indicate indirectly when a PSA was broadcast in a particular market. A burst of calls to the hotline from one particular market in the country between 7:15 and 7:30 p.m. on a particular evening would almost certainly mean that one of the campaign PSAs was broadcast in that market between 7:00 and 7:15 p.m. A few simple questions posed to hotline callers could verify the broadcasting station's number or call letters; this information in turn could be linked with Nielsen data to generate estimates of the size and composition of the viewing audience for that station at that time.

Unfortunately, data on viewers, which are necessary for any comprehensive assessment of implementation, are weak for most television markets because they are based only on diary samples that are obtained during designated "sweep" weeks each year. Programming options tend to be unique during these weeks; as a result, it is not clear that information obtained through these diaries is characteristic of the markets at other times of the year. Furthermore, even if these data accurately reflected the number of people viewing a particular program on a particular station, they provide no information on whether the PSAs captured the attention of the audience. As noted above, the only feasible way to resolve these problems is to carry out a coincidental telephone survey in which a random sample of television households are contacted shortly after the broadcast of a PSA. Brief interviews with respondents can determine whether they were viewing the station on which the PSA was broadcast and, if so, whether they watched the PSA.

Telephone coincidental surveys are not totally without difficulties, however. Their main drawback is that they require enormous coordination to know when a PSA will be broadcast on a particular station in a particular market. Although this kind of information is available for paid advertisements, it is not for most PSAs, making it nearly impossible to implement the strategy of coincidental phone calls nationally. Fortunately, the AIDS hotline could be used to help resolve this problem. The same strategy of monitoring hotline calls to determine indirectly when a PSA was broadcast in a particular market could allow interviewers working in conjunction with the hotline to pinpoint markets for random-digit-dialing coincidental interviews. A small team of no more than 3 or 4 interviewers added to the 68 who are already answering hotline calls could phone random households in areas with PSA broadcasts reported during the prior 30-minute period. Ongoing assessment of this sort could provide valuable information on the clarity of the message and the attentiveness of the audience. These strategies are relatively modest in terms of the resources required for their implementation.

Resources and Aspirations

It is important to recognize that the evaluation of an ongoing set of PSAs brings a media campaign to a critical decision point: whether to continue broadcasting these advertisements, to take them off the air, or to introduce a new set of PSAs. The strategy that has just been described, which involves parallel monitoring of trend information from the national telephone hotline and from telephone coincidental surveys, could prove to be the most useful evaluation tool for this purpose. Indications that particular PSAs have been seen so many times that they no longer provoke thoughtful attention and no longer evoke the same serious responses (as indicated by calls to the AIDS hotline) provide strong, face-valid evidence that it is time to introduce another set of messages.

To monitor the success of a media campaign's implementation, however, it is necessary to obtain more detailed information than is currently available regarding how often the campaign messages are broadcast on television stations throughout the country. Probably the best way to get this information is to supplement BAR data with an ongoing telephone survey of scheduling managers in a probability sample of television stations that have received the PSAs. A survey of this kind would require no more than the equivalent of one full-time telephone interviewer and some administrative support to help design the sampling frame and the plan for systematic sampling in a rolling panel design.

In addition, more use could be made of the AIDS hotline in the variety of ways suggested above. First, consideration should be given to augmenting the hotline protocol with a brief set of questions. We recognize that although this suggestion sounds and should be simple, the situation is complicated by current policy that disallows questioning of hotline callers. We urge that present policy be amended to allow a short, approved list of questions that are carefully crafted to maintain a caller's confidentiality. These questions should cover where and when the caller saw the PSA, which PSA the caller saw, and whether the caller would be willing to participate in a follow-up assessment of the campaign. In addition, a content code should be developed to record the nature of the questions posed by the caller. Given the enormous number of calls handled by the hotline, the selection of a random sample of callers to receive these more detailed questions would be adequate. The resources needed for this activity would include two people: a project manager who is capable of designing a brief series of questions and a sampling scheme to embed these questions in hotline interviews, and a computer programmer capable of augmenting the telephone control system associated with the hotline. The augmented telephone system would record the time of calls and the telephone exchange of callers: that is, the area code and 3-digit prefix identifying the telephone exchange, *not* the entire telephone number. Both of these pieces of information can be recorded mechanically.

The panel also considers it potentially important to implement an ongoing telephone coincidental survey in parallel with the hotline system. As noted above, this survey could involve as few as 3 or 4 additional telephone interviewers working together with the current 68 hotline personnel. The same project manager recommended in the previous paragraph could develop an interview schedule and coordinate the design of this ongoing survey, as well as monitor trends in the data. The interview data obtained in such a survey could be managed by a computer-assisted telephone interview system, thus avoiding any need for data entry.

Costs for all of the resources noted in this section should not exceed 2 percent of the total cost of the campaign. The total cost includes the donated air time for PSAs as well as any other in-kind costs from all sources.

OUTCOME EVALUATION: DOES THE CAMPAIGN MAKE A DIFFERENCE?

Once a campaign has been implemented on a broad scale, any outcome evaluation that is done attempts to answer the question "Does it work?"—that is, Is it effective as it was actually implemented? The answers to this question are usually less clear than the answers to the efficacy question ("*Can* the campaign make a difference?") because the level and integrity of a campaign's implementation may vary widely. Thus, if a campaign does not work very well, it is difficult to determine whether it was because it was not well implemented or because it was not efficacious—that is, it could not have been effective even if it had been well implemented. The previous section discussed determining the efficacy of a campaign. This section considers the panel's recommended approach to determining the effectiveness of a campaign.

Randomized Experiments

As discussed in Chapter 1, the panel recommends randomized experiments to determine the effectiveness of AIDS media campaigns. Several strategies are possible for the conduct of such trials. The ideal approach would be to implement the campaign in one-half of the national media markets—randomly selected—and delay implementation in the other half for six months or more. (This approach is analogous to wait-list controls in clinical trials.) Another alternative would be to implement a "phased roll-out" of the campaign; that is, implement the campaign in several randomly selected markets each month over a 6- to 12-month period. Still another approach would be to implement two very different campaigns with different objectives at the same time and then switch them after six months (a switching replication design). For campaign components that have different objectives, it might be possible to deliver different components to different markets for 3 to 6 months and then switch them (again, the switching replication design). This evaluation approach would be particularly valuable for determining whether specific media campaign strategies were effective in achieving their specified objectives.

Effectiveness evaluation is more complex than efficacy evaluation because it requires an assessment of the extent to which changes in measured outcomes can be linked to PSA exposure. One way to assess this linkage is by means of time-series analyses that monitor trends in these outcomes over the course of the campaign period. The National Health Interview Survey (NHIS), a weekly survey of samples of 800 respondents in the United States, has been used for this purpose—specifically to evaluate the effects of the *America Responds to AIDS* campaign. Unfortunately, the data cannot be interpreted with any confidence because respondents were not randomly assigned to exposure to the campaign or to a nonexposure control condition.

National campaigns like *America Responds to AIDS* make it possible to analyze naturally occurring variations in campaign exposure by comparing aggregate trends in the outcomes across television markets that differ in their frequencies of airing the PSAs. One should recognize, however, that the determinants of this variation in exposure need to be introduced as explicitly as possible into the analysis and the interpretation of results to evaluate the possibility of spurious associations. It is plausible to expect the greatest changes in the outcomes in areas of the country in which the PSAs were shown most often; however, it might be that the decision to air the PSAs frequently was a response by local station officials to the fact that knowledge or attitudes were *not* changing in their communities, in which case one could well find exactly the opposite aggregate pattern. Owing to this problem, caution is needed in drawing conclusions about campaign effectiveness from simple analyses of this sort.

A number of data sources are readily available for use in effectiveness evaluations. The panel comments on three of them here: the NHIS, as an example of population surveys that can be used in evaluation, the AIDS hotline, and other archival sources.

The National Health Interview Survey

The National Health Interview Survey, can be a particularly useful source of data for the analysis of aggregate trends, because it has included AIDS-related items since August 1987. Data are collected from 800 adults per week. Questions are designed specifically to "provide estimates of public knowledge and attitudes about AIDS transmission and prevention and AIDS virus infection . . . for monitoring educational efforts, e.g., the series of radio and television public service announcements entitled *America Responds to AIDS* and the brochure *Understanding AIDS"* (Dawson, 1988). The current version of the NHIS includes questions on the following:

- sources of AIDS information;
- self-assessed level of AIDS knowledge;
- basic facts about the AIDS virus and how it is transmitted;
- blood donation experience;
- awareness of and experience with the blood test for the AIDS virus;
- perceived effectiveness of selected preventive measures;
- self-assessed chances of getting the AIDS virus;
- personal acquaintance with persons with AIDS or the AIDS virus;
- willingness to take part in a proposed national seroprevalence survey; and
- a general risk behavior question.

The National Center for Health Statistics publication *Advance Data* No.163 provides comparisons of the August 1987 and August 1988 responses. By 1988, population knowledge and attitudes had improved significantly in many respects, although there were still misconceptions held by a large proportion of the population.

In addition to the questions that already appear on the NHIS, a small number of items could be added from time to time to assess particular knowledge, attitudes, and beliefs. For example, seven new items were added to the May, June, and July 1988 surveys to evaluate the receipt and use of the brochure mailed out in the May-June period of Phase II of the media campaign. The results indicate that the brochure was received by 63 percent of households, read by someone in more than one-half of those households, and discussed with others by about one-third of those who read it. This type of approach can constructively be used for any new campaign phase.

The panel recommends that items be added to the National Health Interview Survey to evaluate exposure to, recall of, responses to, and changes resulting from a new phase of the media campaign.

Hotline Calls

In a similar way, it is relatively simple to log the number of AIDS hotline calls received per month. As discussed above, additional information could be easily obtained from the hotline.

The panel recommends that CDC increase the usefulness of hotline data for media campaign assessments by collecting evaluation-related data such as the caller's geographic location, selected caller characteristics, issue(s) of concern, and counselor responses.

Each of these types of information could then be related to the issues addressed in the campaign and the regional variations that may have been used in the campaign's implementation.

For Phase IV of the *America Responds to AIDS* campaign, possible exposure to the PSAs should also be related to whether the caller is an adolescent, the parent of an adolescent, or an educator. Because the campaign is specifically directed toward these groups, one would expect more calls from people in these groups than from other people. To the extent that calls from the general population do increase, such a trend might indicate success in reaching the general population. The collection of additional detailed data on the type of question the caller asked and the type of written material (if any) mailed to him or her would further improve the ability to link campaign activities to population behavior. Following up some callers—with their prior permission—would allow for an assessment of subsequent knowledge and behavioral changes.

Other Archival Sources

Evaluators of national AIDS prevention campaigns should collect or monitor data on several other AIDS-relevant archival indicators—such as condom sales and reports of STDs of all types—and use them to aid the interpretation of other evaluation data. These examples and others are all possible indicators of changes in societal norms and behaviors, at least when considered in combination. The limitations in their ability to indicate such changes are discussed in the following section on methodology.

Methodological Issues

As noted earlier, evaluating the effectiveness of a PSA campaign is extremely difficult. To attribute observed changes to a particular campaign requires randomized tests of alternatives or of lagged implementation. This being the case, it is useful to distinguish between problems in effectiveness evaluation of current campaigns and phases, and problems in the evaluation of future campaigns and phases.

Effectiveness Evaluation of Current Activities

There are three levels of analysis that may be undertaken to judge the effectiveness of current campaign activities: aggregate analyses, partially disaggregated analyses, and disaggregated analyses. Each has methodological problems that may limit its use. As noted above, aggregate analyses of campaign effectiveness provide trend information that could be explained on the basis of determinants other than exposure to the campaign. Partially disaggregated analyses—comparing differential trends in outcomes across geographic areas that vary in intensity of campaign exposure—are subject to biases introduced by selection factors. Disaggregated analyses are difficult to perform because measures of individual differences in exposure to the campaign are usually unreliable and often systematically biased. The best one can hope for in a situation of this sort is to make a concerted effort to examine trends on all three of these levels and obtain as much information as possible about potentially important selection factors. The documentation of consistent findings across the three different levels of analysis, coupled with evidence that the trends persist in the face of adjustments for potentially important selection factors, can be taken as strongly suggesting that an association between exposure to the campaign and outcomes of interest is likely to be causal.

The combination of trend monitoring through the AIDS telephone hotline and the parallel implementation of a telephone coincidental survey in an ongoing fashion could also help to provide evidence about effectiveness. The combination of these data would allow an evaluator to determine whether the hotline continues to be used by the same percentage of people who are exposed to the campaign over the course of time. This information is more relevant to determining whether a campaign continues to be effective in calling attention to the availability of additional information through the hotline than it is to the overall effectiveness of the campaign; nevertheless, the issue of continued effectiveness is critical in a campaign that self-consciously defines itself as having a series of phases. Given the seriousness of the AIDS epidemic as well as the expense of mounting a media campaign to slow its transmission, one type of evaluation should be used to determine how long each phase should be maintained (instead of relying on anecdotal evidence about the "typical shelf life" of PSA material, as is currently done). Monitoring hotline calls, and particularly the trends in these calls that can be associated with different PSAs, as well as trends in the types of information requested in the calls, could provide extremely useful information on when particular messages begin to lose their effect or their purpose.

Separating the effects of any national campaign from other national or local campaigns is difficult, but it is particularly so when there are numerous other campaigns in operation, as is often the case with AIDS. It is just as important, and just as difficult, to separate the effects of a national media campaign from national news coverage about AIDS. Nevertheless, the monitoring of other associated activities needs to be an integral part of outcome evaluation for the campaign. Evaluators need to determine to what extent observed changes in knowledge, attitudes, and beliefs are the result of the national mass media campaign and not the accumulated effects of news coverage or of a great many local campaigns. For example, it is impossible to attribute changes in knowledge from August 1987 to August 1988 to either the mailed brochure or the PSA campaign. With hindsight, it is apparent that one possibility for causal attribution would have been a nonequivalent dependent variable approach: that is, a study could have been designed so that some knowledge, attitudes, or beliefs would have been changed by the brochure but not by the PSAs or anything else; some would have been changed by the PSAs but not by the brochure or anything else; and some would not have been changed by either the brochure or the PSAs or anything else. Additions to the NHIS could easily have been designed with this approach in mind, as could future surveys, for example, to contribute to the evaluation of Phase IV of the *America Responds to AIDS* campaign. Another possible method of causal attribution would entail mapping any patterns of increased knowledge collected by the NHIS along with patterns of PSA airings. If the two patterns tracked fairly well, competing explanations for change could be discounted.

A further possibility for evaluating the effectiveness of the brochure is to identify geographic regions that differed significantly in the date of delivery of the brochure. A several-week lag would be required to detect similarly lagged changes in self-reports of brochure receipt and changes in knowledge, attitudes, and beliefs.

Effectiveness Evaluation of Future Activities

For future phases of the *America Responds to AIDS* campaign or for new campaigns, a much more accurate assessment of effectiveness could be obtained by staggering the implementation of the new activity in a randomized sample of markets. The selection of early-exposure markets should be based on the degree to which they are typical of the entire country and on their lack of "spill-out" (picking up television signals in one market from adjacent markets).[6] A systematic variation of this sort, if followed throughout subsequent stages of the campaign, would make it possible to use the analysis of interrupted time-series to evaluate effectiveness.

In this approach, change in the time trend of outcomes associated with the introduction of a new intervention could be interpreted as the result of the intervention rather than the result of other contemporaneous changes in the larger environment. By staggering the introduction of new campaign phases, the validity of this assumption could be assessed by determining whether parallel trend changes occurred in early-exposure and later-exposure markets (separated by perhaps 6-12 months). If parallels can be documented, an evaluator can discount the otherwise plausible concern about influence other than the campaign leading to the change. If parallels cannot be found, then the evaluator should be aware that idiosyncratic influences other than the campaign are likely to be involved. When combined with the use of naturally occurring variations (noted above), this approach maximizes an evaluator's ability to accurately assess campaign effectiveness.

Problems with Sources of Data

The NHIS and Other Surveys. Ongoing surveys have great value in that they can provide data that are useful for conducting some types of trend analysis. Their major limitation, however, concerns the relevance of the collected data: the closer the relation of the questions being asked to the campaign being evaluated, the more useful the survey. The NHIS is obviously of greatest relevance to the AIDS media campaigns in that a series of AIDS-related items has been included since August 1987. These items are limited to fairly general constructs, however, and cannot be used to evaluate focused objectives.

The one advantage of the NHIS over all other federally supported surveys is the ability to insert new items from time to time. To provide more relevant data, new AIDS-related items should collect focused attitude and behavioral information rather than exposure and immediate-use information only (the data collected on the mailed brochure). These items should also be incorporated in the NHIS for a longer period of

---

[6]This approach relies on the compliance of station managers to air the test PSAs. This type of evaluation would be easier to implement if air time were purchased rather than donated.

time, including several months prior to a new campaign, to make some type of trend analysis possible. The NHIS is far too valuable a resource to be limited to items that assess exposure only over a short time frame.

To maximize its usefulness, the NHIS should also be used as the vehicle for the nonequivalent dependent variable approach (described above; see Cook and Campbell, 1979). Under this approach, three types of items would be included: items that should show change as a result of a specific campaign; items that should change as a result of other concurrent campaign(s); and other items (albeit related) that should not be changed by any ongoing campaign.

Ongoing surveys are most useful when the campaign under evaluation is directed toward the general population; whenever a campaign has a more restricted focus (e.g., high-risk women, parents of adolescents, adolescents, school personnel), national surveys become less valuable. How much less valuable depends on how restrictively the selected population is defined. The narrower the population description, the less the selected population will be represented in the survey sample. In such cases, oversampling of the selected population is necessary. For example, CDC could support oversampling of the groups (adolescents, parents of adolescents) that are the focus of Phase IV of the *America Responds to AIDS* campaign.

Hotline Calls and Other Archival Data. Currently, the logging forms for AIDS telephone hotline calls permit only the assessment of the number of calls from month to month, possibly by region. This limitation could and should be removed.

There are two major inferential issues with other archival data: What do observed changes mean? Can they be attributed to a particular campaign? Changes in the indicators listed above need to be interpreted with care. For example, increased sales of condoms have been viewed as an indication of a reduction in unsafe sex; however, the validity of this indication depends on how many of the purchased condoms were actually used, a fact that remains unknown. The meaning of fewer condom sales would be similarly unclear: if the new campaign succeeded in increasing the acceptability of abstinence, it might lead to a decrease in overall sexual activity (provided such a decrease had not already occurred) and to a concurrent decrease in condom sales.

Reductions in reported STDs of all types, in pregnancies among teenagers, and in the number of babies born with HIV could all indicate lower rates of sexual activity or safer sexual practices. As discussed in Chapter 2, these measures do not, by themselves, indicate which is occurring, although in combination with figures on sales of prophylactic and contraceptive devices or materials (e.g., condoms and spermicides), they might. Lower rates of STDs together with lower sales would suggest less sexual activity. In the absence of improved STD treatment, lower rates of STDs together with higher or unchanging condom and spermicide sales would suggest the increased use of safer sexual practices. Archival data must be used with great caution and in combination, without relying on any single indicator.

Despite the valuable information provided by archival data, they offer no evidence on whether observed changes are due to a particular media campaign. Are the changes suggested by such indicators the result of the CDC campaign, some other campaign, or combined campaigns? Would they have occurred even without any campaign? From a public health perspective, it might not matter: the important point would be that sexual practices were becoming safer (and HIV infection should subsequently decrease). From a cost-effectiveness policy or perspective, however, it is critical to determine what caused the changes. If they would have occurred without the CDC campaign, the cost of the campaign was then a waste of resources that might have been used for something more valuable (the opportunity costs). From a policy perspective, it is obviously important to determine whether a particular campaign produced the effects attributed to it. The limitations that must be confronted and the resources necessary to make such a determination are discussed below.

Resources and Aspirations

Outcome evaluation of an ongoing national campaign such as *America Responds to AIDS* is limited by a number of factors. First, the analysis is based on a sample of one case. Second, the environment may vary in ways that induce changes in the target population that are parallel to the effects sought by the campaign, thus making it difficult to attribute trends in outcomes uniquely to campaign effects. Third, CDC does not control variations in exposure to the campaign either over time or over different television markets. NAIEP staff have indicated to the panel that the national media campaign is expected to continue into the foreseeable future; the panel believes strongly that unless randomized tests of alternatives or of lagged implementations are conducted, there is little hope for anything more than educated guesses about the meanings of any observed trends.

Outcome evaluation may also be limited by funding and staff availability. Although CDC has substantial resources for the media campaigns, resources for the evaluation of these activities are much more difficult to determine. Although special AIDS-related items have been and will be added to the NHIS, CDC needs to have adequate staff resources to design these added items to be of optimal value in an outcome evaluation or analyze the resulting data in depth. Another example involves the AIDS hotline. CDC established the national AIDS hotline in 1982 and contracted with the American Social Health Association in 1987 to operate it, but there is little evidence of efforts to determine its effects or effectiveness beyond showing how many calls came in. Information on the number of calls received is useless without knowledge of who is calling, what type of questions are asked, how they were answered, what other information or services were provided to callers, and with what effects. The National Cancer Institute provides an example of better ongoing evaluation of a hotline (Stein, 1986). Another evaluation opportunity involves regional variations in media implementation and exposure. There have been no attempts to analyze the effects of these natural variations.

Conducting randomized tests of media campaigns is expensive but not prohibitively so. For example, a randomized test of delayed implementation would require surveys of randomly selected samples from media markets that receive a campaign first and from markets in which implementation is delayed. A national survey is appropriate as long as items about a respondent's region and exposure are included for all participants. As noted above, this could be done through added items on the NHIS, although a separate national survey would be preferable. A national survey of 5,000 randomly selected respondents, repeated three times, might cost from $500,000 to $750,000. For some campaigns or some phases of campaigns that are directed toward more specific populations, costs might double or triple because of the extensive screening that would be necessary to identify the sample. Randomized tests of alternative campaign strategies are more expensive, but only marginally so. The only additional cost is the production of alternative campaign materials; all other costs of campaign implementation and evaluation are the same as for the delayed implementation model.

Even for the most expensive approaches, the costs of outcome evaluations for media campaigns will not exceed the costs of program development and will be only a small fraction of the total costs of the campaign. Adequate resources for determining campaign effectiveness are estimated to be at least 5 percent of the expected total campaign cost (including donated or in-kind costs from all sources).

A final note is in order on the potential impact of changes in AIDS treatments and social phenomena. Any changes in treatments for AIDS, prevalence rates or infection patterns, public attitudes, or legislation regarding the social treatment of people with AIDS will have implications for public education. The panel urges that the developers of national AIDS prevention campaigns continuously monitor new developments and news reports and consider the implications of new findings, treatments, or vocabularies for future surveys and media campaigns.

REFERENCES

Cook, T., and Campbell, D. T. (1979) *Quasi-Experimentation: Design and Analysis for Field Settings*. Boston: Houghton-Mifflin.

Dawson, D. (1988) Knowledge and attitudes for May and June 1988. *NCHS Advance Data* 160:1-24.

Flay, B. R. (1986) Efficacy and effectiveness trials (and other phases of research) in the development of health promotion programs. *Preventive Medicine* 15:451-474.

Flay, B. R., and Cook, T. D. (1981) Evaluation of mass media prevention campaigns. In R. R. Rice and W. Paisley, eds., *Public Communication Campaigns*. Beverly Hills, Calif.: Sage Publications.

Government Accounting Office (GAO) (1988) *AIDS Education: Activities Aimed at the General Public Implemented Slowly*. GAO/HRD-89-21. December. Washington, D.C.: U.S. Government Printing Office.

Joseph, J. G., Emmons, C. A., Kessler, R. C., Wortman, C. B., O'Brien, K., Hocker, W. T., and Schaefer, C. (1984) Coping with the threat of AIDS: An approach to psychosocial assessment. *American Psychologist* 39:1297-1302.

Joseph, J. G., Montgomery, S. B., Emmons, C. A., Kessler, R. C., Ostrow, D. G., Wortman, C. B., O'Brien, K., Eller, M., and Eshleman, S. (1987) Magnitude and determinants of behavioral risk reduction: Longitudinal analysis of a cohort at risk for AIDS. *Psychology and Health* 1:73-96.

McCusker, J., Stoddard, A. M., Mayer, K. H., Zapka, J., Morrison, C., and Saltzman, S. P. (1988) Effects of HIV antibody test knowledge on subsequent sexual behaviors in a cohort of homosexual men. *American Journal of Public Health* 78:462-467.

McKusick, L., Horstman, W., and Coates, T. J. (1985) AIDS and sexual behavior reported by gay men in San Francisco. *American Journal of Public Health* 75:493-496.

Morgan, D. L., and Spanish, M. T. (1984) Focus groups: A new tool of qualitative research. *Qualitative Sociology* 7:253-270.

Office of Cancer Communications (1983) *Making PSAs Work*. Washington, D.C.: National Cancer Institute.

Office of Cancer Communications (1984) *Pretesting Television PSAs*. Washington, D.C.: National Cancer Institute.

Palmer, E. (1981) Shaping persuasive messages with formative research. In R. R. Rice and W. Paisley, eds., *Public Communication Campaigns*. Beverly Hills, Calif.: Sage Publications.

Stein, J. (1986) The Cancer Information Service: Marketing a large-scale national information program through media. In D. G. Leather, G. B. Hastings, K. M. O'Reilly, and J. K. Davies, eds., *Health Education and the Media*, Vol. 2. London: Pergamon.

Valdiserri, R. O., Lyter, D., Leviton, L. C., Callahan, C. M., Kingsley, L. A., and Rinaldo, C. R. (1988) Variables influencing condom use in a cohort of gay and bisexual men. *American Journal of Public Health* 78:801-805.

Wright, P. (1979) Concrete action plans and TV messages to increase reading of drug warnings. *Journal of Consumer Research* 6:256-269.

4

Evaluating Health Education and Risk Reduction Projects

This chapter focuses on CDC's new direct grants program to fund health education/risk reduction projects of community-based organizations (CBOs). In the past, CDC's Center for Prevention Services (CPS) has provided funding to CBOs via two mechanisms: cooperative agreements with states and a cooperative agreement with the U.S. Conference of Mayors. Now CPS is poised to launch a program that will directly fund CBOs. The national objectives for the CBO projects are the same as those for CDC's counseling and testing program: behavior change, surveillance, and public education (CDC, 1988). An additional purpose for direct funding to CBOs is to reach hard-to-reach groups.

Evaluation of community-based projects presents both conceptual and practical problems that are quite different from those encountered in evaluating the media campaign or the HIV testing and counseling program. The major conceptual difficulty arises from the diversity of the activities that are offered by the projects; the major practical difficulty is the present scarcity of comprehensive information describing the projects themselves.

BACKGROUND AND OBJECTIVES

The traditional CPS instrument for implementing its funding priorities is a state cooperative agreement.[1] Since 1985, when agreements for funding

---

[1] For specific and well-defined products, CDC has occasionally executed cooperative agreements with professional organizations such as the American Public Health Association, the U.S. Conference of Local Health Officers, the National Association of County Health Officers and the Association of Teachers of Prevention Medicine.

CBOs were instituted, 59 states and localities have had rather broad discretion in the allocation of federal dollars consistent with an approved state plan; the ultimate recipients of these dollars have numbered in the hundreds. In addition, CPS has an "arms length" relationship with dozens more CBOs through a cooperative agreement with the U.S. Conference of Mayors. The states and the Conference of Mayors have been responsible for accepting proposals from CBOs, selecting projects for funding, and providing project oversight and administration.

This arrangement contrasts with the new direct grants relationship that CPS is now implementing to fund minority and other community-based organizations, which is focused on organizations in 27 major metropolitan areas. Approximately 400 proposals have been submitted by CBOs under this program, and CPS expects that between 55 and 65 projects will soon be funded at an annual support level of $50,000-$225,000 per year for 3 years.

The new direct grants program is designed to afford greater access to high-risk individuals as well as to permit CDC a direct link through which it can provide hands-on technical assistance to organizations for refining and evaluating their intervention projects. Moreover, the new program will permit CBOs to address problems that they and CDC jointly identify as important and that can be dealt with most effectively through local organizations.

Although CPS has not yet had any experience dealing directly with CBOs, another branch of CDC has. Since August 1988, the National AIDS Information and Education Program (NAIEP) has extended grants or contracts to 33 minority CBOs. Some evaluation data have been collected from these projects during two or more site visits by project officers, whose main task has been to lend technical assistance to the grantees, and through the filing of an annual report (not standardized) by each CBO. Process evaluations are in progress, but no outcome evaluations have been conducted of the NAIEP program. Consequently, the new direct grants program presents a special challenge to CPS to work with the diversity represented by CBOs and the specific contextual frameworks that define who is proposed to get what services, when, by what means, and to what end. As one example of the extent of this challenge, the management information systems that have been developed for monitoring, tracking, and evaluating official health agency project activities are likely to be of limited usefulness when applied to the broad range of CBO activities.

CBOs tend to be narrowly focused with respect to their mission, primary constituency, and target population. The feature that distinguishes them from other organizations is their evolution from and their involvement with the community they propose to serve. Seldom, however, does any single CBO evolve to a point where it can mobilize all of the relevant local resources because communities, especially urban inner-city communities, are complex, diverse entities that are segmented by race, ethnicity, sexual orientation, and other individual and social characteristics.

Thus, the CBOs that have been grantees through the Conference of Mayors agreement, for example, are quite diverse in both the primary constituencies they serve and the activities they propose to undertake. Constituent groups vary by race, age, sexual preference, religious orientation, language, addictive behavior, occupation (e.g., farm workers, migrant workers, prostitutes), and other factors (e.g., runaway and "throwaway" youth). In terms of project activities, panel members identified at least 18 different types of activity, including conducting educational seminars and workshops to train AIDS educators; compiling, publishing, and distributing printed material; developing counseling sessions; engaging in parades and street fairs; sponsoring AIDS-related performing arts activities; establishing focus groups; and producing videos and PSAs.

Given their emphasis on service delivery, the CBO projects that have been funded have not paid much attention to evaluation. Thus, there is little evidence on the relative effects that such interventions have had on the target populations. At present, none of the CBOs can demonstrate the effectiveness of the interventions they have implemented.

To address this lack in the new program, CPS called for the formulation of an evaluation plan as one of the criteria (worth 15 points of a possible 100) to be used in selecting projects for funding under its new direct grants program. The CDC guidelines on grant preparation appear to advise applicants to produce evaluation plans for both process and outcome evaluation. CDC staff informed the panel that although preapplication workshops were held to provide guidance in developing the plans, the evaluation designs submitted by the CBOs were generally inadequate.[2]

The panel does not find this result surprising. CBOs are not, in general, in the business of doing evaluation research. They are unlikely to employ the methodologists and statisticians required to develop a competent research design to demonstrate the effects of their programs. Furthermore, the panel's own struggle with this task led it to conclude

---

[2] In addition to running preapplication workshops, CPS's project officers continue to provide extensive technical assistance to CBOs after they are funded. Their work is especially critical in the first 3 to 6 months when, through telephone and site visits, project officers encourage a focused approach to CBO interventions, help practitioners establish realistic goals and work plans, cultivate input from their communities, and document the project's delivery processes.

that designing adequate evaluations for these programs is a challenging task—even with expert personnel. In the rest of this chapter the panel presents and discusses its strategies for the important and difficult task of evaluating the health education and risk reduction projects that will be undertaken by community-based organizations.

WHAT SERVICES ARE DELIVERED?

There are three evaluation strategies to be considered in determining what activities were planned by a project and what activities actually took place: case studies of individual projects, gathering data through a standardized administrative reporting system, and conducting a census or sample survey.

Case Studies of a Sample of Projects

Case studies can be immensely helpful in describing an activity and learning about the process involved in conducting it. The major limitation of a case study is that, without a supplemental statistical study of a sample of projects, the generalizability of the information cannot be known. Well-conducted case studies, however, can improve the design of a statistical study of such projects. Indeed, when the universe of projects being studied is diverse or not well understood by researchers, case studies will be a prerequisite for other research (by survey or other methods) since they can identify the questions that ought to be asked.

After reviewing abstracts of the CBO projects presently under way, the panel concluded that descriptive case studies are required and should be undertaken as a first step in evaluation. The case studies should focus on identifying the major approaches to health education and risk reduction that are being undertaken in these projects, developing a better understanding of the basic project components and processes, and better specifying the specific outcomes that are anticipated.

The strategy that seems most sensible to the panel is to use case studies with a small sample of sites as a first step, and subsequently to develop survey questionnaires or administrative reporting forms for systematic data collection from all projects (or a large sample of projects).[3] For the sake of concreteness, the panel provides below an example of

---

[3] The design suggested in the text is a stratified sample. Stratifying projects by type and then randomly choosing sample projects ensures that results will effectively be applicable to all of them. A certain amount of ambiguity will remain with regard to unique project types that fall outside the sampling scheme. When projects are quite diverse and few in number, however, case studies can be conducted of all of them. Each design choice has its virtues: studying a sample is less costly and less time-consuming; studying all the sites is more precise.

the way in which case studies might be used to provide descriptive information.

Our example focuses on identifying the approaches to health education/risk reduction currently being provided to IV drug users. In order to identify the approaches that are currently in use, preliminary case studies might be conducted of prototypical projects funded by CDC and the National Institute on Drug Abuse (NIDA). As noted above, the objectives would be to identify the major approaches for evaluation; to develop an understanding of the basic project components and processes; and, since CBO projects differ by type, to prepare a set of protocols appropriate for different types of interventions and target audiences as a basis for more rigorous evaluation. In addition, such case studies could enhance understanding of:

- the target groups and subgroups being served;
- how individuals learn about services and what other services are available to them;
- how a CBO learns about and reaches out to individuals, engages them in receiving services, and limits attrition from the project;
- what services or educational material are delivered, by whom, how often, to whom, and in what context;
- the accuracy and timeliness of the education or risk reduction information selected groups receive; and
- how funds are used.

Key elements in the design of such a study would include the selection of a sample of sites for case studies, the collection of data during site visits to each project, and the analysis and interpretation of the data.

Sample

The sample of projects selected for study might be stratified by seroprevalence rates among IV drug users in the community, (e.g., high or low); the setting in which activity is conducted (e.g., street outreach or treatment program); and target group (e.g., IV drug users themselves or those at high risk of HIV infection by sexual contact with IV drug users). These three stratification variables produce a $2 \times 2 \times 2$ matrix of candidate projects—requiring case studies of a minimum of 8 programs if one project is chosen from each cell of the matrix.[4] Whenever feasible,

---

[4]Some cells of this matrix might, of course, be empty. For example, there might be no street outreach programs to the sexual partners of IV drug users established in low prevalence areas. If there are empty cells in the matrix, the number of case studies required would be smaller.

however, the panel believes that more than one project should be selected for each cell in order to provide a crude indication of the variation that exists between projects. In selecting projects within the cells, priority should be given to projects on the basis of the replicability (in theory) of the treatment offered in the project; the local feasibility of doing a study; and the representativeness of the program or site category.

Data Collection

To collect data from the projects, site visits of 3 to 4 days would be conducted by a team of 3-4 persons. The project team should include an AIDS education specialist, an expert on the risk behavior of IV drug users, and an evaluation design specialist. (If needed, a person to abstract project records should also be available.) The site visit team would conduct open-ended interviews with key project staff, other program personnel, key individuals in programs or communities, and at least 5-10 program participants, or potential participants. The interviews would focus on program activities, opinions about those activities, and the identification of key content, process, or structural elements that may determine the success of a program.

Analysis

All project team members would prepare individual case study reports covering the process evaluation topics noted above. A summary report would then be prepared outlining the major findings of the team and identifying the elements of the project that appear appropriate for further data gathering using other procedures.

Standardized Administrative Reporting

The Center for Prevention Services plans to gather data from the direct grantees in two ways: site visits made by CDC project officers and quarterly narrative reports provided by the sites. Of the three topic areas for the quarterly narratives, one asks CBOs to describe their progress toward meeting project objectives. This section is intended to elicit information about activities offered to date and about the target audience. Site visits are intended to monitor services and audiences. (Program staff may also code the data gathered from site visits and narratives and enter it into a data base.)

We encourage data collection on the progress towards goals and the proposed establishment of a data base. However, we believe it would be more desirable to develop a standardized administrative reporting form for CBOs. Such a form could solicit more comprehensive periodic data on a number of program elements, including:

- the project goals and primary target group;
- characteristics of the services delivered (type, to whom, how often);
- nature of the quality controls for the delivery of services;
- number of voluntary and paid staff;
- staff qualifications; and
- staff turnover.

This is a very preliminary list of the information that should be obtained, but we believe that it is more extensive and will be more consistent than data collected by quarterly narratives. In addition, comprehensive and standardized data are more amenable to coding than elements offered in a narration. The panel anticipates that substantial refinement to the list will be possible after the proposed case studies are completed.[5]

The panel notes that obtaining information about project goals is especially important, and it is likely to require careful probing. A health education/risk reduction project might readily assert that its primary goal is "education." However, the information that would be most helpful is much more specific: for example, the project might be using street outreach workers to educate Hispanic persons who use IV drugs about (1) the opportunities for drug treatment that are available in their community, (2) the risks posed by sharing of injection equipment, and (3) methods for sterilizing injection equipment. Similarly, "risk reduction" might take the form of providing bleach or condoms. The intensity, duration, and character of these risk reduction activities might also vary; for example, bleach might be available at any time or only 2 hours a day. Knowing only that a project's goal is "education" or "risk reduction" will not be sufficient to allow a detailed classification of projects or ultimately to learn which intervention strategies work best.

The information gathered by an administrative form (together with the results of case studies and site visits by project officers) could provide a reasonably accurate, up-to-date, and comprehensive description of the services being provided by CBOs. In implementing such an administrative reporting system, the panel cautions against introducing too much complexity in its design and operation. The purpose is elementary

---

[5]Case studies of street outreach projects should include examinations of the sometimes free-form daily logs in which outreach workers record their activities on the streets. Such analysis will further the development of forms amenable to the sometimes esoteric characteristics of service delivery made by outreach projects.

description rather than micromanagement, and the level of complexity of the system should reflect that purpose. The panel notes that CPS has developed a standardized reporting system to monitor the counseling and testing projects the agency supports. The experience CPS has acquired in developing that system in the counseling and testing arena might be exploited for CBO projects, although they are admittedly more varied and so will be more difficult to describe.

A Census or Sample Survey

If simple administrative reports of the kind just described existed and were completed regularly by CBOs—covering goals, strategies, and other program elements (and on the changes that occur in them)—they would be useful to CDC to understand what is planned and what is under way. To the extent that the reports are well circulated among the CBOs, they might help other CBOs learn which organizations are engaged in similar activities and to build networks that facilitate mutual education. However, different, in-depth information, obtained independently of the project itself, would enhance CPS's and the public's understanding of what actually occurs in projects. In part, the need to obtain such independent information arises from the fact that no project is ever delivered quite as advertised. In addition, when projects continue over time, goals, plans, and delivery methods may change as what has been learned is used to improve the intervention.

Detailed independent information may be obtained through a census or sample survey. A census or sample survey of projects can provide a more informative statistical description of activities than is generated by administrative reports. In the case of CDC's direct grants program, a census of 60 projects may be feasible. However, a sample survey of, for example, 30 projects would probably be sufficient for generating basic statistical information on a number of questions:

- What services are provided and to whom?
- When, how often, and for how long are services provided?
- In what context are these services delivered?

A census or sample survey might also gather information on client flow, and it could probe more deeply than an administrative reporting system into project objectives, characteristics of the services delivered, and other program elements. Responsibility for such a survey might be assigned to CDC's project officers, who already conduct semiannual or more frequent site visits to lend technical assistance and monitor progress.

The additional information generated by a census or sample survey might be helpful in describing projects to the public and to Congress and in identifying projects that appear to have good potential for use in other locales. In addition to such uses, the statistical information produced by such a survey or census might be useful locally, especially if the CBOs assist in designing questions that are of special interest at the local level.

Recommended Combination of Strategies

Of the three strategies the panel considered to answer the question, "What project activities are planned and undertaken?", a census or sample survey seems the least attractive simply because it is premature. At least some routine administrative data and some description or "scouting" of the projects—of the sort embodied by case studies—is essential for the design and execution of a good survey. Thus, while we endorse the notion of quarterly narrative reports and site visits, we go a step further.

The panel recommends that a simple standardized reporting system for health education/risk reduction projects be developed and used to address the question of what activities are planned and under way.

The panel also recommends the expanded use of case studies.

In making these recommendations, the panel believes that an administrative reporting system can provide broad statistical information; the case studies can provide enriched descriptions of program processes, character, and target groups, and they can aid in the design of further studies to collect statistical information. Regardless of which strategies are selected, the panel believes it will be sensible to sequence their use so that each strategy can take advantage of the information generated earlier in the sequence. In most circumstances, case studies should be attempted prior to other techniques since they will provide helpful insights about the topics that should be covered by surveys or administrative reporting systems.

Methodological Issues

The methodological problems involved in the two recommended strategies (case studies and administrative reporting) are not unusual. For instance, the design of a simple administrative reporting system would have to take into account the diversity of the health education/risk reduction projects being undertaken by the CBOs and the limited interest of the CBOs in providing such reports. As noted above, CDC's experience in developing a standardized reporting scheme for testing and counseling sites and its experience with the AIDS demonstration projects are both likely to be helpful. Even a simple reporting system should have a quality control component, however. For the type of reporting system the panel recommends, this component might include at least rudimentary checks, by telephone or in other ways, of a small sample of the reports that are submitted.

Conducting good case studies of a small sample of health education/risk reduction projects to understand project activities engenders somewhat different problems. The diversity among the projects will make the organization of results difficult. Moreover, it may be anticipated that some sites may object to being "scrutinized." The panel believes, however, that obtaining the cooperation of the projects should not be a major problem if it is made clear that the studies are not being conducted to determine the success or failure of the projects.

Obtaining an adequate number of suitable persons to do the site visits might be a problem. The number of individuals expert in such studies, especially in the context of minority and other community-based organization efforts, is relatively small, and implementing this approach may require the assistance of experts from outside CDC. Some people might be recruited from the pool of researchers engaged in work on CBO efforts in manpower (see Boruch, Dennis, and Carter-Greer, 1988), drug use prevention and treatment (see Hubbard et al., 1988), and other areas.

Resources and Aspirations

Some of the resources needed to exploit the two recommended options may already be available through specialized work that CDC has been supporting in other program areas. In the next chapter we note CDC's experience in developing an administrative reporting system for its counseling and testing program. Similarly, CDC's efforts in documenting and evaluating the activities of the AIDS community demonstration projects (CDC, 1989a), using survey methods and ethnographic approaches, may prove helpful.

The development and installation of an administrative reporting system, including technical support for quality control, can of course be done through a contract. Some related systems have been developed for more specialized CBO efforts, notably in experimental tests of manpower programs (see Betsey, Hollister, and Papageorgiou, 1985). Moreover, the case studies suggested above may help in the development of a system.

With regard to time, the panel believes that the case studies could probably be accomplished within 1 year. Major expenditures would be for project staff, case study personnel, and travel costs. Each case study, which would include staff preparation and write-up time, would require about 40 person-days per site and travel costs of $3,000-$4,000. The case studies would be relatively inexpensive, at a cost of $15,000 per site, and one to three full-time staff persons would be required for coordination.

For the money, this type of study provides a substantial amount of descriptive information. For example, it would help give some structure to a fairly diverse set of approaches and programs. The information provided through the case studies is essential before controlled studies or even useful surveys or management information systems can be developed.

DO THE PROJECTS MAKE A DIFFERENCE?

CDC has been encouraged to estimate the relative effectiveness of its various projects—that is, to determine whether the projects make a difference. Such an estimation requires some basis for comparison. One commonly proposed basis uses the before-and-after design.

Before-and-After Evaluation Designs

CDC's guidelines for evaluation of the new CBO projects propose the use of a "baseline" preprogram measure as a basis for estimating change that occurs as a consequence of these projects (CDC, 1989b). The panel believes that the nonexperimental, before-and-after evaluation design is useful in the context of process evaluation, (i.e., for looking at the scope and quality of a project's services); however, when the design includes pretest and posttest measures of attitudes and behaviors in the context of outcome evaluation, its usefulness is more limited.

The evidence produced by before-and-after comparisons of a project is often ambiguous at best and misleading at worst because no control groups are involved. The inference of cause and effect from such designs alone is generally not sustainable, and competing explanations for changes in attitudes and behaviors cannot ordinarily be ruled out.[6] The panel notes that there are typically a large number of AIDS-related activities and events occurring in any given locale, which makes any attribution of behavior change in a population (i.e., any "difference") to a specific project unconvincing.

While the design is thus limited, it might still be usefully applied in an evaluation that aims to test the null hypothesis that no change occurred (regardless of cause). When it can be confidently assumed that the uncontrolled factors (e.g., other programs in the community, media,

---

[6]The design invokes *post hoc, ergo propter hoc* arguments.

etc.) should increase the amount of change reflected in a posttest, not reduce it, a before-and-after design that shows no change has occurred between pretest and posttest is informative. Such negative findings might, in fact, be useful information at the first stage of program design and implementation, and so the design could serve a purpose in a formative evaluation. If change does occur, however, the evaluation design must be supplemented with additional research because the extent of the change that can be attributed to the program—rather than other events or activities—cannot be reliably inferred.

The panel recognizes that some local projects may consciously apply quasi-experimental methods to design nonrandomized evaluations that produce evidence that may be defensible under certain assumptions (see Campbell and Stanley, 1966). Indeed, at least one manual has been drafted to assist AIDS prevention programs in the design of quasi-experiments (Mantell and DiVittis, in press). When evaluation results are available from well-executed quasi-experiments, the panel believes they should be reviewed and, if the results are of sufficient importance to warrant the effort, the evaluation could be repeated using a randomized design.

Because of the inferential problems that affect nonexperimental designs such as before-and-after studies, the parent committee's earlier report urged that serious consideration be given to randomized experiments to estimate the relative effects of AIDS prevention projects. This advice is extended in the discussion that follows about practical strategies to determine whether CBO projects make a difference.

Randomized Field Studies

There is ample evidence that randomized experiments designed to understand whether new projects make a difference are sometimes feasible. Past examples of these studies include:

- schools being randomly assigned to alternative programs in studies of which programs best prevent high-risk behavior;
- small groups of clients being randomly assigned in comparative tests of different kinds of counseling programs; and
- individuals being randomly assigned to program or control conditions in studies of teacher training, hospice care for the terminally ill, and home or hospital care.

The randomized study option is more feasible for new projects than for ongoing ones. New projects can justify a control condition in which the new services are not offered when the following conditions prevail: (1) resources are scarce and cannot provide the new services to everyone; (2) showing that the project works or does not work relative to scientific standards will lead to better approaches or to more money for approaches that have been shown to work, or both; and (3) related services are available elsewhere, so that having a no-treatment control group is not problematic.[7] The panel recognizes that opportunities to conduct such studies may be few, but they should be pursued wherever possible.

One such study is now under way to test the effectiveness of a counseling intervention and to explore more efficient approaches to providing counseling. This study involves a community-based AIDS risk reduction program sponsored by the National Institute of Mental Health, in which researchers are using randomized experiments with delayed-treatment controls. In the first part of the study, Kelly and colleagues (1989) randomly assigned individuals to an experimental or control group to measure the effects of an intensive 12-week counseling program. In the second half of the study, researchers are trying to replicate the positive effects found in the first half with a shorter, 6-week counseling component.

It is much more difficult for ongoing projects to create a new control condition, except when the demand for program services exceeds the supply. Then, providing limited service on a random basis to equally deserving individuals or organizations can be justified and implemented, and it does not conflict with professional and social ethics (Riecken et al., 1974; Federal Judicial Center, 1981). At the present time, the panel does not believe it would be appropriate to interfere with the ongoing operations of the CBO projects funded through the states and the Conference of Mayors in order to impose "control" groups. In reaching this conclusion, the panel was impressed by the practical difficulty of such a strategy, particularly given the relatively modest levels of funding that have been provided to these projects. However, for projects that are just now being funded (or that may be funded in the future), the panel recommends that randomized field studies be attempted. The panel considered two options for conducting these studies: conduct evaluations of all CBO projects as a funding requirement or select a sample of CBOs for evaluation and provide incentives to elicit the cooperation of those CBOs.

The panel rejects the first option of requiring that all CBOs undergo evaluation using randomized field assignments. The recent history of

---

[7] Availability of services also means accessibility. Thus, a given CBO intervention that is uniquely accessible to members of a community would not meet the condition for withholding the service.

field studies in the social sciences suggests that requiring randomized studies of all projects in a program, even in cases in which the projects are designed to be uniform, is not reasonable. Sample sizes in some projects may be too small to use in randomized studies except through a cooperative, multisite effort. Moreover, many sites will not have the capacity, regardless of technical support, or the willingness, regardless of incentives, to cooperate in controlled tests. In addition, not all projects have activities and purposes that lend themselves to comparative tests. Finally, not all projects will be "important" enough to evaluate (in the sense of estimating their effects): that is, the investment of evaluation resources may not be justified, given the small size, limited replicability, or idiosyncratic nature of the project.

The panel therefore argues for the second option of evaluating a sample of CBO projects. To proceed with this approach, the panel suggests four steps:

1. Identify those CBO projects that are important enough to justify the costs of studies and that are technically appropriate for comparative randomized assignment. The selection criteria for such projects should include the replicability (in theory) of what is offered in the project; the local feasibility of doing a study; and the representativeness of the project or site category.

2. Develop incentives, notably funding, for the selected CBOs to encourage their cooperation in comparative randomized tests.

3. Use an independent evaluation team to design the experiment in each site, execute the randomized assignment of participants, monitor the integrity and maintenance of the assignments, and analyze results. The evaluators must be both technically able and capable of working with CBOs. The evaluators will also be responsible for analyzing data, estimating the relative effects of the project on the groups, and reporting to CDC.

4. Establish an advisory board to oversee the evaluations, perform periodic, simultaneous secondary analysis of the data produced by the projects, and conduct cross-site analyses. The cross-site analyses are likely to be essential given the expected diversity of even 10-20 projects.[8]

---

[8]Where increased confidence is wanted–such as in decisions to deploy an intervention nationwide–error can be reduced by repeating the experiment in other settings. The resulting cross-site distribution

The feasibility of such strategies has been demonstrated in a variety of areas. The cross-site oversight approach to independent projects, for instance, has been used in the multisite experiments on police handling of domestic violence being conducted by the National Institute of Justice (1989). The single-team approach to evaluation design and execution has worked well in recent assessments of training programs for a variety of vulnerable populations in projects supported by the Ford Foundation, U.S. Department of Labor, Rockefeller Foundation, U.S. Department of Education, and others (Turnbull, 1989).

Methodological Issues

The methodological problems that will be encountered in carrying out randomized field studies for health education/reduction projects are likely to be similar to those encountered in other social science experiments. They include:

- determining eligibility criteria;
- identifying and recruiting individuals and ensuring samples of sufficient size;
- random assignment and quality controls on the integrity of assignments;
- tracking individuals;
- using sufficiently sensitive measures to assess response to the project; and
- coping with missing data problems and fallible measurements.

However, the diversity typical of health education/risk reduction projects that are developed by CBOs will multiply these problems. For instance, working with a sample of 20 or more projects might be appropriate in order to span the range of activities being conducted by the CBOs, but the practical difficulties of coping with 20 different kinds of response variables may make a sample of this size impossible to handle.

Dealing with these problems requires considerable skill, but such skills are available, as are standard approaches to resolving some of the issues. For example, past experience with similar research indicates

---

of effect sizes will show the range of effects likely to be encountered when the program is implemented nationwide. Moreover, cross-site analyses of obtained effect sizes can be tested for homogeneity (the consistency of effect of an intervention), a measure of robustness. No criteria exist for the number of repetitions needed to be secure about results; rather, judgment on the part of the analysts ought to suffice.

that pre- and posttest behavior should be assessed by self-reports of participants to interviewers or ethnographers who are independent of the project being evaluated. Experience in AIDS-related research on sexual behavior and IV drug use[9] will be helpful in designing measurement procedures for obtaining complete information on risk behaviors, and cognitive pretesting should be beneficial in the refinement of these procedures (see Lessler, Tourangeau, and Salter, 1989). To maintain credible samples, it would appear that tracking by name may be necessary—although O'Reilly reports some success using an approach that preserves respondent anonymity (CDC, 1989a). If names are used, experience indicates that periodic recontacting of the sample facilitates tracing of persons who change residence and reduces sample attrition.[10] Similarly, appropriate confidentiality guarantees and compensation (in some form) appear to be critical to achieving high levels of cooperation and low levels of sample attrition over time.

Resources and Aspirations

Controlled experimentation of the kind the panel suggests is a labor-intensive effort. It should only be undertaken when there is a clear understanding of the major, active components in health education/risk reduction project or projects at issue and where there is a commitment of support for the 3 or more years necessary to design, execute, and analyze such studies.

To carry out evaluation using controlled field studies will require a joint commitment by the projects, federal agencies, and the research team. Success will hinge on the compatibility of the collaborators and the leadership and scientific support provided by CDC and by the oversight board.

The skills needed to conduct high-quality randomized studies of new projects are not commonly found among CBO administrators and staff. The requisite technical skills are more common in academic environments, although experience doing AIDS prevention through CBOs is not. These facts suggest that joint efforts involving CBOs and academic researchers will be required to carry out randomized studies that produce high-quality evidence. CDC's (1989a) experience with the AIDS community demonstration projects may be helpful in developing these joint efforts insofar as they involve demonstrations with strong ties to academic institutions. The types of collaborative linkages that would be useful to

---

[9]See Chapters 2 and 3 of Turner, Miller, and Moses (1989) for a review of this research.

[10]Such periodic recontact is done for the purpose of staying in touch with sample persons and not necessarily to gather data.

develop between the evaluator and the service provider in private or public community organizations are well described elsewhere: see, for instance, Bangser (1985) on tests of programs for the adult mentally retarded; Boruch, Dennis, and Carter-Greer (1988) on tests of programs for minority female single parents; and Garner and Visher (1988) on randomized field experiments to learn how to reduce domestic violence most effectively.

Finally, with regard to the aspirations for such evaluations, the panel concluded that some projects fielded by CBOs cannot be evaluated— in the sense of discovering whether they make a difference.[11] Some organizations will not be able to commit the resources of their staffs to lengthy study; some will not be willing to participate; some will be too small (have too few potential clients), and so on. This does not mean, however, that such projects are ineffective. To be credible, judgments about whether a project makes a difference must be based on evidence, and in some projects such evidence may simply be impossible to generate.

WHAT WORKS BETTER?

The preceding section proposed that a small sample of the new projects to be funded under CDC's direct grants program to CBOs be tested against control conditions. The object of such a test is to understand whether the project "works," that is, has beneficial effects. A similar strategy might be used in the context of either new or ongoing projects to determine which of two or more approaches to a problem works better.

Such comparative tests might take a number of forms. One example might involve augmenting existing or standard approaches in ways that arguably are at least as effective as the standard—for example, tripling the time dedicated to certain education activities or increasing the number of outreach staff—to determine whether, indeed, the additional resources lead to remarkably better results. Another possibility might be comparative tests that involve adding new elements—for example, distribution of bleach, condoms, or other material assistance purported to reduce risks—to understand whether these materials produce an effect. Alternatively, the new regimen might involve changes in the type of staff made available to serve the community's needs, the frequency of service or outreach, or other aspects of service delivery.

Although such testing will ultimately be valuable, the panel concludes that it would be premature to begin developing strategies to conduct such tests at the present time. Attempts to test the relative efficacy

---

[11] On the other hand, in the sense of discovering what is being delivered, process evaluations of all projects can be conducted (whether they all should be evaluated is another question).

of different intervention approaches mounted by CBOs should await the completion of the first phase of field studies outlined above. The results of those experiments and the experience gained in conducting them should guide subsequent efforts to test the relative effects of alternative interventions. In reaching this conclusion the panel also notes that when individuals are randomly assigned to alternative regimens within a site, a distinctive problem arises in addressing the question "What works better?" This problem concerns the capacity of CBOs to run side-by-side variations and the ability of the evaluator to ensure that individuals assigned to each variation continue within that variation. The panel believes that, in many cases, CBOs will find it difficult to provide two different educational regimens. Furthermore, maintaining a separation between the two groups or regimens can present difficulties. The separation is essential to a fair comparison between the groups, but it may be subverted if individuals assigned to one regimen interact often with individuals assigned to the other. The type of interaction that can affect comparative tests (e.g., exchanging information or sharing risk reduction material) is arguably low for some selected audiences such as IV drug users in areas in which there is no well-established user community. Interaction may be great, however, within some groups (the "sharing" of doses of drugs in some medical clinical trials has been reported), which may diminish the ability to detect differences between the effects of program A and program B.

REFERENCES

Bangser, M. R. (1985) *Lessons from Transitional Employment: The STETS Demonstration for Mentally Retarded Workers.* New York: Manpower Demonstration Research Corporation.

Betsey, C. L., Hollister, R. G., and Papageorgiou, M. R., eds. (1985) *Youth Employment and Training Programs: The YEDPA Years.* Report of the NRC Committee on Youth Employment Programs. Washington, D.C.: National Academy Press.

Boruch, R. F., Dennis, M., and Carter-Greer, K. (1988) Lessons from the Rockefeller Foundation's experiments on the minority female single-parent program. *Evaluation Review* 12(4):396-426.

Campbell, D. T., and Stanley, J. S. (1966) *Experimental and Quasi-Experimental Designs for Research.* Chicago: Rand McNally.

Center for Disease Control (CDC) (1988) Announcement No. 901. September 20. *Federal Register* 53(182):36492-36493.

Centers for Disease Control (CDC) (1989a) *AIDS Community Demonstration Projects Progress Report: 1989.* Atlanta, Ga.: Centers for Disease Control.

Centers for Disease Control (CDC) (1989b) *Cooperative Agreements for Minority and Other Community Based Human Immunodeficiency Virus (HIV) Prevention Projects.* Announcement Number 908. Washington, D.C.: U.S. Department of Health and Human Services.

Federal Judicial Center (1981) *Experimentation in the Law*. Washington, D.C.: Federal Judicial Center

Garner, J. and Visher, C. (1988) Policy experiments come of age. September-October. *NIJ Reports* 211:2-6.

Hubbard, R. L., Marsden, M. E., Cavanaugh, E., Rachal, J. V., and Ginzberg, H. M. (1988) Role of drug-abuse treatment in limiting the spread of AIDS. *Reviews of Infectious Diseases* 10:377-384.

Kelly, J. A., St. Lawrence, J. S., Hood, H. V., and Brasfield, T. L. (1989) Behavioral intervention to reduce AIDS risk activities. *Journal of Consulting and Clinical Psychology* 57:60-67.

Lessler, J., Tourangeau, R., and Salter, W. (1989) Questionnaire design in the cognitive research laboratory. *Vital and Health Statistics* 6(1): May, 1989.

Mantell, J. E., and DiVittis, A. (In press) *Evaluating AIDS Prevention Programs: A Guidebook for the Health Educator*. New York: Gay Men's Health Crisis, Inc.

National Institute of Justice (1989) *Spouse Assault Replication Project Review Team*. Washington, D.C.: U.S. Department of Justice.

Riecken, H. W., and others (1974) *Social Experimentation: A Method for Planning and Evaluating Social Programs*. New York: Academic Press.

Turnbull, B., ed. (1989) *Meeting the President's Mandate for Accountability of Education Projects: Report to the U.S. Department of Education*. Washington, D.C.: Policy Studies Associates.

5

Evaluating HIV
Testing and Counseling Projects

In this chapter the panel outlines strategies for evaluating CDC's widely disseminated program of funding HIV testing and counseling services. Goals for this program are similar to those discussed for CBOs: behavior change, HIV surveillance, and public education (CDC, 1988). Strategies for evaluating the counseling and testing program are somewhat different, however, because the most credible research design for answering, "Does the program make a difference?" is not appropriate here: that design is the randomized experiment in which some people (controls) receive no services. In the case of counseling and testing for HIV, the panel believes strongly that having a no-treatment control group—that is, denying access to information that could have important consequences for people's personal planning and medical management of infection—would be unethical.

BACKGROUND AND OBJECTIVES

In terms of expenditures—$100 million in fiscal year 1989—CDC's support of counseling and testing services is its largest AIDS intervention program. At present, the Center for Prevention Services (CPS) channels funds for such programs through 62 cooperative agreements with states, territories, and a handful of major cities to support this widescale program. Grantees provide HIV testing and counseling services free of charge in a variety of health care settings.

Through the program, individuals are offered a dual AIDS intervention: confidential (frequently anonymous) HIV testing and pre-and posttest counseling. In addition, in cases of seropositivity, a third service may be available: partner notification and referral. CDC encourages infected individuals to notify their partners of their exposure risk and to refer them to testing and counseling; if clients refuse, CDC recommends that a well-trained site practitioner do the notification. However, partner notification is not mandatory.[1]

From discussions with program staff, the panel learned that the purpose of the counseling and testing program has evolved and may still be evolving. One of the original motives for the program was to divert individuals from using blood banks to learn their antibody status. Accordingly, shortly after the licensure of the ELISA test in March 1985, a program was initiated to deploy a series of what was called alternative test sites around the country. Since then, the demand for counseling and testing services has increased dramatically. In March 1986, CDC recommended that infected but asymptomatic individuals be encouraged to come in for counseling (CDC, 1986), and services were expanded beyond alternative test sites to other health facilities.[2] In the next year, demand grew threefold when the Surgeon General recommended testing for heterosexually active individuals and recipients of blood products.

There has been widespread support in the public health community for expanded programs of voluntary testing for all those who may have been exposed to HIV (see, for example, IOM/NAS, 1988:74). In establishing new HIV testing and counseling sites, priority has been given to projects that serve those segments of the population that are most likely to be infected or that engage in behaviors that risk HIV transmission (CDC, 1987:510). Halfway through 1989, there were more than 1,600 counseling and testing sites nationwide, and that number is expected to grow to 2,000 by the end of the year.

HOW WELL ARE SERVICES DELIVERED?

As noted above, the overall objectives for the counseling and testing program are surveillance, promotion of behavior change to reduce the risk of infection, and public education. In addition, one of CDC's internal documents on process performance indicates that "quality" counseling is

---

[1]For example, the 1987 CDC (1987: 513) guidelines for counseling and testing note that persons who are antibody positive should be instructed in how to notify their partners and to refer them for counseling and testing. If they are unwilling to notify their partners or if it cannot be assured that their partners will seek counseling, physicians or health department personnel should use confidential procedures to assure that their partners are notified.

[2]The shift in emphasis from testing to counseling was accompanied by a change in nomenclature to refer to the sites as counseling and testing sites.

a goal, which introduces a new concept to be evaluated.[3] Finally, from the history of CDC's repeated recommendations to encourage various populations to take advantage of counseling and testing, along with the ever-widening deployment of testing sites, the panel inferred that accessibility was also an implicit goal of the program.

To address these goals, the panel believes that five aspects of service delivery need to be evaluated. To do so, a number of information gathering methods can be used.

The panel recommends that data be gathered from multiple sources—including testing sites, clients, groups at increased risk of HIV infection, and independent observers—to evaluate five aspects of service delivery: the adequacy of the counseling and testing protocol, the adequacy of the counseling that is actually provided, the proportion of clients that complete the full protocol, the accessibility of services, and the nature of the barriers, if any, to clients seeking and completing counseling and testing.

The rate of completion of the program and the identification of barriers to participation in the program are subsumed under "adequacy" and "accessibility."

We use "adequacy" to mean correspondence with client needs. In terms of the testing protocol, client needs include confidentiality; reasonable waiting periods; secure linkage between counseling and testing; provision of test results; and, possibly, partner notification. In terms of counseling, client needs include support; risk assessment; and accurate and appropriate information about the transmission of the virus, risk factors, risk reduction behaviors and techniques, coping skills, and the meaning of test results. In the case of seropositivity, client needs also include information and counseling about the medical and psychological management of infection and partner notification. We realize that assessing adequacy and accessibility involves judgment on the part of an evaluator; nonetheless, we believe a system of cataloguing the fulfillment of needs can be implemented. CDC has in fact developed a prototype "HIV Disease Intervention Skills Inventory" for managers that could be useful in the evaluation of adequacy (CDC, n.d.).

There are four sources of information on the various aspects of service delivery: the administrators and staff of testing and counseling sites; the clients who use the service; specific population groups who should

---

[3] In addition to any "calculable results" from the program, counseling efforts are to "be judged by . . . the quality of the process performance" (CDC, n.d.).

TABLE 5-1 Four Sources of Information about Delivery of Counseling and Testing

SOURCES OF INFORMATION

SERVICE ASPECT	Sites	Clients	Population Groups	Observers
Protocol adequacy		X		X
Counseling adequacy		X		X
Client completion	X	X		
Accessibility	X	X	X	
Client barriers		X	X	

use services (but may not); and independent observers who visit the sites. Table 5-1 identifies the sources of information that are most likely to be useful for evaluating each feature of HIV testing and counseling service delivery. Each of these sources of information can be translated more or less directly into a method of data collection or study design. In the following sections, the panel suggests several designs for collecting data from each of these information sources. Note that these designs are not mutually exclusive; rather, they are complementary, as each provides a different perspective on the adequacy and accessibility of services.

A Site Services Inventory

A typical setting for counseling and testing is a local health department, but services are also offered in institutional facilities, health clinics for the treatment of sexually transmitted diseases or drug use, family planning clinics, and other settings. Because clients of these other sites often have non-HIV related reasons for their visits, they may not be motivated to return for test results and posttest counseling. Thus, the setting in which testing and counseling services are delivered may be a significant factor to be taken into account in analyzing data collected from project sites.

As a first step, the panel believes CDC should prepare an inventory of the various services that are delivered by HIV testing and counseling sites. Although recipients of CDC funding for testing and counseling are required to provide quarterly summary data about their services, we believe these data are insufficient to describe the range of testing and counseling activities now being undertaken at the 1,600 CDC-supported sites across the country. The 62 grantees funded by CDC have no uniform method for reporting data from their counseling and testing sites, and the level of detail provided on any particular service may be inconsistent from one grantee to the next. These inconsistencies preclude cross-tabulation or any detailed analysis of how and to whom services are delivered.

A promising solution to these problems would be the widespread adoption of an enhanced version of the data management system developed by CPS last year. The central feature of this system is the HIV Counseling and Testing Report Form, an electronically scannable record of each visit to a testing and counseling site (see Figure 5-1). The form offers the advantages of uniform reporting and relatively easy data analysis. It assigns an identification number to and elicits data on each counseling intervention, recording the type and date of the site visit as well as visitor demographics and risk factors. These data can then be used in four ways: to link test data with type of service site; to identify the demographic distribution of clients and determine trends in client utilization of the site; to link test data with risk behavior and demographic data to assess trends in seropositivity; and to link test results with posttest information to determine trends in return rates for results, counseling, and partner notification and referral. The data gathered with this form would also allow analysis of variations among project sites and geographic regions.

The panel believes that the value of this inventory can be enhanced and that it would be valuable to augment the current form to collect information on other relevant variables (such as counselor characteristics, length of counseling session, whether the session is an initial or repeat visit).[4] Furthermore, the panel believes that the *required* use of this form by *all* HIV testing and counseling sites funded by CDC and other government agencies would permit the development of uniform and manipulable data bases that could be used for the evaluation of testing and counseling projects. Some states have developed and are using alternative forms and are already building data bases. To avoid requiring these states to modify their efforts, it may be feasible for CDC to furnish technical assistance to make state data sets compatible with the federal form.

Client Surveys

The mere presence of clients indicates that the testing and counseling intervention has been successful in *attracting* people to receive services. The gross number of individuals served, however, does not tell us whether

---

[4]The form could also provide an indicator of the socioeconomic status of clients. It has been postulated but not proven that, increasingly, the AIDS epidemic is becoming lodged in the most disadvantaged segments of the American population. Until now, such arguments have been based on trends in the race and ethnicity of new AIDS cases—which does not provide a wholly appropriate analysis. To track trends in the socioeconomic status of persons served by counseling and testing projects, the panel suggests that a question on education level be added to the form.

★ U.S. GOVERNMENT PRINTING OFFICE:1990—734-539

HIV COUNSELING AND TESTING REPORT FORM A

IDENTIFICATION NO.

PROJ AREA

SITE TYPE
- ① HIV CTS
- ② STD
- ③ DRUG TRMT
- ④ FAMILY PL
- ⑤ PRENAT/OB
- ⑥ TB
- ⑦ OTHER HD
- ⑧ PRISON
- ⑨ COLLEGE
- ⑩ PRIV MD
- ⑪ OTHER
- ⑫ UNKNOWN

SITE NUMBER

DATE OF INITIAL VISIT
MONTH DAY YR.
- ○ JAN
- ○ FEB
- ○ MAR
- ○ APR
- ○ MAY
- ○ JUN
- ○ JUL
- ○ AUG
- ○ SEP
- ○ OCT
- ○ NOV
- ○ DEC

LOCAL USE ONLY

RESIDENCE

STATE   COUNTY   ZIP CODE

AGE

REASON FOR VISIT?
(mark all that apply)
- ○ REQUESTING HIV TEST
- ○ FOLLOW-UP TO STD VISIT
- ○ STD EXAM/TREATMENT
- ○ REF BY HIV+ SEX PARTNER
- ○ REF BY STD SEX PARTNER
- ○ REF BY HEALTH DEPT/HIV
- ○ REF BY HEALTH DEPT/STD
- ○ REF BY PMD/BB/HOSP
- ○ REQ IMMIGRATION
- ○ PRENATAL
- ○ TB INFECTION/DISEASE
- ○ SYMPT HIV/AIDS DISEASE
- ○ ASYMPT, WORRIED ABOUT AIDS
- ○ OTHER
- ○ NOT STATED
- ○ UNKNOWN

RISK EXPOSURE GROUP
(mark all that apply)
- ○ MAN WHO HAD SEX W/A MAN
- ○ IV DRUG USER
- ○ PERSON WITH HEMOPHILIA
- ○ BLOOD RECIPIENT, 1978-85
- ○ HETEROSEXUAL
- ○ SEX PARTNER OF HOMOSEXUAL/BISEXUAL
- ○ SEX PARTNER OF IV DRUG USER
- ○ SEX PARTNER OF PWA/+HIV
- ○ SEX PARTNER OF PERSON WITH HEMOPHILIA
- ○ EXCHANGED DRUGS/MONEY FOR SEX
- ○ NO KNOWN RISK EXPOSURE

RACE/ETHNICITY
- ① WHITE
- ② BLACK
- ③ HISPANIC*
- ④ ASIAN/PACIFIC ISL
- ⑤ AM INDIAN/AK NATIVE
- ⑥ OTHER
- ⑨ UNDETERMINED

SEX
- ① MALE
- ② FEMALE

PRETEST COUNSELED
- ⓪ NO
- ① YES

MONTH DAY YR.
- ○ JAN
- ○ FEB
- ○ MAR
- ○ APR
- ○ MAY
- ○ JUN
- ○ JUL
- ○ AUG
- ○ SEP
- ○ OCT
- ○ NOV
- ○ DEC

← **DATE POSTTEST COUNSELED**

POSTTEST COUNSELED
- ⓪ NO
- ① YES

PARTNER NOTIFICATION (Positives Only)
- ① PATIENT ALREADY REFERRED PARTNERS
- ② PATIENT WILL REFER ALL PARTNERS
- ③ HD WILL REFER ALL PARTNERS
- ④ PATIENT/HD EACH TO MAKE REFERRALS
- ⑤ ALL PARTNERS UNKNOWN/UNLOCATABLE
- ⑥ PATIENT DECLINES PARTICIPATION
- ⑦ SUBJECT NOT RAISED WITH PATIENT

* **IF HISPANIC, SPECIFY**
- ① MEXICAN/MEX AMER
- ② PUERTO RICAN
- ③ CUBAN
- ⑧ OTHER
- ⑨ UNDETERMINED

REFERRED FOR TB TEST
- ⓪ NO
- ① YES

REFUSED HIV TEST   ○ YES

RESERVED
1 2 3 4 5 6 7 8 9 10

LAB TEST RESULTS

ELISA
- ⓪ NEGATIVE
- ① REPEATEDLY REACTIVE

WESTERN BLOT
- ⓪ NEGATIVE
- ① POSITIVE
- ② INDETERMINATE

OTHER CONFIRMATORY
- ⓪ NEGATIVE
- ① POSITIVE

FIGURE 5-1 HIV Testing and Counseling Report Form

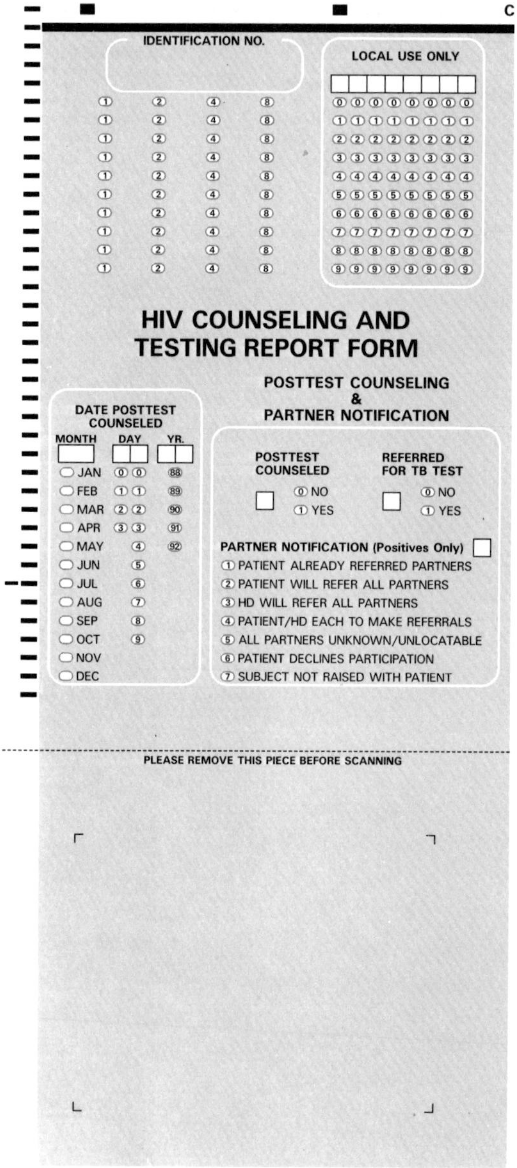

FIGURE 5-1 HIV Testing and Counseling Report Form (cont'd)

the intervention is providing satisfactory services to the groups that need them. A survey of the clients of a testing and counseling site can:

- provide specific information on the accessibility of the site and its services to specific populations;
- reveal problems with the intervention as it is currently delivered;
- elicit information about users' experiences in obtaining the service, such as how long it takes to get an appointment or to get test results, etc.;
- gather data on the scope of the counseling clients receive: the extent of pertinent information provided about HIV infection and AIDS, the time spent with and the emotional support lent by the counselor, the nature of referrals for medical and other support; and
- gather information about whether the respondent completed the testing and counseling protocol, and if not, why.

While the reliability and validity from such surveys must always be considered, information from such surveys might also be helpful in designing more inviting and accessible settings for testing and counseling (e.g., "attractive" physical surroundings, "convenient" locations for services), understanding what aspects of the pretest counseling session encourage clients to return to learn tests results, assessing the optimal content and timing of a posttest counseling session and the provision of referral services, and specifying the profiles of the more effective counselors for different circumstances.

Population Surveys

Another way to evaluate how well services are delivered is to conduct surveys of populations that include potential and actual clients to determine whether counseling and testing services are accessible to all who need or want them. This strategy can be used to evaluate barriers to access. The surveys can be directed toward the general population, toward particular neighborhoods or communities, or toward high-risk or hard-to-reach groups. They can be used to measure the proportion of the specific population that has had experience with counseling and testing and the proportion of the population that wants services but cannot get them (or has chosen not to seek them). Data from such surveys could be analyzed according to demographic and risk factors to identify groups that are not adequately served and the barriers that need to be overcome to make the services more accessible to those groups.

Such surveys present other opportunities as well. They could be used to identify the testing and counseling services that are desired or expected by a given population and could help project administrators better understand the service needs of these individuals. They might also afford insight into the group's awareness of the availability of services and the perceived cultural relevance of the project to users and nonusers alike. Based on this information, efforts might be made to publicize the availability of services and to modify as necessary such project characteristics as location, hours, site design, esthetics, informational materials, and counselor sensitivity. This kind of survey could also gather useful information on the group's concerns about the confidentiality (or anonymity) of HIV testing and counseling and other concerns or fears about the test procedure.

Case Studies Using Direct Observation

The direct observation of interactions at testing and counseling centers is the panel's final suggested study design. This design could be implemented by both nonparticipant observers as well as "professional customer" participants.[5] This method mainly provides qualitative data, although quantitative data can be gathered as well.

The panel is aware that CDC already employs regional monitors and public health advisers to conduct oversight and quality assurance activities for the counseling and testing centers.[6] Nevertheless, the panel believes that case studies using direct observation might identify those factors that produce testing and counseling environments that are particularly supportive of clients and that provide effective contexts for educational messages. In selecting the project sites for case studies, choices should be spread across different types of facilities (e.g., public health departments, clinics for sexually transmitted diseases, drug treatment centers, etc.) and regions of the country, both geographically and by level of HIV prevalence.

Methodological Issues

As noted above, the four separate options for assessing service delivery are not mutually exclusive. Indeed, the approaches suggested are complementary to one another, and all might be undertaken to yield the most

---

[5] As noted in chapter 1, the panel believes that project administrators should be given advance notification that professional customers will be visiting their sites for counseling and testing services, and prior consent should be solicited before this method of data collection is used.

[6] Its document on process performance standards covers a series of steps its counselors are to take in providing counseling and partner notification, and it provides a skills inventory to be used by managers in evaluating counselors performance (see CDC, n.d.).

comprehensive information. Gaps in coverage by an individual study design can be filled in by data from research using another design.

Although a services inventory could show who is using testing and counseling services and could monitor trends in this use over time, some caution is warranted in interpreting inventory data. The main methodological problem will be the accuracy of the project site's reporting. Inaccurate reporting may occur through errors and it is also possible that inaccurate reports may be made purposely to convey a false picture of site activities. But the most plausible threat to accurate reporting will probably be the burden the forms place on the counselors. In the course of a busy day with much "real" and pressing work to do, it is virtually inevitable that filling in forms will not receive high priority. Furthermore, where testing is anonymous, repeat testers could be counted multiple times. This problem can be avoided by adding a question to the scannable form that asks whether a client has been previously tested.

A major concern about client surveys is the reliability and validity (or meaningfulness) of the measurements that are obtained with this method. Clients who are surveyed, for example, may have little or no experience with counseling. Consequently, they may have unrealistic expectations of what and how services should be delivered, expectations that may color their responses.[7]

Surveys can be conducted to gather data from two levels of society: specific, high-risk groups and the general population. To conduct surveys of high-risk populations, probability samples should be used whenever possible. When such a sampling frame is not feasible, replicable convenience samples could be used (see the discussion in Turner, Miller, and Moses, 1989:150-153). However, this latter method will not provide estimates that will be generalizable to the population of persons in the specific high-risk groups. As discussed in the section on client surveys, the reliability and validity of the responses obtained in group surveys will always be a matter of concern. The panel notes, for example, that respondents in such surveys may have unrealistic expectations of what and how services should be delivered.

The general population is of lesser interest than specific high-risk groups, but a large enough sample can provide important information about certain subpopulations. To this end, the panel suggests that CDC take advantage of the National Health Interview Survey (NHIS) sponsored by the National Center for Health Statistics. As described in Chapter 3, the NHIS is a weekly household interview survey of a probability sample

---

[7]For discussions of these complexities, see Bradburn and Sudman (1979); Smith (1984); and Turner and Martin (1984).

of the civilian noninstitutionalized adult population of the United States. Since August 1987 the NHIS has included questions about respondents' knowledge of HIV transmission and their experience with HIV testing; it has also collected limited information on behavioral risk factors.

The panel recommends that the NHIS be periodically augmented with several questions about accessibility and barriers to HIV testing and counseling services.[8]

Given its large size (approximately 50,000 households a year), the NHIS can provide samples of reasonable size, even of relatively rare populations, as long as they are found in households. For example, the September 1988 NHIS estimated that approximately 3.5 percent of the total U.S. population (exclusive of those tested during blood donation) expected to have an HIV test in the next 12 months.[9] Given the annual sample size, this means that 1,750 respondents intended to seek a voluntary HIV test.

To conduct case studies, a site visit team might conduct open-ended interviews with key project staff and 5 to 10 clients. The interviews should focus on counseling and testing activities and materials, opinions about activities and materials, and the identification of key content, process, and organizational elements. Alternatively, *with prior informed consent from site administrators*, "professional customers" can pose as clients of the projects to gather information unobtrusively. A mix of seronegative and seropositive "customers" could be recruited to gather information about the adherence of sites to counseling protocols much in the same way that public health monitors do. For the purposes of case studies, the panel notes that projects are evolving entities; changes may occur in personnel, organizational structure, project instrumentation and goals, and so on. Because of such developments, case studies cannot be conducted once and considered done. Instead, frequent studies are necessary to ensure good results.

The panel members did not agree about whether such site visits would be well received. Some members believe that site staff would welcome the opportunity to demonstrate their projects; others believe that staff would feel overly scrutinized. If there are strong negative reactions on the part of project staff, it may be necessary to spend considerable time

---

[8]The panel understands from program staff that planning is under way at the National Center for Health Statistics to add questions of this nature.

[9]Fitti (1989:8) reports that 7 percent of the sample responded "yes" to the question, "Do you expect to have a blood test for the AIDS virus in the next 12 months?" Moreover, 51 percent of those who responded "yes" said the test would be "voluntarily sought" when they were asked, "Will it be part of a blood donation, voluntarily sought or part of some other activity that requires a blood sample?"

convincing local staff of the need for case study research. If local staff cannot be satisfied that the research is needed and beneficial, it may be quite difficult or impossible to conduct. If the alternative of using professional customers to gather information is considered, it may be desirable to ask for a site's informed consent before that site is funded for HIV testing and counseling services.

Resources and Aspirations

An inventory system requires record-keeping by personnel at the counseling and testing sites. It also requires a centralized professional staff to ensure the completeness of reporting, conduct data analyses, and disseminate results. Other costs of the inventory option should be relatively low because the data management system is based on personal computers, and the use of a scannable form minimizes labor costs for data entry. The panel believes an inventory system could be implemented program-wide within 6 months.

The aspirations for this type of evaluation research are somewhat limited. Although a services inventory would provide data on individuals who avail themselves of services, it cannot identify people who need or want those services but who do not receive them. Another limitation of the system is that it does not provide data on the counseling and testing services provided by private physicians or clinics, blood banks, insurers, and other non-CDC funded sources. This lack is regrettable because such information could bear on an evaluation of CDC-funded services, such as whether a client completes a protocol at CDC-funded sites, or seeks services elsewhere.

The major advantage of client surveys is that they provide information on most of the program aspects that must be assessed to determine how well testing and counseling services are being provided. An additional advantage, when compared with other methods of data collection, is that information can be gathered on other intervention activities to which clients have been exposed. Furthermore, the client survey option is one of the least expensive methods of obtaining information about testing and counseling services. Nevertheless, it will require the involvement of personnel who are trained in survey research design and familiar with its methodological problems.

To survey the general population, the NHIS could be expanded at periodic intervals to measure people's needs for HIV testing and counseling services on a national basis. (The NHIS cannot be used for local information.) This option would require some staff time for data tabulation and analysis on the part of the personnel responsible for the household survey, but costs should be relatively low. Population surveys are somewhat limited, however: for example, the NHIS does not permit access to homeless or institutionalized populations, which may include higher proportions of individuals at risk for HIV than are included in the household population.

For a number of reasons, surveys of samples of high-risk populations are more expensive and more difficult than adding questions to the NHIS. These surveys are labor intensive; in addition, they must be repeated at regular intervals in order to monitor changes in the need for counseling and testing services. Furthermore, this kind of research requires highly trained personnel to design and administer the surveys.

Conducting case studies requires special skills and knowledge. Expertise in AIDS prevention and in evaluation design is desirable, as is knowledge of the particular risk factors that are addressed in the setting being studied (e.g., drug treatment centers). A team of two or three site observers is preferable to a single observer because of the range of knowledge desired—evaluation methodology, counseling expertise, and any other site-specific expertise. Using more than one observer also makes it possible to assess the reliability of several reports. Site visits of 3 or 4 days would be required for each study site. Major costs include observer salaries and their travel expenses. Each case study would require about 40 person-days per site. Case studies can provide a rich and in-depth look at some aspects of service delivery for a subset of testing and counseling sites, which will in turn be important for developing studies that evaluate comparative effectiveness.

OPTIONS FOR EVALUATING WHETHER HIV TESTING AND COUNSELING SERVICES MAKE A DIFFERENCE

The panel weighed several options for addressing the question, "Does the policy of providing free HIV testing and counseling services make a difference?" As noted above, the panel seriously considered the feasibility of randomized tests with a no-treatment control group. One approach would be to use a randomized experiment at the site level in which individuals who sought services were randomly assigned either to an intervention condition or to a control condition in which they received services from alternative sources or no services at all (e.g., they were put on a waiting list). The individuals in both groups would be measured and compared on the relevant outcome variable to test the effects of treatment. Although conducting such an experiment is the usual desired strategy to evaluate effectiveness, the panel rejected it as unethical and infeasible. In the context of a deadly epidemic, it is indefensible to withhold this treatment in the interests of conducting an experiment from any individual who desires it. In addition, follow-up for such a group would be extremely difficult as they would have little incentive to cooperate, and locating a diversely situated group would be difficult.

The panel also considered a variation of a randomized experiment that would capitalize on delays in the implementation of projects, but concluded that such an experiment would not usually be feasible. This design variation assumes that lags occur in the deployment of counseling and testing projects because of scarce resources; as funding becomes available for some projects, sites can be randomly assigned to receive the intervention or to continue waiting. However, such a design is not very practical. First, there are already a large number of sites throughout the country, and it is unlikely that a waiting list of homogeneous centers is available. Second, the recruitment of control sites would be problematic because sites on the waiting list would have to be offered strong incentives to participate in data collection.

Alternative strategies for assessing effectiveness (e.g., simple before-and-after designs that establish that a change has occurred or not occurred) do not suffice because they do not control for rival explanations of changes in behavior, knowledge, or serostatus. Other competing explanations for such changes may include natural history (the adoption of change regardless of exposure to counseling and testing), the self-selection of program participants, and the effects of conducting research.

The suitability of such research designs for answering the question, "Does it make a difference?" is so low as to invite the investment of evaluation resources in more tractable areas, especially as the value of counseling and testing has been so widely accepted. Indeed, the panel noted some presumptive evidence that HIV testing and counseling do have a positive effect. There is, for example, increasing evidence that testing can result in individual medical benefit among persons infected with HIV by enabling them to monitor their immune function and initiate early prophylaxis for *Pneumocystis carinii* pneumonia. Furthermore, an individual's knowledge about serostatus can be an important factor in making decisions about sexual behavior, needle sharing, and childbearing. For example, one study found that gay and bisexual men who were tested for HIV and received pretest and posttest counseling were more likely than those who did not to reduce their incidence of unprotected anal intercourse (Coates, Morin, and McKusick, 1987).

When HIV testing is performed, the panel believes that testing should be accompanied by counseling, both before the test is administered and after the test result is given to the individual. The need for such counseling and the ethical and practical motivations for providing it are discussed elsewhere (see, e.g., IOM/NAS, 1986, 1988; Presidential Commission on the Human Immunodeficiency Virus Epidemic, 1988:73-75). At a minimum, pretest counseling is ethically mandated to ensure that individuals give informed consent. Posttest counseling is appropriate to ensure that individuals who are distressed by the results of their tests are comforted and that all individuals are warned about the risk of transmission through their future behaviors.

Although the panel found that the question of effectiveness should not be experimentally tested, it did not find the question uninteresting. On the contrary: the panel discussed current research efforts that study the sequelae of HIV testing.[10] One impetus for such studies has been the emerging indications that testing may have negative as well as positive effects (see Chapter 2). Although the evidence is sparse, these studies point to the need to monitor potentially negative as well as positive effects of HIV testing and counseling.

WHAT WORKS BETTER?

The heart of the question "What works better?" is how to maximize the beneficial effects of testing and counseling. The way to learn what these effects are is through well-controlled studies that test two or more approaches to delivering the intervention. As recommended in Chapter 1, the panel's preferred strategy for comparative tests is randomized experiments. For the "What works better?" question, the control group is assigned not to nontreatment but to an alternative treatment. So, for example, each individual who agrees to participate might be randomly assigned to one of two (or more) programs of counseling and testing that are thought to be effective but whose relative effectiveness is unknown. Because the groups are composed randomly, the comparison of outcomes—such as client return rates—for clients receiving regimen A or regimen B is then a fair one.

In some circumstances, HIV seroconversion may be a helpful outcome measure for evaluating the effectiveness of different counseling and testing projects. Yet the use of more proximate outcomes is desirable because seroconversion will *not* be informative regarding behavioral

---

[10] The particular approach taken in these research efforts is the natural history study. Using longitudinal cohorts, researchers have attempted to estimate the effect of testing and counseling, compared with other factors in a person's life, on behavioral change. Such studies of gay men and IV drug users are currently under way. For example, among the cohorts of gay men, seroconversion rates and behavioral changes in men who have not been tested for HIV are compared with: (1) those who have been tested but do not know their antibody status and (2) those who have been tested and do know their status. Unfortunately, natural history studies do not lead to fully adequate, testable models of behavior, but when there appear to be consistent effects, those effects should be noted.

change among persons whose initial test result is positive. Similarly, in populations in which HIV is not heavily seeded, seroconversion may be a rare event even though the population frequently engages in risky behaviors. Thus, experiments can assess how well different versions of an intervention work to increase a person's willingness to return to a site for test results, to increase his or her knowledge of risks, or to reduce risky behavior. Furthermore, experiments can assess the effectiveness of various regimens in reducing identified side effects, such as psychological distress.

With clear outcomes such as these in mind, alternative approaches to testing and counseling, based on theory and the perceived effectiveness of past approaches, can be evaluated through randomized experiments. After a brief discussion of the unit of assignment and experimental regimens, the next section presents appropriate study designs for answering the question, "What works better?"

Randomized Experiments of Alternative Treatments

Unit of Assignment

As noted in Chapter 1, the unit of assignment in a field experiment may be a large organizational unit such as a community, a smaller organizational unit such as a project (i.e., all of the clients of a project), or individual participants. There are several factors involved in the choice of treatment units (see Chapter 1). The panel suggests consideration of three types of assignment:[11]

- random assignment of individual testing and counseling sites to alternative regimens;
- random assignment of project staff members at a given site to the use of alternative regimens; and
- random assignment of individual clients to alternative regimens at a site.

In cases of random assignment of sites, we recognize that some facilities, such as those whose primary mission is not HIV-related, may not be amenable to being randomly assigned to provide different interventions. However, service providers in a large city with several counseling and testing sites may be more flexible and should be encouraged to participate in controlled experiments. When the preferred design is the random

---

[11] See Turner, Miller, and Moses (1989:Chapter 5) for a discussion of precedents in other areas regarding the random assignment of entities (e.g., sites) to alternative regimens.

assignment of individuals within a project to alternative regimens, the panel believes that at least two or three projects in different communities should be encouraged to cooperate in uniform tests. Because detectable relative differences may be small but important, the number of clients and sites involved in the tests must be large enough to estimate relative differences with confidence.

Experimental Regimens

There are a variety of experimental regimens that might be tested, but in designing randomized experiments of alternative counseling and testing treatments, it is best to test alternatives in which one regimen is not obviously better than the others. In the three examples noted in this section (below), the unit of analysis varies. These regimens test the effects on behavior of alternative modes of providing counseling and testing. Some of the alternatives fall into the category of structural variables. For example, the setting in which testing and counseling is delivered may have an effect on whether an individual returns for test results and follow-up counseling. As noted above, a client's initial purpose in visiting a site may not be HIV testing; similarly, some sites and their staffs may be geared primarily to providing services other than counseling and testing (a drug treatment facility is one such example). Particular service delivery aspects of sites may also produce different effects. For example, Rugg and colleagues (1988) found that higher return rates for HIV test results were associated with such site characteristics as a shorter wait for testing and the comfort and nature of the setting. The number of sessions as well as the content of counseling may have an effect on cognition and behavior. Other process variables that may influence return rates involve the adequacy of services in terms of emotional support and medical service referral.

> **The panel recommends that evaluations of "What works better?" focus on the comparative effectiveness of testing and counseling services that (1) are delivered in different settings, (2) have different content, duration, and intensity, and (3) are accompanied by different types of supportive services.**

Service Delivery Setting. As discussed above, the accessibility and suitability of testing and counseling projects are critical issues. Projects now exist to serve gay men, IV drug users in treatment, and users of general public health agencies such as STD or family planning clinics. These projects are widely distributed, but they are not necessarily accessible in all communities or equally accessible for all types of individuals.

In addition to assessing whether particular projects serve more of the individuals who desire testing than other projects, it is important to understand whether particular service settings are more effective contexts for providing testing and counseling to different types of clients.

Content, Duration, and Intensity of Counseling. The experimental regimen could consider a number of potentially more effective intervention approaches, including more frequent, longer, or intensive counseling. The content of counseling messages could be varied, too: for example, the elimination of risk behaviors or the adoption of protective behaviors could be stressed. Other enhancements may include the use of support groups, the involvement of partners, and outreach services for individuals who continue to engage in high-risk behavior. As the standard protocol for counseling and testing evolves and is improved, experiments can examine the increased effectiveness of enhanced programs compared with the costs of their implementation.

Additional Services. The third major area for exploration is the effect of providing services beyond the basic counseling and testing intervention now being offered. Increased relapse prevention services for IV drug users in treatment who become seropositive are a good example. A common reaction to stress by IV drug users is to seek and use drugs for stress reduction. Relapse prevention projects address this issue in general and could include components that are specially geared toward seropositive clients. Another example of potentially risk-reducing services is psychological counseling (beyond the counseling provided with HIV test results), which might help diminish adverse stress reactions.

A creative evaluator is likely to identify many more interventions whose effectiveness can be assessed using alternative regimens (e.g., videotapes, group sessions, cognitive interventions, etc.). Yet not all sites will be suitable for testing augmented regimens. Consistent with the overall recommendations, the panel believes that sites should be selected for randomized trials on the basis of their willingness to cooperate and the potential effectiveness and replicability of the augmented intervention programs they would offer.

Methodological Issues

Conducting randomized experiments can present various problems, including cost, impediments to random selection of treatment units, and difficulties in collecting complete data from participants and to retaining participants in the study.

As noted in Chapter 1, offering alternative services to individuals within a project deserves a special note of caution. Problems can arise in that both clients and project staff may be uncomfortable with random assignment, and this discomfort could preclude randomized assignment. A practical solution in such cases is making the site the unit of assignment: that is, all clients at site 1 receive service regimen A, all clients at site 2 receive regimen B, etc.

Data collection poses another challenge to study designers. Although eliciting sensitive information may seem feasible given the confidentiality assurances available under Section 303 of the Public Health Service Act, data gathering at HIV testing and counseling sites may be difficult. At sites that offer anonymous testing, it will not be possible to do follow-up interviews unless either the clients agree to confidential (rather than anonymous) data collection or the study uses a follow-up method that preserves client anonymity. In the latter regard, O'Reilly (CDC, 1989) has reported recontact rates of between 50 and 80 percent using one scheme that preserves client anonymity. These recontact rates are certainly impressive, but they leave considerable room for uncertainty about the effects of attrition on the outcome measures. Although these uncertainties are troubling, the panel points out that some important crucial outcome measures—e.g., the proportion of clients that return for HIV test results and subsequent stages of the protocol—can be known with certainty even in an anonymous testing program.

Although the panel recommends that a skilled evaluation team carefully design and conduct randomized studies, the evaluation team and the sponsoring agencies should be prepared for a certain number of failures in carrying out experiments. In the panel's opinion, a failure rate of 20 percent or more should not be surprising. In the event of a failure (e.g., the contamination of individuals at the point of their selection, substantial attrition from the study) it will be useful to have a fall-back position. For example, if the randomization of individuals fails, a randomized experiment might still be conducted at the clinic level. Such a redesigned experiment may not be as "clean" as one that uses individual participants, but it might still provide useful information.

The panel's experience with counseling and testing sites suggests that sites will be willing to cooperate in experimental studies if they have substantial involvement in the implementation of new approaches and of the evaluation strategy. Most administrators are sophisticated enough to understand the need for evaluation in the interest of improving interventions, even if they do not necessarily understand the statistical aspects of such studies.

Resources and Aspirations

Three types of personnel resources will be beneficial to conduct randomized field experiments of testing and counseling interventions: (1) a qualified team of behavioral, social, and statistical scientists to design and conduct the studies; (2) an independent scientific oversight group for quality control (as recommended in Chapter 1); and (3) appropriately trained CDC staff to design and conduct the studies and to monitor studies undertaken by outside groups (also as recommended above).[12] The first type of personnel, the individual investigator or investigative team, would be responsible for developing and implementing interventions. A university-based or non-public health system contractor might be a good choice; however, because some elements of the evaluation of HIV testing and counseling will require the direct involvement of the public health system and community-based organizations, personnel from these settings should not be excluded from consideration.

The oversight group should be an academic or other scientific research agency team that is independent of the project investigator or investigators. (Appendix B describes one such oversight approach, the "Project Review Team.") This oversight body can be used at the outset to facilitate consensus on evaluation protocols and to approve or develop outcome measures. Further along in the evaluation process, it can provide strong, centralized oversight and quality control of the work. Past experience with large-scale, decentralized social research and evaluation programs indicates that without vigorous oversight the research may be of poor quality. This problem seems to occur for a variety of reasons, including a lack of coordination together with the inherent difficulties of conducting methodologically rigorous research in the context of a social action program (see Betsey, Hollister, and Papageorgiou, 1985).

Finally, evaluation studies that are carried out as randomized trials by outside experts will require appropriately trained CDC staff to interact with the investigators and to interpret study results. In addition, CDC's personnel expertise and workload should also permit staff to conduct evaluation studies themselves. The types of staff needed for such tasks are behavioral, social, and statistical scientists trained in evaluation research (see Chapter 1).

---

[12] Still a fourth resource for a sponsoring agency would be an interagency coordinating body to draw upon the expertise of the federal agencies that are knowledgeable in relevant areas (e.g., CDC, the National Institute of Mental Health (NIMH), the National Institute on Drug Abuse (NIDA), etc.). A body of this kind could draw on one agency's expertise—for instance, that of NIDA in the field of HIV prevention with IV drug users—and on CDC's expertise in providing services. Together, such a body could facilitate the development of creative interventions that are theoretically based and that could then be empirically tested.

In addition to personnel and funds, conducting experiments requires time. Results will not be available quickly; indeed, when positive effects are found, they will need to be measured again at intervals to guard against erosion. Consequently, investigators and policy makers alike must find the patience needed to carry out such research and a commitment to using evaluation research as a tool for the long-term improvement of testing and counseling programs.

The panel also notes that advances in the treatment of asymptomatic HIV-infected individuals may increase the demand for testing and counseling services. Recent research suggests that some early treatments of persons infected with HIV may postpone the onset of AIDS and decrease morbidity and mortality from opportunistic infections. Thus, there may be a substantial increase in the demand for HIV testing—as well as for medical monitoring of seropositive persons. In a rapidly changing environment, an ongoing program of evaluations will be essential to assess progress toward both the goal of adequate service delivery and the goal of reduced HIV transmission. In keeping with its general recommendations, the panel urges that evaluation of HIV testing and counseling be an ongoing activity and that selected projects be reevaluated periodically to monitor their continued effectiveness.

REFERENCES

Betsey, C. L., Hollister, R. G., and Papageorgiou, M. R., eds. (1985) *Youth Employment and Training Programs: The YEDPA Years.* Report of the NRC Committee on Youth Employment Programs. Washington, D.C.: National Academy Press.

Bradburn, N. M., and Sudman, S. (1979) *Improving Interview Method and Questionnaire Design.* San Francisco: Jossey Bass.

Centers for Disease Control (CDC) (1986) Additional recommendations to reduce sexual and drug abuse-related transmissional human T-lymphotropic virus type III/lymphadenopathy-associated virus. *Morbidity and Mortality Weekly Report* 35:152-155.

Centers for Disease Control (CDC) (1987) Public Health Service guidelines for testing and counseling to prevent HIV infection and AIDS. *Morbidity and Mortality Weekly Report* 36:509-514.

Centers for Disease Control (CDC) (1988) Announcement No. 901. *Federal Register* 53(182):36492-36493. September 20.

Centers for Disease Control (CDC) (1989) AIDS Community Demonstration Projects Progress Report 1989. Centers for Disease Control, Atlanta, Ga.

Centers for Disease Control (CDC) (n.d.) Prototype: Process Performance Standards for Personnel Performing HIV Disease Intervention (Counseling and Partner Notification). Centers for Disease Control, Atlanta, Ga.

Coates, T. J., Morin, S. F., and McKusick, L. (1987) Behavioral consequences of AIDS antibody testing among gay men. *Journal of the American Medical Association* 258:1889.

Fitti, J. E. (1989) AIDS knowledge and attitudes for September, 1988. *Advance Data.* No. 164. DHHS Pub. No. (PHS) 89-1250. January 3.

Institute of Medicine/National Academy of Sciences (IOM/NAS) (1988) *Confronting AIDS: Update 1988.* Committee for the Oversight of AIDS Activities. Washington, D.C.: National Academy Press.

Presidential Commission on the Human Immunodeficiency Virus Epidemic (1988) *Final Report of the Presidential Commission on the Human Immunodeficiency Virus Epidemic.* Washington, D.C.: U.S. Government Printing Office.

Rugg, D., Sweet, D., Hovell, M., and Fagan, R. (1988) Factors Affecting the Decision to Learn HIV Test Results. Paper presented at the Fourth International AIDS Conference, Stockholm, June 12-16.

Smith, T. (1984) Nonattitudes: A review and evaluation. In Turner, C. F., and E. Martin, eds. *Surveying Subjective Phenomena.* Vol. 2. New York: Russell Sage Foundation.

Turner, C. F., and Martin, E., eds. (1984) *Surveying Subjective Phenomena.* 2 vols. New York: Russell Sage Foundation.

Turner, C. F., Miller, H. G., and Moses, L. E., eds. (1989) *AIDS, Sexual Behavior and Intravenous Drug Use.* Report of the NRC Committee on AIDS Research and the Behavioral, Social, and Statistical Sciences. Washington, D.C.: National Academy Press.

6

Randomized and Observational Approaches to Evaluating the Effectiveness of AIDS Prevention Programs

In previous chapters, the panel recommended that randomized controlled experiments be used to evaluate a small number of important and carefully selected AIDS prevention projects. Our reasoning has been that *well-executed* randomized experiments afford the smallest opportunity for error in assessing the magnitude of project effects, and they provide the most trustworthy basis for inferring causation. Notwithstanding this conclusion, we recognize that this strategy will not always be feasible and that nonrandomized studies may be required in some instances.[1] In this chapter the panel reviews a number of observational approaches to the evaluation of the effectiveness of AIDS prevention programs. (In addition, Appendix F presents a background paper for this chapter which provides a detailed treatment of an econometric technique known as selection modeling and its potential uses.)

On January 12-13, 1990, the panel hosted a Conference on Nonexperimental Approaches to Evaluating AIDS Prevention Programs. Fifteen experts from the behavioral sciences, statistics, biostatistics, econometrics, psychometrics, and education joined panelists and federal representatives to discuss the application of quasi-experimentation and modeling to evaluating CDC's three major AIDS interventions. This chapter is an outgrowth of those discussions and the papers presented at this conference (Bentler, 1990; Campbell, 1990; Moffitt, 1990).

[1] Observational designs may convey other practical benefits. For example, such studies avoid the ethical debate that may accompany the withholding of treatment in a randomized study, as discussed in Chapter 5. Observational studies may also be advantageous when an intervention occurs "naturally" or has saturated a community before randomization can be implemented.

OVERVIEW

Determining the effectiveness of an intervention project requires comparing how a project participant (or group of participants) fares with how that participant or group would have fared under a different intervention or *no* intervention. Because such direct comparisons are ordinarily not possible,[2] researchers have developed a number of ways to construct a comparison group that "looks like" the participants. The objective is to make this group as similar as possible with respect to confounding factors[3] that may affect the outcome (other than the fact of the intervention itself).

If participants' selection or reason to enter into a study is *not independent* of the study's outcome variables, however, *selection bias* is introduced. For example, if individuals who enter a counseling and testing project are more highly motivated to change their risk-associated behaviors than individuals who do not choose to enroll in such programs, a selection bias is present, and the effects of the intervention cannot be estimated by simply comparing outcomes among program participants and nonparticipants. Strategies to evaluate AIDS interventions in such instances require the assumption that the effects of such confounding variables can be estimated and adjusted for. (A variant of this problem can also arise in randomized experiments, where the attrition of respondents from experimental and control groups can introduce an analogous selection bias.)

As explained in Chapter 1, selection bias can initially be controlled by the random assignment of individuals to one group or another. When properly implemented, randomization will, on average, create groups that have the similar initial characteristics and thus are free (on average) of selection bias. The chance always remains, of course, that randomized groups are different, but the chance is small and decreases as the sample size increases. Furthermore, standard statistical tools such as confidence intervals can be used in properly randomized experiments to calculate the variability in the effect size associated with the randomization. Thus, well-executed randomized experiments require the fewest assumptions in estimating the effect of an intervention. Notwithstanding this statistical advantage, the panel urges that underlying theory about who an intervention will affect (and how) be sufficiently compelling to justify mounting

---

[2] A few important exceptions arise, such as when the same subject can try two diets or two ointments. But if temporal sequence is important or if memory or attitude is at stake, "you can't go back." Similarly, only one of two alternative surgical procedures will be applied in any one patient, etc.

[3] That is, variables that (1) influence outcomes, and (2) are not equivalently distributed in the treatment and comparison groups.

a randomized trial and sufficiently explicit about the relationship between independent variables and the outcome to allow the analysis of the experimental data if randomization fails and statistical adjustments are needed.

Nonrandomized studies require additional assumptions and/or data to infer causation. This is so because it is seldom safe to assume that individuals who participate in a program and receive its services are similar to those who do not participate and do not receive services. In a few cases, the differences between participants and nonparticipants may be fully explained by observable characteristics (e.g., age, partner status, education, and so on), but often the differences may be too subtle to be observed (e.g., motivation to participate, intention to change behavior, and so on). This is particularly true in the AIDS prevention arena because so little is known about changing sexual and drug use behaviors. Thus, a simple comparison of the risk reduction behavior of participants and nonparticipants in a program can yield a misleading estimate of the true effect of the program.

In addition to randomized experiments, six observational research designs will be discussed in this chapter. These alternatives use a variety of tactics to construct comparison groups.[4] For organizational purposes, the panel clusters the six strategies under two umbrellas that differ in their general approach to controlling bias and providing fair comparisons. One approach involves the *design of comparability* and the other involves *post hoc statistical adjustment*:[5]

- Design approaches develop comparability *a priori* by devising a comparison group on some basis other than randomized assignment. This may be done through:
  - quasi-experiments,
  - natural experiments, and
  - matching.

- Adjustment approaches correct for selection bias *a posteriori* through model-based data analysis. Such approaches

---

[4]Throughout this chapter, *control groups* will refer to the randomly assigned groups that may either have received no treatment or have received an alternative to the experimental treatment. Their nonrandomized counterparts will be referred to as *comparison groups*.

[5]A third type of observational method is the case study, in which evaluators probe individual histories for factors related to outcome variables. Because little comparability is achieved in these studies, the panel will not discuss them, except to note that case studies often yield hypotheses and measures that can eventually be used in the other designs and can yield useful information to help interpret the results of randomized trials that are not optimally implemented.

use models of the process underlying selection or participation in an intervention and of the factors influencing the outcome variable(s). Specific methods include:

- analysis of covariance,
- structural equation modeling, and
- selection modeling.

It should be recognized that the panel's distinction between the two approaches is not absolute. Matching, for example, is sometimes done retrospectively as a method of controlling selection bias, and prospective data can be collected for use in modeling. Furthermore, in some sense, all the approaches involve "modeling"—at least to the extent that they take account of behavioral theories or models to infer causation. Despite some imprecision, the panel finds the general distinction helpful in thinking about the ways that have been developed to estimate project effects from nonexperimental designs.

Choosing Among Strategies

Despite the panel's preference for randomization, we realize that it is not always feasible or appropriate and that its implementation is not immune to compromise. When randomization is infeasible or threats to randomization loom large, we believe researchers should look to alternative strategies and determine which of them, in turn, will be feasible, appropriate, and produce convincing results.

The choice of approach can present itself in many ways: a cohort study, for example, can begin to study all new entrants at a clinic (the *a priori* approach), or it can look back at all entrants who first appeared at that clinic at some time in the previous months—if the clinic records are good enough.[6] Because the data are already in hand, the *a posteriori* approach may permit an apparently faster investigation of the problem. Offsetting this advantage, however—and often outweighing it—are two other considerations. First, retrospectively collected data may not include measures of key variables, and the available data may be difficult to interpret. Planned data collections may profit from steps taken to ensure the availability of information on all variables of interest. Second, design imposes control over the observations of behavioral and psychological variables: planning what data to collect, how to collect them, and what comparisons to make improves the prospects of obtaining valid and

---

[6]Some quasi-experiments and nonexperiments may also offer the choice. If the trigger event is an earthquake, then only the retrospective mode is likely to be available, but if it is the initiation of a new legal requirement at a future date, then the choice of a prospective study is available.

reliable measures of project inputs and outcomes.[7] For these reasons, the panel believes that strategies that build on data collected for the specific purpose of evaluating project effects should, in general, have a greater likelihood of success.

In the case of AIDS interventions in particular, the panel is pessimistic about our ability to correct for bias after the fact because we have at present a poorly-developed understanding both of the factors affecting participation in such projects and the factors that induce people to change their sexual and drug use behaviors (e.g., motivation, social support, and so on). Success through *a posteriori* approaches benefits from a comprehensive understanding of these confounding factors and reliable measurements of them.[8]

Finally, the panel notes that the charged climate that surrounds many AIDS prevention programs can render decision making difficult in the best of circumstances. Research procedures that produce findings that are subject to considerable uncertainties or that provoke lengthy debates among scientists about the suitability of particular analytic models may, in the opinion of this panel, impede crucial decision making about the allocation of resources for effective AIDS prevention programs. These factors underlie the panel's preference for well-executed randomized experiments, where such experiments are feasible. This is not to say that observational strategies do not have a place in AIDS evaluation designs nor that their role must necessarily remain secondary in the future. Rather it reflects the panel's judgment that in the current state of our understanding of AIDS prevention efforts and the state of development of alternative observational strategies for evaluation, overreliance on observational strategies would not be a prudent research strategy where it is feasible to conduct well-executed randomized experiments.

Before reviewing observational strategies for evaluation, the panel provides a brief reprise of the basis for its recommendation that carefully executed randomized experiments be conducted to assess the effects of a small subset of AIDS prevention projects.

RANDOMIZED EXPERIMENTATION

Randomized controlled experiments specify a single group of interest of sufficient size,[9] and then randomly assign its members to a treatment

---

[7]See Appendix C for a discussion of validity and reliability of behavioral data.

[8]Success through design approaches also depends on these things, but careful design allows some of the factors to be controlled. Randomization leads to the most trustworthy expectation that these factors have been controlled, although theory is important to examine whether groups are indeed comparable.

[9]The question of sample size is important because it affects the statistical variance of the estimate of

group or a control group that receives an alternative treatment or no treatment at all. By randomly assigning units (i.e., individuals, schools, clinics, communities) to treatment and control groups, it becomes possible in theory to interpret any resultant intergroup differences as a direct estimate of the magnitude of the effect, if any, induced by the treatment. The method's assumption that selection bias has been controlled is probabilistically hedged by the significance test. In properly randomized experiments, statistical significance tests can indicate whether the observed differences in group outcomes are larger than can be explained by the random differences in the groups.

By providing a statistically well-grounded basis for assessing the probability that observed differences in outcomes between groups are attributable to the treatment, *well-executed* randomized experiments reduce ambiguity in the interpretation of findings and provide the greatest opportunity for producing clear-cut results. This reduction in ambiguity is made possible by the fact that assignment to a particular treatment group is *by definition* independent of all other factors. This inferential strategy requires, however, that the randomization of assignment not be compromised in its execution and that it be maintained through time.[10]

When assignment is not random *or when randomization is compromised,* differences between the treatment group and the control group may result from either the effect of the treatment, or from idiosyncratic differences between the groups, or both. If, for example, members of the treatment group differ from those in a comparison group because they were more motivated and thus more aggressively pursued or stuck with the intervention program, the treatment's success may be overstated. On the other hand, if the treatment group represents those at highest risk, any comparison group would have the advantage of being composed of individuals less in need of the intervention. As such examples illustrate, selection bias can cause the intervention group to perform either "better"

---

treatment effect derived from a given experiment. (Other things being equal, the squared standard error of this estimate will be directly proportional to the square root of the sum of the standard errors of the estimate of the means of the treatment and control groups.) Sample size is discussed in more technical terms in Appendix D, but, in brief, it should be noted that as the size of the sample increases, the variance in the expected distribution of estimated effects will decrease, thus permitting more precise estimates. (In addition to large sample sizes, homogeneous populations will also reduce variance.)

[10]In practice, nonequivalent attrition in the treatment and control groups and other factors can reintroduce the selection biases that randomization excluded. When randomized assignment is thus compromised in execution, the same inferential problems that beset observational studies operate and they may require use of procedures such as statistical adjustments, modeling of attrition bias, and so forth. In such instances, it should be clearly recognized that the inferential uncertainties attending a severely compromised randomized experiment may be just as large (or even larger) than those that attend the use of a purely observational design.

or "worse" than the comparison group. The direction of the bias, let alone its magnitude, is often difficult to predict beforehand.

The Power of Experiments: An Example

History provides a number of examples of the interpretive difficulties that can attend observational studies (or compromised experiments) and the power of a well-executed randomized experiment to provide definitive results. In the infant blindness epidemic at mid-century, for example, well-executed controlled experiments ended an inferential debate that observational studies had fueled instead of extinguished.

In the 1940s and early 1950s, more than 10,000 infants—most of whom were born prematurely—fell victim to a previously unknown form of blindness called retrolental fibroplasia (Silverman, 1977). Over the years, more than 50 hypotheses were offered for the cause of the disease and for effective treatments. About half the hypotheses were examined observationally, but only four were actually tested in experimentally controlled trials.

Before the experimental studies took place, an uncontrolled study had indicated that the application of ACTH (adrenocorticotrophic hormone) would prevent the fibroplasia. A randomized controlled trial showed that this therapy was unhelpful or worse: a third of the infants who received ACTH became blind whereas only a fifth of the control group did.[11]

One hypothetical cause of the observed blindness—based on a study of 479 infants—was a deficiency of oxygen. This proposal was countered by another hypothesis—based on 142 observations—that an excess of oxygen was to blame. (During the period of the epidemic, premature infants were routinely given oxygen supplements at a concentration of more than 50 percent for 28 days.) Once again, a well-controlled randomized experiment put the debate to rest: the group of infants randomly assigned to receive the routine supplemental oxygen had a dramatically higher incidence of blindness than the control group (23 percent versus 7 percent).[12] Observational studies might have finally yielded this same conclusion—at least one small study had suggested excess oxygen as the culprit—but the human cost and the time involved (10,000 blinded children and more than 10 years) were dear indeed.

---

[11] Because neither the cause of nor the cure for the children's blindness were known, the randomized trials reported here met ethical standards for varying treatments.

[12] The results of the study were widely publicized among ophthalmologists, and within a year the practice of providing high concentrations of oxygen to premature infants was largely modified. Subsequent efforts have been made to provide an oxygen concentrate that prevents brain damage but does not cause blindness (Silverman, 1977).

Compromised Randomization

The panel believes that the inferential debates that bedevil the interpretation of nonexperimental studies are largely avoided by well-conducted randomized experiments. In practice, uncertainties may nonetheless attend the inference that a causal relationship exists between the intervention being evaluated and the outcome(s) observed in a randomized experiment. In this section, we discuss four important sources of uncertainty that investigators need to monitor: sample attrition, compliance with treatment, spillover (and diffusion of effects), and compensatory behavior. Note that the first three of these are not solely problems for experiments; they can frustrate observational studies as well. The last, however, is a special risk of randomized experiments.

Attrition

Careful randomization of participants into treatment and control groups is not sufficient in itself to guarantee informative results. Successful experiments also require that sample attrition be minimized. Any such attrition can introduce post-assignment biases in the composition of treatment and control groups.

Two types of attrition can occur, each with different results. With one, participants drop out of the study and cannot be followed up. To the extent that this occurs, the integrity of the experiment is compromised and results are subject to some of the same concerns about selection bias that threaten the results of observational studies. If different plausible ways of analyzing the data lead to qualitatively different interpretations, it is then evident that: (1) the evaluator will have to model the self-selection bias, (2) the conclusions may depend on the model approach chosen, and (3) if no strong basis exists for confidence in the chosen model, the study results must be subject to considerable uncertainty.

A second type of attrition occurs when people do not complete the protocol but are still available for follow-up. In this case a valid interpretable randomized comparison can still be made: outcomes can be compared between all those who *started* on intervention A and all those who *started* on intervention B. This comparison is sometimes meaningful because, in practice, the choice may be to start a participant in one intervention or another, in full recognition that some participants may not stick with it.

If defection rates are high, however, restricting analysis to only those who stay with the assigned treatment would produce wholly biased results. For example, selective drop-out may occur from experimental group A because project participation entails more effort than staying in control group B. This type of drop-out introduces selection bias, with the result being that the outcomes of the experimental group will be artifactually overestimated because the more motivated participants remained.[13] But some members of group B might also have dropped out had they been assigned to the program that required effort on the part of participants.

Where selective attrition occurs, differences in outcome between the two groups are inevitably an unknown mixture of effects related to the actual differences in treatment effects and differences in the kinds of participants who do and do not drop out of the two treatment groups. Even if selective attrition does not occur, the completeness of information may still differ systematically between treatment groups (especially where participant cooperation is necessary to information acquisition); again, bias from self-selection is a risk.

Compliance

Both the first report of the parent committee (Turner, Miller, and Moses, 1989: Chapter 5) and the preceding chapters of this report identify compliance, along with attrition, as major threats to the integrity of experiments. Even in the most carefully designed experiments, a substantial number of individuals may leave the program or fail to comply with the requirements of the experiment and thus not receive the full strength of the intervention. The threat that attrition and noncompliance pose underscores the panel's sense that an essential first step of any outcome evaluation is to analyze the delivery of services before interpreting estimates of project effects. Tracking respondents' compliance with the assigned treatment is essential to ensure that valid inferences can be drawn from the data.

The potential importance of tracking compliance is well illustrated by an example. Clofibrate, a drug intended to treat coronary heart disease, was compared to a placebo in a very large clinical trial, and no significant beneficial effect was found.[14] Upon later analysis, however, it was observed that those patients assigned to Clofibrate who actually took at least 80 percent of their medication had a much lower five-year mortality than those in the Clofibrate group who took less than 80 percent

---

[13] On the other hand, participants may drop out because their transportation falls through or they move away, which, one might expect, would not introduce selection bias. It is, however, the case that *ad hoc* inferences such as these are always open to challenge. "Transportation falling through" may be a polite way for subjects to disguise their lack of interest in a program.

[14] In the trial, 1,103 individuals were randomly assigned to receive the drug, and 2,789 individuals received the placebo.

of their medication. The mortality rates for the Clofibrate compliers and noncompliers were about .15 and .25 respectively. Note that this was not a randomized comparison; the randomization put all these patients on Clofibrate rather than on placebo. These results *appeared* to show an important difference and suggested that the drug had beneficial effects.

Compliance—actual drug-taking—was, however, a matter of self-selection. As it turned out, the group assigned to take the placebo also had "good" compliers (who took at least 80 percent of placebo) and "bad" compliers (who took less than 80 percent). Moreover, their five-year mortality rates *were also about .15 and .25* (Coronary Drug Project Research Group, 1980). The effort to use the information available on the patients to account for this self-selection effect failed; the data in the records were not sufficient to adjust away the mortality difference in either group. Without the randomized control group data on compliance, however, a false treatment benefit could easily have been claimed for those who took 80 percent or more of the Clofibrate.

While this example does not tell us how alternative methods might have been used to resolve the problem, it does clearly illustrate the importance of tracking self-selection and compliance. It also illustrates the usefulness of data from a randomized control group.

Spillover

The diffusion of treatment effects throughout the population can also obscure evaluation results. A major threat to the internal validity of the randomized experiment is "spillover." This phenomenon—the communication of ideas, skills, or even outcomes from the intervention group to the control group—can result in the dilution of estimated program effects in a variety of ways. Members of an experimental group who adopt safer sex skills as a result of an intervention, for example, are likely to come into contact with members of the control group. If both groups are drawn from the same population, the control group may thereby adopt safer sex skills as well, at least when involved with individuals from the experimental group.

Alternatively, an effective intervention may produce the outcome of lower infection rates among the experimental group; this outcome would then spill over into reduced rates among the control group because of the reduced pool of HIV-positive individuals to whom they could be exposed. In these situations, it is plausible that any observed difference between the experimental group and the control group is an underestimate of the program's true effect.[15]

---

[15] It is unlikely that these rates can be adjusted to reflect initial conditions in different communities

Such spillover effects are less of a threat when the unit of randomized assignment is at the organizational level rather than at the level of the individual. As discussed in Chapter 1, the unit of assignment can be a clinic (i.e., the clientele of the clinic), a community, or city, and so on. In fact, when thinking about AIDS interventions, it is apparent that many educational projects, such as the media campaign, are based on a diffusion theory that assumes that interpersonal contacts are made after media exposure. In such cases, organizational units are appropriate to study because spillover *within* units is desired. Nonetheless, spillover *across* units can remain harmful to the evaluation effort, so geographic proximity of treatment and control groups should be avoided.

Compensatory Behavior

A problem unique to randomized designs is the threat that control group members will act in a way that compensates for their having been assigned to the control group (and that is, in fact, different from the way they would have behaved if truly "untreated"). Such compensatory behavior can contaminate the outcomes of an evaluation, and it is difficult to predict the direction of such bias beforehand. For example, if an attractive AIDS counseling project were offered to some participants but not to others (and both groups were aware of this assignment decision) the nonrecipients could react in different ways. They may overcompensate for their exclusion by taking it upon themselves to change their risky behavior or form their own support group. Such overcompensation would diminish the effects of a project detected by an evaluation. Or, nonrecipients may become demoralized and give up, not making any change in their behavior or even backsliding to riskier ways. Such a reaction by the control group would then tend to overestimate the effects of the intervention on the experimental group.

Such effects are particularly worrisome in that they can easily go unnoticed and result in misleading conclusions. Some protection against such missteps may be afforded by blinding the study so that participants are unaware of the alternate treatments—a strategy that may be feasible when randomization is done at the clinic or community level. Use of ethnographic observers (See Appendix C) may also be helpful in recognizing the presence of such compensatory behaviors. Replication of experiments in different milieus may also protect investigators against such experimental artifacts.

---

because we lack reliable data on the prevalence and distribution of HIV in the U.S. population. (See discussion in Chapter 1 of the 1989 report of the parent committee [Turner, Miller, and Moses, 1989].)

Salvaging Compromised Experiments

Extensive data collection can be of some help in salvaging randomized field experiments when the above factors reduce comparability between the treatment and control groups. If the randomized design is compromised, the estimates derived from the data will be subject to bias. For this reason, it can be a wise idea to collect data for randomized experiments as if the experiment were going to fail in one of these ways. Experiments ought to be monitored so that reliable measures of the content of the intervention and relevant characteristics of respondents can be used to advantage in a nonexperimental analysis if systematic attrition does occur. Both attrition and noncompliance will necessarily cause researchers to resort to analyses that use available data and a set of assumptions (a "model") to arrive at conclusions. Note that noncompliance becomes another behavioral variable to be modeled, as in the Clofibrate example given above.

Close monitoring of experiments will enable researchers (1) to test whether the remaining members of the experimental and control groups are comparable on pretest measures, or (2) to use the collected data in a nonexperimental evaluation study where assignment or attrition are modeled. As discussed in more detail in a later section of this chapter and in Appendix D, this approach requires detailed data on project implementation, the project environment, and characteristics of participants and nonparticipants, such as demographic and socioeconomic data. Modeling the degradation of the experiment will, however, raise inferential problems because factors such as motivation to comply will be very difficult to measure.

An alternative to modeling attrition is to try to prevent it in the first place. Given the great investment required for many interventions and their trials, it may sometimes be important to attain high levels of project completion to apply the maximum strength of the intervention. Three approaches can help foster both completion and compliance: a "running-in" period, indoctrination, and outreach.

- To improve compliance a standard intervention could be offered during a running-in period to detect and reject individuals who drop out within the first few days or weeks. Those individuals who stick with the project can then be randomized into an enhanced intervention or the standard protocol. Alternatively, before a study is fully deployed, would-be participants could be screened in a pre-intervention process in which the enhanced intervention is delivered but not evaluated, to see which individuals will comply with treatment.

In either case, only good compliers are allowed into the experiments.[16]

- Indoctrination involves instructing individuals when they enroll in a project about the expectations for the project. By supporting participants early in the project, when attrition rates are usually highest, investigators can often foster the understanding and trust needed to keep participation and compliance rates high and maintain a well-executed experiment.

- Finally, outreach efforts may be helpful to enhance completion and compliance. By reaching out to individuals who have difficulty completing an intervention, investigators can improve compliance and encourage dropouts to resume participation if attrition occurs. The panel suggests that the research protocol include outreach efforts to dropouts and poor compliers.

Such special efforts to induce completion and compliance should be closely monitored. It should be noted, furthermore, that it may not be possible to maintain such special efforts when the intervention is eventually fielded, so effects estimated under the maximum strength intervention may tend to overestimate what will eventually be obtained.

The panel recommends that studies be conducted on ways to systematically increase participant involvement in projects and to reduce attrition through outreach to project dropouts. All trials should assess levels of participation and variability in the strength of the treatment provided.

In addition to providing insight into how to control attrition, these studies may also be important in determining whether a lack of compliance with treatment contributes to its ineffectiveness. For example, a project or treatment could be constructed that, in itself, is entirely efficacious, but it is so unattractive or unpalatable to potential participants that compliance is negligible. A case in point is the treatment of alcoholism with disulfiram (Antabuse), a drug that induces weakness and extreme nausea when combined with alcohol. If taken, the drug works as intended; however, few alcoholics can be convinced to comply with the treatment regularly (Fuller et al., 1986).

---

[16] A disadvantage of this option is that some candidates who would have benefited from the study will not be admitted into the experiment.

When Should Randomized Experiments Be Considered?

The panel repeats its strong belief that, if it is *appropriate* and *feasible,* a well-executed randomized design is currently the most promising design for conducting an evaluation of the effectiveness of AIDS prevention programs. The questions of appropriateness and feasibility are discussed below.

Is a Randomized Experiment Appropriate?

Whether and when a randomized experiment is appropriate have to do with the research question being asked and whether an intervention project has reached the stage where such questions are timely.

What Is Being Asked? In a process evaluation, when the question is "What is being delivered?," randomized designs are unnecessary because no comparisons need to be made. In a formative evaluation (e.g., testing the persuasiveness of a set of story boards, as described in Chapter 3), experiments can be quite helpful, but other designs are certainly possible. Conversely, when the question is "What works better?," randomized experiments are particularly appropriate. Such cases involve the evaluation of relative effects, such as assessing different versions of a campaign message, educational project, or counseling regimen. The panel has endorsed randomized experiments for such evaluations. Under clearly defined conditions, the panel has also endorsed randomized field experiments to answer the question "Does the project work?" This question requires that the control group not receive an intervention or receive it later than the experimental group. (Note that the latter design cannot be used when it would involve denying or delaying a treatment that is known to be efficacious. Ethical concerns are discussed at greater length in Chapter 5 and Appendix D.)

Timeliness. The panel has previously recommended that process evaluation occur before an outcome evaluation of an intervention is attempted. A site is simply not ripe for outcome evaluation using randomized controlled experiments until the project's implementation is understood and is essentially stable. Moreover, an experimental trial of an intervention is premature until reasonable grounds exist for believing that it may make a difference. It would be a mistake to commit precious resources to a rigorous study undertaken without sufficient theoretical or empirical grounds for hypothesizing the type of effect likely to result from a given intervention. Where theory is insufficient and an empirical base needs to be established, quasi-experimental studies and statistical models will be useful for initially assessing an intervention and providing some data against which to suggest treatment effects. Such preliminary work could be especially important to provide a strong basis for experimentally manipulating large social systems, such as communities. Thus, process evaluations and observational studies of proposed interventions can and frequently should precede a true experiment.

Is It Feasible?

The merits of the *well-executed* randomized experiment for evaluating project effects are not a subject of much debate; however, the feasibility of such experiments is debatable. A randomized experiment is feasible if it is affordable, acceptable to the community, and random assignment is logistically possible. The panel addresses each of these issues below.

Affordability. The cost of an evaluation design depends on the scope of the planned research. The scope, in turn, includes such factors as the number of alternate treatments to be studied, the number and geographic dispersion of the sites, the number of study participants, the amount of information to be collected from each participant (and the difficulty involved in collecting that data), and the difficulty of the analysis. Cost involves dollars, personnel, and time—as well as lost opportunities to improve human welfare—and is obviously an important consideration for the sponsor of research.

The panel recognizes that high-quality evaluations can consume substantial resources. Although it may appear that nonexperimental designs can save on costs, we believe this is not necessarily the case. The level of rigor, not the approach chosen, is the foremost determining factor of the cost of evaluation research. In addition, nonexperimental studies often incur cost beyond those of experimental studies. The cost of inconclusive nonexperimental studies during the infant blindness epidemic is illustrative. Because considerable uncertainties attend the interpretation of the results of nonrandomized experiments, firm inferences of causality may require additional labor on the part of investigators to rule out competing explanations, and widespread acceptance of the study's conclusions may be difficult to obtain.

Even when an intervention's desired outcome is distant in time, the properly executed randomized experiment can save time and can provide widely accepted answers to controversial questions. A case in point is the treatment of breast cancer, for which survival rates are measured at some time distant from the intervention. In the late nineteenth century, Halstead introduced a form of surgery designed specifically to reduce the local recurrence of the disease by removing regional lymph nodes in addition to the cancerous breast. Because of its dramatic success in reducing the local recurrence of tumor, the surgery was widely adopted and extended to the treatment of axillary lymph nodes. This "radical" mastectomy prevailed as the standard treatment of breast cancer for nearly 70 years, despite the fact that it was a disfiguring operation, required a lengthy recovery period, and in some cases, resulted in a prolonged disability.

In 1971, a randomized trial involving close to 1,700 patients was initiated to compare radical mastectomy with a less extensive form of surgery called total mastectomy. For 20 years prior, scattered anecdotal information was reported about the value of less extensive surgery, but the studies were sufficiently flawed as to only increase the controversy about the effectiveness of radical mastectomy in improving survival rates. The randomized trial demonstrated conclusively that radical mastectomy offered no survival advantage. This approach has changed dramatically the way patients are now treated and also has changed the scientific understanding of the nature of the disease (Fisher et al., 1985).

Resources for Evaluation. Because the practical benefits of evaluation may accrue in the long term, the near-term perspective on evaluation —especially during a health emergency such as AIDS—may be short-sighted. A commonly held viewpoint is that current allocations for evaluation consume money that could be used to run additional AIDS prevention projects, a perception that can foster the resentment of evaluation efforts among practitioners, sponsors, and recipients. To avoid this kind of resentment and the pressure to forgo evaluation in the near term so that projects can be deployed, we believe that the responsibility for funding evaluation should be separated from the responsibility for running the programs.[17]

The panel recommends that the Office of the Assistant Secretary for Health allocate sufficient funds in the budget of each major AIDS prevention program, including future wide-scale programs, to implement the evaluation strategies recommended herein.

Finally, the panel repeats its advice that, to limit the resources needed for evaluation, evaluation efforts be concentrated on projects that are believed to be important and that are technically appropriate—i.e., they are representative of an intervention type, replicable in theory, and locally feasible to implement. (These criteria are discussed in Chapter 4.)

---

[17] Because the resources for fighting the epidemic are certainly limited, project costs are also important. It may be tempting to deliver inexpensive alternatives rather than their more expensive versions but, ultimately, an evaluation that demonstrates which project has the highest dividends ought to lead to a more economical allocation of funds.

Acceptability. Community acceptance of evaluation varies. The panel recognizes that evaluation research of any kind may be suspect in some communities. In such situations, communities may single out randomized experimental designs as particularly unattractive, for several reasons. Because of a diversity of community viewpoints, a number of ways may have to be tried to make randomization more palatable.

One objection to experimentation may involve perceptions that investigators are unmindful of the needs and constraints of project administrators and, as a result, the affected community. A way to improve an experiment's quality and at the same time increase its acceptability is to involve project administrators and practitioners in its design. Enlisting practitioners' insights into a project's goals and operations ought to lead to better research by ensuring that its design is implemented as planned, by understanding if—and how—a design needs to be altered, and by communicating goals to project participants. Such a strategy should go a long way toward: (1) improving the research, (2) building up pools of evaluation expertise, (3) engendering support and derailing misunderstandings that could otherwise lead to nonrandomized assignments, and (4) allaying perceptions of a project's or community's "guinea pig" status.

Another major objection to the use of controlled trials is the public perception that eligible populations are being denied services. Yet, when resources are scarce *and need is widespread,* assignments made on a random basis (e.g., through a "lottery") should be less objectionable than assignments made on almost any other systematic basis. In addition, the need for an intervention can be taken into account. Randomization does not necessarily mean that every respondent has to have an *equal* probability of assignment to treatment; rather, stratified random assignment or other probability-based allocation can be used.

Stratification involves dividing a population into mutually exclusive groups, or strata, and randomly selecting sample units from among them. This procedure ensures that certain strata theoretically related to an outcome are included in a sample in sufficient numbers to analyze them statistically. For example, a community intervention to educate gay men in the negotiation of safer sex may stratify its clients according to whether or not they are in stable relationships, if theory predicts that pre-existing relationships are important. Half of the clients in each stratum might then be assigned at random to group A or group B.[18] When outcome data are analyzed, variance attributable to stratum membership can *then* be controlled and reduced because the organization of the population into homogeneous subsets reduces sampling error.

[18]Note that treatment and control groups need not be of equal size.

At the same time, stratification can also be used to favor groups with greater needs in a way that tips the probability of treatment assignment to them, thus making randomization more attractive. Stratification can delineate groups with greater needs—e.g., those who inject cocaine instead of or in addition to opiates[19]—and attach a probability of assignment greater than .50 that they will receive a treatment or an enhanced intervention. For example, a stratum of cocaine injectors might be favored at .75, so that three quarters of its members receive the enhanced intervention, whereas the odds of assignment could be reversed (i.e., .25) for the stratum that inject opiates only.[20]

Providing alternative or delayed treatment is another way of increasing the acceptability of randomization, as the panel has pointed out in previous chapters. A recent example of alternative treatments is provided by Valdiserri and colleagues' (1989) evaluation of the effects of two peer-led interventions to reduce risky sexual behaviors. A sample of gay men in Pittsburgh was randomly assigned to receive either a lecture on safer sex or a lecture and a skills-training intervention in which safer sexual encounters could be rehearsed. Men who received skills training had a higher rate of condom use at follow-up than men who received information only in the lecture.

An evaluation design such as Valdiserri's answers the question "What works better?" but not "Does it work?" To increase the acceptability of randomization to answer the latter question, the panel has suggested delayed project implementation. A wait-list condition, which only temporarily withholds treatment or services from control group members, may be more palatable to some project administrators or their target audiences than no treatment at all. For example, Coates and colleagues (1989) used a delayed treatment condition in their evaluation of a project designed to reduce risky sexual behavior. Investigators recruited 64 seropositive gay men meeting certain study criteria and randomized half to receive stress management training and the other half to a waiting list. They found that the experimental group reported a mean of 0.50 sexual partners at post-treatment, compared with 2.29 partners for the control group (baseline means were 1.41 and 1.09 partners, respectively).

Some people have suggested that withholding or delaying treatment is unprincipled. The objection to withholding services assumes, of course,

---

[19] A New York study indicates that cocaine is injected more frequently than opiate drugs because of its relatively short-lived effect; in addition, it is thought that needle hygiene decreases over the course of an injection session (Friedman et al., 1989).

[20] When program effects are estimated from strata with different probabilities of assignment, the estimates will require weighting by the inverse of the selection probability if one wishes to generalize the estimate of effect back to the population that was randomized.

that the services are known to be effective. The panel has already stated its position that withholding *effective services* is unethical; testing whether services are effective, however, is ethical. (The ethics of randomized experiments are discussed in Chapters 4 and 5 and Appendix D; the related question of confidentiality is also discussed in Appendix D.)

A final suggestion to increase the acceptability of a randomized study involves offering new or improved services to participants as integral parts of research and demonstration projects. By making grants or contracts available to fund such services with a rigorous, well-designed controlled trial, the demand for increased services can be linked to the need to gather convincing evidence of their effects. Successful examples of this linked approach are projects funded by the National Institute on Drug Abuse and the National Institute on Alcohol and Alcohol Abuse: e.g., a psychotherapy trial for cocaine abuse, two research and demonstration projects for drug treatment improvement, and collaborative trials of patient-treatment matching.[21] These initiatives provided substantial funding for services that are part of a research protocol. The panel believes that by coordinating such grants to require replicable service protocols and standard instrumentation, these collaborative studies will provide opportunities to systematically investigate more services and combinations of services than would be possible with typical single-site, single-investigator models.

The panel recommends that new or improved AIDS prevention services be implemented as part of coordinated collaborative research and demonstration grants requiring controlled randomized trials of the effects of the services.

Such randomized trials would be affordable and would address the right kinds of questions—i.e., "Does it work?" and "What works better?" The panel believes that broad and insurmountable ethical barriers to randomized experiments do not arise except when the use of no-treatment controls is considered; we note that any particular study, however, may raise idiosyncratic ethical questions that must be resolved before this recommendation can be implemented.

Logistics of Randomized Assignment. The logistics of randomization entails the careful assignment of study participants to subsets that receive a treatment or its alternatives in such a way that every participant

---

[21] The National Institute on Drug Abuse details the cocaine psychotherapy trial in announcement DA-90-01 and the drug treatment research and demonstration projects in DA-89-01 and DA-90-05. The National Institute on Alcohol and Alcohol Abuse details the patient-treatment matching trials in announcement AA-89-02A.

has a known and nonzero chance of being assigned to a given subset. For example, if two equally-sized subsets are going to be constructed, participants can be assigned by tossing a fair coin—if the toss is heads, he or she is assigned to group A; if it is tails, he or she is assigned to group B. If there are more than two subsets, a die might be tossed, cards may be shuffled, spinners may be turned. Alternatively, a random number list or computerized random number generator can be used to assign participants to different subsets depending on whether odd or even numbers turn up.

A possible pitfall of the randomized controlled trial is faulty implementation. This trap can open up by misassignment of project participants at the beginning of a study, which can occur in a number of ways, both inadvertently and intentionally. Sometimes the randomization mechanism is simply faulty or its use misunderstood.[22]

Perhaps a greater threat is intentional misassignment. Efforts are needed to forestall the opportunity for anyone involved with the randomization —investigator, administrator, participant—to change the assignment in any way (or to influence it in advance). These opportunities can occur when the interviewer and/or the participants are aware of the details of the experiment. In medical trials, the experiments should be "blinded"—i.e., participants should not be aware of the condition for the experiment, and the health care provider should either be unaware of the treatment condition or of who is receiving the treatment.[23] Blinding is not always possible in social experimentation, but attempts should be made to avert the possibility of clients' knowing and changing participant assignment or behaving in a "socially desirable" way. Take, for an example, the train-the-trainers interventions that are frequently offered by CBOs. In such cases, a desired outcome could be subsequent knowledge or behaviors of the trainers' clients; to avoid the appearance of specialness, the clients should not know whether their trainer received the intervention or not.

Another logistical problem has to do with the eligibility of participants. Obviously, the feasibility of a randomized experiment is greatly diminished if a candidate population has already been exposed to the

---

[22]The device used to randomize assignments should be tested, understood, and correctly used. For example, researchers must comprehend how to use published random number lists, or if a computerized random number generator is used, a new seed must be selected every time a new list of numbers is created.

[23]Blinding can also be successful at reducing the effects of knowing participation status and the ensuing "Hawthorne effect" (see, e.g., Maxwell and Delaney, 1990). As mentioned in Chapter 1, this is the psychological effect of knowing that one is participating in an experiment, which may cause people to behave differently than they would in a natural setting.

program in question or to a similar program, thus thwarting the prospects of a control group. For example, if a community-wide AIDS intervention project has already "saturated" the community, the random assignment of individuals or communities to experimental and control conditions is virtually precluded. (If records are good enough, however, another evaluation design may be possible—such as the interrupted time series analysis, to be discussed in the next section on quasi-experiments.)

It is because randomized experiments are not always feasible or appropriate that we look to alternative methodologies. Despite some inferential ambiguity with their results, the panel believes it is often preferable to pursue a nonrandomized study—if carefully conceived and implemented—than to forgo an evaluation because randomization is not possible. As discussed earlier, we divide the alternative approaches to outcome evaluation into two camps: those that design comparison groups on an *a priori*, nonrandomized basis and those that develop comparability through *post hoc* statistical adjustments of the data. We turn now to the group of strategies that design comparison groups on a nonrandomized basis.

DESIGNING COMPARABILITY
INTO NONRANDOMIZED STUDIES

One general nonexperimental approach to control selection bias is to build group comparability into a research design before collecting and analyzing the data. In such planned comparisons, the panel believes it may be possible to control some of the confounding factors that could otherwise produce spurious outcome differences between groups. The panel cautions, however, that the usefulness of such designs in evaluating AIDS projects may be hobbled by inadequate information about the relevant determinants of outcomes and the factors that affect selection into projects.

In this section, the panel addresses the use of quasi-experiments, natural experiments, and matching for the outcome evaluation of AIDS prevention programs. Potential sources of data for nonrandomized designs will also be discussed in this section.

Quasi-Experiments

When randomized assignment to treatment is not appropriate or feasible, it may be possible to use quasi-experimental designs to estimate the direction and approximate magnitude of project effects.[24] These studies attempt to build comparability into comparisons through a deliberate design that *may* permit the inference of a treatment effect along with estimates of its size, given some assumptions that may not be too difficult to justify (see Campbell and Stanley, 1966, and Cook and Campbell, 1979). In the following section the panel discusses the conceptual foundations, assumptions, data needs, and possible inferences of time series and regression displacement/discontinuity designs. (Some of the time series and regression examples used here involve the analysis of "natural" events; natural experiments will be further discussed in a later section.)

Interrupted Time Series

In the interrupted time series design, a number of observations are made over time on an outcome measure of interest for a well-defined group. During the course of the measurements, the intervention (i.e., "the interruption") is introduced, and the schedule of observations continues. The resulting time series can then be examined for shifts in the outcome measure, the crucial question being whether an effect appears simultaneously or soon after the treatment or interruption.[25] In this case, the group who receives the intervention acts as its own comparison group, i.e., by comparing the group's records before and after the intervention.

In some cases, the timing of the interruption is controlled by the investigator, who can then design the quasi-experiment around the manipulated interruption. This option may apply in the evaluation of some AIDS prevention projects. In other cases, the interruption occurs naturally—that is, a situation arises in which some individuals will receive an intervention and others will not, for reasons apparently unrelated to the outcome variable. Although investigators cannot control such "natural" interruptions, they can sometimes anticipate them (as in the case of pending legislation) and begin to collect relevant data before the event occurs. Other times the natural interruptions are unforeseen; if records are good enough in these cases, time series analyses may be feasible.

A good way to describe the interrupted time series design is by illustration. One example is provided by the national 55 Mph speed

---

[24]In Chapter 4, the panel noted that a quasi-experiment might be useful to test the null hypothesis that no change occurs when it can be confidently assumed that uncontrolled factors will have a positive effect on outcome, if they have any effect at all. We should caution that a quasi-experiment that does not reject the null hypothesis has not in fact settled the issue of whether an intervention is effective. If good theoretical grounds exist for believing that the intervention should make a difference, a randomized experiment may still be needed to test effects.

[25]A good test for identifying a distinct change in the series of measurements is given in Box and Tiao (1965).

limit adopted by Congress in 1974. Shortly after this legislation was enacted, investigators in Texas estimated its effects using a time series model of state highway fatalities. Examining monthly records from 1972-1974, investigators found a 57 percent reduction in Texas fatalities attributable to the new law (Transportation Research Board, 1984). This analysis could be made only because suitable records were available from previous periods, although this analysis did not take into account competing hypotheses for change.

A related design is the multiple time series approach. This method uses one or more comparison groups or areas where the intervention is not introduced. Outcome measurements are made of the treated area concurrently with outcome measurements of the comparison areas. This method works better than the single-site approach at ruling out competing hypotheses for any observed changes. Consider, for example, a multiple time series that was applied in the 1970s after a methadone maintenance clinic was closed in Bakersfield, California. Investigators took advantage of this involuntary "intervention" by following up the clients of the defunct treatment center for two years and comparing them with clients of a clinic that continued to function. Both groups were measured for readdiction, arrest, and incarceration. Investigators found that clients of the closed clinic fared more poorly than clients of the open clinic (McGlothlin and Anglin, 1981).

A more recent study used both single-site and multiple time series analysis to test the effects of anonymity on the number of gay men seeking HIV testing. Prior to December 1986, all public HIV testing in Oregon was done confidentially. At that point, clients of public testing centers were offered a "new" intervention—anonymous testing. In the first four months following the intervention, the demand for HIV testing increased by 125 percent on the part of gay men. By comparing the number of test takers on a pre/post basis, a time series was constructed that used the history provided by pre-intervention observations as a way to rule out other explanations for observed changes. Second, by comparing the number of individuals seeking HIV testing across several sites, investigators were able to test the hypothesis that demand among gay men would have remained constant had anonymous testing not been available. Natural comparison groups that did not receive the new intervention were users of anonymous private test sites in Oregon, anonymous public sites in California, and confidential public sites in Colorado (Fehrs et al., 1988).

Assumptions. When no comparison groups are used, the history provided by the before-treatment observations becomes a control mechanism, allowing estimates of the outcome that might have been measured without the treatment. The validity of inferences from the interrupted time series design rests on the assumption that no competing hypotheses plausibly explain the shift in the time series that occurs after the intervention (competing explanations include historical events, maturation of individuals, changes in record keeping, the sensitizing effects of testing on participants, and so on).[26] This assumption of a good control is vulnerable when compared to well-executed randomized experiments.

Alternative hypotheses, for example, had to be considered in evaluating the effects of the national 55 Mph speed limit law. Using a time series method to analyze the effect of the legislation *nationwide,* investigators examined national statistics of highway fatalities between 1970 and 1979. Their initial analysis indicated a reduction of 10,400 fatalities per year, an estimation that was later substantially revised downward. The magnitude of effects was significantly reduced when the following competing explanations for change were observed: (1) a concurrent historical decline in fatalities which was discovered when a longer time series was used, (2) a reduction in discretionary travel coinciding with the Arab oil embargo and ensuing fuel shortages, and (3) improvements in highway and auto safety. Taking these other factors into account, the speed limit law appears to have saved about 3,200 to 4,500 lives per year rather than the 10,400 lives initially estimated (Transportation Research Board, 1984).

Data Needs. Compared to randomized experiments, interrupted time series designs typically require more data to infer causation. Particularly in the context of AIDS preventions, a wide range of data may be needed to test for the effects of changes in project recruitment, of other AIDS programs, and of contemporaneous events. Information about these types of changes occurring during the study is essential because such changes may provide alternative explanations for a shift in a time series. Information about them also helps to model the behavior of the time series and may serve to reduce the size of the error term in the statistical model. In the presence of such confounding factors, it may not be possible, however, to disentangle the effects of a particular intervention in a quasi-experiment from other events that occur at the same time. To circumvent this problem, the panel suggests, whenever feasible, collecting data on multiple comparison groups, multiple indicators of an outcome, multiple interruptions, and multiple measurements over time.

Multiple comparison groups may be used to rule out history and various forms of selection bias as plausible explanations for changes in

---

[26]With the multiple time series design, the use of multiple comparison groups helps to verify that history is not a plausible explanation for change.

the outcome variable. Multiple indicators—or "nonequivalent dependent variables," as they are sometimes known—refer to variables that are expected to be changed by a particular intervention as well as variables that theory predicts should *not* be changed by the intervention. For example, a neighborhood project that distributes bleach and teaches safer injection practices can anticipate (1) changes in methods of cleaning drug paraphernalia, but not (2) changes in the frequency of drug use. If the investigator measures both indicators, however, and the time series indicates changes in (1) and not in (2), it would provide a clearer inference that the project—and not some other intervention or historical trend—was leading to change. This strategy of measuring multiple indicators will not always be possible, but it is worth trying when feasible.

Analysis of multiple interruptions can provide additional certainty in inference; although multiple interruptions are not typical, they should be exploited whenever possible. For example, Hennigan and colleagues (1982) were able to devise a time series with two separate interruptions to add plausibility to their surprising finding of the effect of television on crime. Using an interrupted time series design with "switching replications,"[27] investigators discovered increased larceny rates following two separate local introductions of television in 1951 and 1955. Because of a freeze on new broadcasting licenses ordered by the Federal Communications Commission, television was introduced in this country on a staggered basis: some communities gained access to television before the freeze was initiated, and others had to wait until the freeze was lifted. Although investigators found no increase in violent crimes, burglary, or auto theft, they did find consistent increases in larceny with the introduction of television, both in prefreeze locations relative to postfreeze locales and again in the postfreeze locales relative to the prefreeze areas. This increase was observed for both the communities that received television in 1951 and again for the communities that received television in 1955.[28]

Multiple measurements over time may also increase our confidence in the results of a quasi-experiment. Emmett (1966) notes that in evaluating radio and television messages, repeated measurements before and

---

[27] A switching replication design usually involves two groups acting as comparison groups for one another: two interventions are provided the two groups at the same time, and the interventions are switched after a prescribed period of time. (The design used by Hennigan and colleagues can also be said to involve switching replications.)

[28] Content analysis of early television indicated a preponderant depiction of upper- and middle-class lifestyles, the preponderant advertisement of consumption goods, and a subordinate portrayal of larceny relative to violence in crime shows. The authors tentatively attributed the increase in larceny to factors theoretically associated with viewing high levels of consumption—i.e., explanatory theories of relative deprivation and frustration—rather than to factors associated with the social learning theory of larceny.

after a broadcast are a good way to increase the confidence that changes are attributable to the broadcast and are not short-lived. Data collection in such designs may begin many months before the intervention starts and continue for several months or even years after the project's conclusion in order to obtain a series of baseline and post-interruption measurements. It should also be added that time series design requires stable instrumentation to avoid misconstruing changes in measurement procedures with changes in outcomes.

Inferences. In interrupted time series analysis, the comparison group is the same community as it was in the recent past, and any systematic changes in the outcome variable are modeled as a time series (possibly a nonstationary series—i.e., one that exhibits a secular trend). Potential problems that may arise in such time series analysis include autocorrelated error,[29] the effect of repeated measurements on the sample, too few data points in the time series, and the fitting of overly complicated models to the data.

The shortness of either time series (before or after the intervention) lessens the strength of the inference, and modeling becomes more difficult. For example, Boruch and Riecken (1975) found that an evaluation of nutrition and education programs in Cali, Colombia produced "drastically" biased estimates of program effect because it was based on an overly short time series. In this case (see McKay, McKay, and Sinisterra, 1973), the time series estimate of the program's effect on children's cognition was half the size of the effect estimated in a randomized test. The reviewing authors posited that the bias would have been smaller had a longer time series been available.

To increase one's ability to model the process, multiple time series analysis is preferred. By using another area that does not receive the intervention as an additional comparison group, a (partial) control on the effects of history is added. In the context of AIDS research, the panel believes that multiple time series analysis may provide a useful method for evaluating the effects of community projects or the media campaign when randomized experiments are not feasible.

Regression Discontinuity or Regression Displacement

These quasi-experimental designs are similar in concept to the interrupted and multiple time series designs discussed above, but they do not require

---

[29]In a regression equation, the error term represents the difference between the real value of the outcome and its predicted value. Autocorrelated errors occur when the error term at time 1 is correlated with the error term at time 2, and so on.

the same assumptions about selection factors because the basis for selection is deliberately designed into treatment eligibility. In both regression designs, a group is assigned to an intervention on the basis of a decision variable that may or may not be related to the outcome variable, and the other group or groups are assigned to be the comparison.

Campbell (1990) provides a helpful example of the regression displacement design.[30] As shown in Figure 6-1, he looked at the effects of a "natural" intervention–Medicaid–on the number of times individuals visit physicians, comparing the number of doctor's visits made by six groups of individuals with varying levels of income (data reported by Wilder [1972] and Lohr [1972]). Individuals earning $3,000 or less were entitled to Medicaid; the others were not (thus delineating the decision criterion). When compared with visits made by the other groups (for whom the number of doctor's visits increased as income increased), the number of doctor's visits by the poorest group was "displaced" after the intervention was introduced.

In regression displacement analysis, a *single* regression line is fit for the comparison groups, which excludes the experimental groups or areas from the analysis. The regression line is fit after the intervention by regressing posttest scores on pretests.[31] A test is then made to see if the experimental group belongs along the regression line or is significantly "displaced" from it. In regression discontinuity analysis, *separate* regression lines are fit for the groups' outcomes; if the intervention has an effect, a "discontinuity" between the lines should appear at the decision point. (See Mood [1950] for a *t* test of the significance of a regression displacement point and Cook and Campbell [1979] for a significance test for regression discontinuity.)

It should be clear that many regression displacement and regression discontinuity designs completely confound their treatment (e.g., Medicaid) with a particular level of the sorting variable used to determine eligibility for the treatment (e.g., incomes below $3,000). In theory it is possible that post-intervention evidence of "displacement" or "discontinuity" could reflect the influence of the sorting variable and not the intervention. Evidence to rule out such counter-hypotheses can of-

---

[30] Regression displacement is a new name coined by Campbell (1990) for an old but largely neglected design. Cook and Campbell (1979:143-146) called the method the "Quantified Multiple Control Group, Posttest Only Design," and Riecken and Boruch (1974) called it the "Posttest-Only Comparison Group Design." Fleiss and Tanur (1973), Ehrenberg (1968), and Smith (1957) were also among the methodological progenitors of the design.

[31] The regression of posttest on pretest measures is not strictly necessary. Any variable can be used to set a decision point between comparison groups as long as it is theoretically related to the outcome variable of interest.

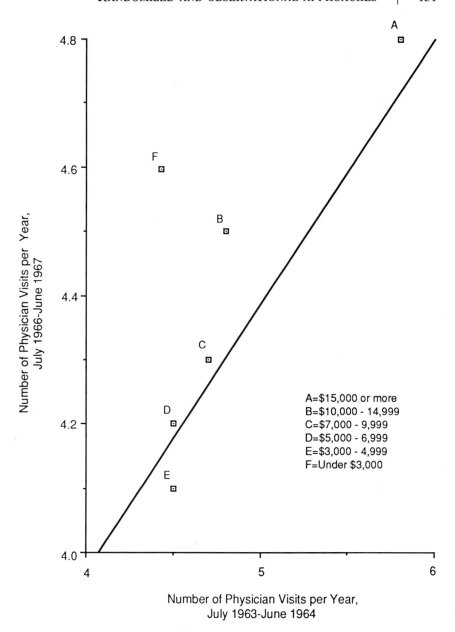

FIGURE 6-1 Regression displacement analysis of the effects of the introduction of Medicaid in 1964. SOURCE: Data points by Wilder (1972); displacement analysis by Campbell (1990).

ten be adduced from pre-intervention studies (see, for example, Lohr, 1972). The inference that the treatment itself is causing the displacement or discontinuity will be clearest when the same function fits both the pre-intervention data and the untreated portion of the post-treatment data.

Although regression discontinuity and displacement designs have not been frequently used to evaluate large-scale social programs, some attempts have been published. For example, Berk and Rauma (1983) employed a regression discontinuity design to evaluate the effects that paying unemployment benefits had on recidivism of ex-offenders. The decision point for receiving benefits was based on the number of hours an ex-offender had worked in prison. Using this method, the authors found that the group receiving the intervention had a significantly lower recidivism rate. To the best of the panel's knowledge, no evaluations using these designs have been made of AIDS prevention programs, so their value has not been established in this area.

Assumptions. Regression discontinuity and regression displacement designs assume that the intervention group and comparison group or groups come from the *same population* so that, except for their intervention eligibility, idiosyncratic differences between individuals are distributed more or less equally among the population. The assumption that selection is thereby controlled is not verifiable, and the panel warns that other factors may vary between the groups, and they may be important determinants of the outcome. Both regression displacement and regression discontinuity designs also rely on the usual assumptions underlying typical regression models, including homogeneity of error variance, stability of the regression coefficients over the time period, and the adequacy of functional specification. These assumptions cannot, in many circumstances, be verified.

Data Needs. In regression discontinuity and regression displacement designs, additional data are required to make a causal inference plausible. Moreover, it is important to have reliable measures of the decision variable that is used to determine a cut-off or demarcation point between treatment and comparison groups. Measurement is crucial because an individual's score on the decision variable decides his or her participation in the intervention. Unfortunately, scoring is fallible, which means that the basis for an individual's selection into a project can be mistaken. For example, in the Medicaid study, scoring could be invalidated if persons underreported their incomes in order to participate in the program.

Inferences. If the assignment mechanism is known and measured, it becomes more plausible that intervention effects can be isolated. It is important that the point of demarcation be fixed between the intervention and comparison groups in regression discontinuity and displacement designs, because any mixing of the groups about the decision point makes inference more difficult. Note, however, that a purported advantage of these designs—their ability to target an intervention to those areas in greatest need—can be a disadvantage to the extent that the effects of the intervention are not generalizable to groups with different levels of need. Further, as previously noted, the confounding of the assignment variables and the intervention requires that other evidence be adduced to support the inference that it is the intervention that is inducing the displacement or discontinuity.

Another potential problem with the designs is that competing hypotheses for change cannot always be convincingly ruled out. In the Medicaid illustration shown above, for example, potential sources of selection bias included, among other things: (1) the underreporting of income to be eligible for the program, (2) a disproportionate demand for medical care among the poorest group, and (3) the effect of a program requirement for medical consultations. Such potential sources of bias can be checked against archival records, *if* the data are good enough (in this case, data on medical visits collected before and after Medicaid came into effect was able to rule out the hypothesis that the poorest group had a disproportionate demand for medical attention (see Riecken and Boruch, 1974)).

Furthermore, the true functional form of the relationship between the decision variable and the outcome variable in these designs cannot be verified, as will be shown in a hypothetical plot shown in the next section. Nonadditive effects (interactions) of the selection variable and other unmeasured variables may, for example, underlie the observed bivariate association. Multiple studies undertaken prior to the introduction of the intervention may help, however, to verify the functional form of the relationship.

Notwithstanding these inferential problems, the panel believes that these designs are worth trying if multiple studies can be made. Regression displacement or regression discontinuity might be useful designs, for example, to evaluate prevention projects such as those conducted by community-based organizations. To ensure that their interpretation goes more securely, however, we advise that such studies should be replicated elsewhere to provide some test of the robustness of their conclusions.

Existing Data Sources for Use in Quasi-Experimental Designs

The panel believes that quasi-experimental and nonexperimental designs may be useful in the event that randomized experiments are not feasible.

In this section, the panel discusses some existing data sources that might be used in quasi-experimental studies. Such current efforts to collect data on HIV infection and on the public's knowledge, attitudes, and beliefs about AIDS provide observations that might be used to support interrupted time series or regression displacement designs.

The Neonatal Screening Survey. CDC/NIH's newborn screening survey may offer an opportunity for a local quasi-experimental evaluation of the effectiveness of a media or community health education project. The newborn survey, now being implemented in 44 states, the District of Columbia, and Puerto Rico, conducts blinded HIV antibody tests on heel stick blood specimens obtained from 50 to 100 percent of newborn infants (depending on the state). The resulting data provide evidence of the level of HIV infection among the population of women giving birth because a newborn infant carries maternal antibody to HIV whether or not the infant is infected. The great advantage of the newborn data is that they provide an unbiased estimate of HIV prevalence among all women who bear children in a particular time period. (They do not, however, reflect rates among women who abort their pregnancies or successfully practice contraception.) If the newborn infant seroprevalence survey is expanded, as currently planned, to gather data on 100 percent of hospital births, the quantity of data should permit estimates of infection to be made for even relatively small communities and for different age groups and separately for blacks, whites, and Hispanics within the community.[32] These estimates may then allow relatively narrow geographic areas to be targeted for intervention.

It is reasonable to expect that expanded data from the survey will reflect variations in the overall patterns of HIV transmission that occur via heterosexual sex and drug use in a community. However, as noted in Chapter 2, HIV prevalence rates are less than ideal indicators in some respects. They do not provide, for example, *rapid* signals that protective changes in sexual or drug use behavior are occurring, and they provide little or no information on communities where the HIV virus is not well seeded in the population.[33] Furthermore, these data will not reflect HIV transmission among men who have sex with men. Thus, although the newborn seroprevalence survey may provide important opportunities for quasi- and "natural" experiments, the range of its application will be somewhat narrow.

---

[32] Sufficient precautions must be taken to prevent the inadvertent identification of individuals from the survey; e.g., by masking data in small non-zero cells.

[33] In a *closed* population with a zero prevalence rate, prevalence will remain unchanged whether or not protective behavioral changes are adopted.

The panel also has some misgivings about using seroprevalence rates as the outcome measure of any AIDS prevention project because, among other things, a long interval of time is required to net enough occurrences of seropositivity to be able to test project effects (see Chapter 2).[34] On the other hand, the panel believes that such rates may be useful in evaluations of community education projects aimed at reducing *pregnancies* among HIV-positive women (for example, health education projects delivered in community family planning clinics and through local, highly visible media campaigns). These data are more attractive because the interval between the intervention and the indicator of its effectiveness is shorter (nine months) and because the rates could reflect the desired outcome—a reduction in pregnancies. Analysis would, of course, require controls for age. So, for example, if the survey were to include mother's age to the nearest year, the prevalence of infection in this year's 18-year-old mothers could be compared with the prevalence among next year's 18-year-old mothers. The effectiveness of a campaign might manifest itself in a lower prevalence of infection in locales with high-intensity education projects than in locations without such projects and in a lower rate of births to women who were HIV seropositive.

It may be possible to use data from the CDC/NIH newborn survey to evaluate such an intervention with a regression displacement design, for example. A decision point for which communities receive the intervention can be established on the basis of the incidence of HIV infection found from the newborn survey. Following the intervention, seroprevalence rates can be examined to detect the effect of the intervention on the treated groups. The comparison groups in such a regression displacement design would be those locales that did not receive the intervention.

The following is a simple, hypothetical illustration of such an evaluation; the illustration does not take into account the possibly nonlinear growth rates of HIV infection. In this hypothetical example, the average heel stick seroprevalence rate for communities with populations of 500,000 or more is 3.0 per thousand (i.e., 3 babies with antibody to HIV per 1,000 births). An intensive community health education intervention is targeted to reduce pregnancies among women at high risk for HIV in communities where the heel stick rate is 3.0 to 3.9 per thousand. Communities A, B, and C have rates of 3.0, 3.4, and 3.8 per thousand, and

---

[34]Rates of HIV depend not only on behaviors but also on the amount of infection seeded within a population or locale and other factors that can make incidence rates specious indicators of project effectiveness. It is unlikely that these rates can be adjusted to reflect initial conditions in different communities because there is a lack of reliable data on the prevalence and distribution of HIV in the U.S. population. (See discussion in Chapter 1 of the 1989 report of the parent committee [Turner, Miller, and Moses, 1989].)

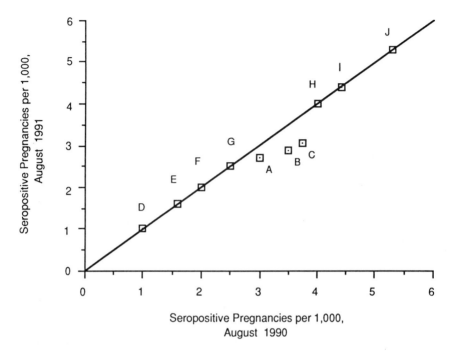

FIGURE 6-2a Hypothetical example of regression displacement analysis of the effects of a contraception campaign aimed at women at high risk for HIV.

they receive the intervention in August 1990. Communities D-J have heel stick rates of 1.0, 1.6, 2.0, 2.5, 4.0, 4.4, and 5.3 per thousand, so they do not receive the intervention. Twelve months later, heel stick specimens are reexamined: the antibody rates for HIV do not change in the untreated communities, but the rates in communities A-C decline by 15 to 20 percent. As illustrated in Figure 6-2a, these rates are clearly below the regression line fitted for the communities D-J.

This example is clear and simple; however, effects are rarely so evident. Another example will illustrate the problem of determining the functional form of the relationship. In this example, we assume that rates in untreated communities will *not* be unchanged but will fluctuate from year to year. We also assume that the communities with the highest antibody rates will be targeted (communities H, I, and J). Figure 6-2b plots the rates of communities H-J in 1990 against post-intervention rates that decline by 15 to 20 percent. The 1990 rates of communities A-G are plotted against post-intervention rates that fluctuate, untreated, by 0 to (plus or minus) 5 percent. Results are much more difficult to interpret because the data can be fitted not only linearly but also curvilinearly.

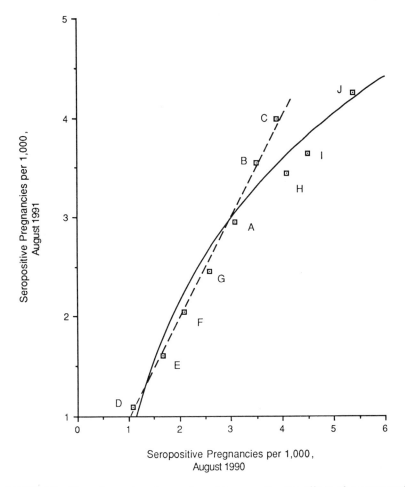

FIGURE 6-2b Alternative pre/post-intervention plots suggesting the effects of a contraception campaign aimed at women at high risk for HIV.

Thus, we believe that a healthy amount of caution should be exercised in accepting the plausibility of the assumptions of regression displacement designs.

The National Health Interview Survey

A second, perhaps more promising, source of data for quasi-experimentation is the National Health Interview Survey conducted by the National Center for Health Statistics. As discussed in earlier chapters, this is a weekly probability sample of the adult population of the United States. Since August 1987, the survey has provided cross-sectional data on the population's knowledge of HIV transmission, experience with HIV testing, and other matters related to AIDS. It is conceivable that new items might be added to this survey to measure other variables of interest to evaluators. Such additional items might then allow the use of multiple nonequivalent indicators, which would help improve the prospects of conducting convincing observational studies.

In Chapter 3, the panel recommended using the Health Interview Survey to evaluate aggregate trends in knowledge and attitudes about AIDS following exposure to phases of CDC's media campaign, particularly its public service announcements. The evaluation design proposed was a time series analysis that would monitor trends in desired outcomes over the course of the campaign period. In order to minimize the effect of the competing explanation for change—history—an extension of the measurement period before and after the broadcast could be combined with the randomized staggered implementation of the campaign as discussed in Chapter 3. Even if the assignment cannot be randomized across markets, staggered implementation of the campaign would be of use in a time series design. It might also enable the use of a regression discontinuity design to model effectiveness, using scores on the Health Interview Survey as the decision criterion for selecting particular markets.[35]

The panel recognizes that staggered implementation of the media campaign would create extra demands on CDC's personnel and contract agency administrators because it would affect the approval process for a public service announcement campaign. Such implementation would require extending the period between approval and release of some phases of the campaign. In addition, it would require changes in the expectations held by the consortium set up by the National AIDS Information and Education Program to disseminate its public service announcements. (The current expectation is that they will receive new broadcast "spots" every six months.) However, the panel feels strongly that if the desire for evaluation is real, some changes in logistics must be initiated. We urge that policy makers within CDC accept the need to change the distribution schedule of public service announcements to enable the collection of data useful for a meaningful evaluation. Policy makers and staff will have to encourage patience and cooperation within their consortium of media outlets and to make these outlets understand why scheduling changes are desirable and to make the changes acceptable.

---

[35] The feasibility of this approach may be constrained by the sample size of roughly 50,000 households per year. Some markets might be represented by too few respondents to allow sufficiently precise estimates of the level of knowledge in that market.

The panel recommends that CDC initiate changes in its time schedules for the dissemination of public service announcements to facilitate the evaluation of the media campaign. To enable the staggered implementation of television broadcasts, changes are needed in (1) the distribution schedule of public service announcements within the National AIDS Information and Education Program's consortium of media distributors and (2) the period of time between Public Health Service approval and release of new phases of the campaign.

The panel also recognizes that adding questions to the National Health Interview Survey is not a simple matter. All such items must undergo a somewhat lengthy approval process by the National Center for Health Statistics and the Office of Management and Budget. Second, the panel understands that lengthy delays may occur in getting access to the data once they have been collected. The panel is concerned about both of these problems and urges greater cooperation on data sharing between the National Center for Health Statistics and other divisions of CDC.

The panel recommends that CDC initiate changes in its data collection and data sharing activities to facilitate the evaluation of the media campaign. To generate needed data, changes are needed in (1) the period of time for internal approval of data items for the National Health Interview Survey and (2) expeditious data sharing between the National Center for Health Statistics and other divisions of CDC.

Natural Experiments

As discussed earlier, one way to increase the number of situations in which a comparison group is feasible is to take advantage of natural experiments. A natural experiment occurs when membership in the treatment (versus comparison) group comes about for a fortuitous reason that makes it unlikely that selection biases could operate.[36] The panel has mentioned several evaluations that have used time series analysis or

---

[36] Judgments as to what is truly "fortuitous" will be open to challenge. One can, however, imagine natural experiments that arise from situations that are indeed equivalent to a true randomized experiment. In the extreme case, one might imagine, for example, that a computer anomaly caused the IRS to mistakenly add $500 to the tax refunds of persons with Social Security numbers that ended in the digit 5. In such a fanciful event, one would have (with only some trivial assumptions) a random experiment with which to assess the impact of small, accidental windfalls upon the behavior of taxpayers.

regression displacement to estimate the effects of an intervention that has occurred exogenously. (Later we will discuss the utility of natural experiments in our discussion of selection modeling.)

A "natural laboratory" can also be established if one is willing to restrict the experiment to special subgroups. For example, the effects of alternative interventions were compared between natural comparison groups by Ziffer and Ziffer (1989). These investigators delivered alternative AIDS education courses to students enrolled in one-semester courses at the same college. They were not able to randomize who attended the different courses, but by restricting the intervention to a discrete pool of possible participants they obtained some plausible comparisons. (For example, investigators found that the course offering a "values and attitudes" component had a significantly greater effect on attitude change than the basic "facts" course.) Contaminants to this research design are clearly possible: for example, students choosing an early morning class might be different from those choosing to meet in the afternoon, or students enrolling in an AIDS course offered by the psychology department might be different from those enrolling in a biology department course. Still, design flaws such as these might be handled by keeping the alternative courses as parallel as possible in their contexts.

Identifying Natural Experiments

Finding a natural experiment or natural laboratory takes resourcefulness in identifying, defining, and recruiting the groups under analysis, as well as a bit of luck and patience. The panel believes that it is useful to be aware of and to search for situations in which natural experiments might arise. One such situation occurs when AIDS-related legislation is pending or has passed in a given state, creating a natural laboratory of persons affected by a "treatment" as well as a neighboring pool of people not so affected. For example, Florida requires that women convicted of prostitution undergo screening for a variety of sexually transmitted diseases, including HIV; women who are found to be infected must submit to treatment and counseling as a condition for release (Gostin and Ziegler, 1987). In this case, the relevant outcomes of testing and counseling might be compared between convicted, involuntarily "treated" women in Florida and their counterparts in states that do not mandate such intervention.[37]

---

[37] In choosing this example, the panel does not wish to imply our endorsement of mandatory testing; rather, we support the idea of recognizing natural experiments when they occur.

Assumptions of Natural Experiments

Although the search for natural laboratories or experiments is an important way of reaping the benefits of a control group, pitfalls do occur. The investigator employing natural experiments, for example, typically has no control over selecting and implementing interventions and little control over measuring and managing controls. The unverifiable assumption is that the comparison group is identical to the treatment group except for the lack of the intervention, and except (perhaps) for statistical adjustments that might be made for differences in observable characteristics of the comparison and treatment groups.

Data Needs of Natural Experiments

It will not be possible to confirm the assumption that groups are identical except for the intervention. It would help, however, to at least partially corroborate the assumption by examining data on pre-intervention differences between two or more sites. The natural experiment of anonymous HIV testing in Oregon described earlier is a good illustration because investigators there used not only pre-post measures of the Oregon testing sites but also multi-site comparisons with neighboring states.

Matching Without Randomization

Matching is the third type of research design the panel considered for developing group comparability before data are collected for a study. Under *some* circumstances, matching is done retrospectively; moreover, it is sometimes done in conjunction with a type of statistical adjustment called analysis of covariance, which we will discuss in the following section on statistical adjustments and modeling. (Matching can also be used in a randomized experiment; if matching on factors known to have an important effect on outcome were possible, one of each pair might be randomly assigned to a project.)

Comprehensive knowledge about selection factors is crucial before matching is attempted. Although matching can control *known* sources of bias, other variables may influence the outcome. This approach assumes not only that the matching procedures are effective in eliminating the biasing effects of matched variables but also that these other confounding variables do not exist.

When participants in a singly constituted study group can be matched in pairs, and only one of the pair receives an intervention, some extraneous variables may be effectively controlled (e.g., individual motivation for inclusion in the study). For example, suppose members of a cohort study are offered a support group meeting on Tuesday evenings to practice social skills associated with safer sex practices. Individuals who are unable to attend meetings on those evenings can be matched with those who do join the support group. (Note, however, that even in this example, the group that cannot attend on a certain night may still differ in important respects from the group that can attend.)

Prospective Nonrandomized Matching

In the prospective nonrandomized matched study, the group assigned to receive an intervention is matched with a comparison group that does not receive it. For example, it might be possible to identify four communities that are about to receive funding for CBO projects and then match them with four similar communities.[38] In such designs both the treatment group and the comparison group are often given a pretest and a posttest. It is useful to recognize this design as a special case of the multiple interrupted time series design, where the series is constituted by only two points in time.

Another strategy for developing comparable treatment and comparison groups is the use of matched groups in an ongoing cohort design. In such a design, pairs of individuals may be identified as matched on independent variables that are assumed to be strongly correlated with the outcome of interest, such as baseline behaviors. The individuals might, for example, be matched on the level of the outcome variable at two or more points *prior* to the intervention. This option is attractive because the cost of data collection on an intervention's effects is minimal since baseline data will already have been routinely collected. Other matches can be made based on factors predicted by the underlying behavioral theory to affect outcomes.

Even in cases when matching does not provide a convincing control for contaminating factors, prospective cohort studies can help generate hypotheses about which interventions are effective. These hypotheses might later be tested in a quasi-experimental or experimental setting.

Retrospective Nonrandomized Matching

The more typical matched study involves nonrandomized retrospective matching, wherein an investigator attempts to find an untreated group that, in some important respects, "looks like" a group that has received

---

[38] This research design was used, for example, to evaluate the effects of the Youth Incentive Entitlement Pilot Projects. For a project aimed at reducing school dropout rates and providing work experience for teenagers, four communities were selected as pilot sites and were matched with four communities that did not receive the program (see Betsey, Hollister, and Papageorgiou, 1985).

an intervention. The comparison group frequently is constituted from existing pools of individuals and institutions—e.g., areas served by different hospitals, separate cities or counties, and so forth. Sometimes a comparison group is constructed from the same cohort that intervention members belong to; the comparison group are the respondents who do not, for whatever reason, receive an intervention. Unlike prospective matches, retrospective matches do not provide the opportunity to do pretesting and multiple pre-intervention measurements that are individually tailored to the needs of the evaluation design. Such retrospective designs yield more convincing results when data are available to permit matching of respondents on baseline behaviors. The designs are also obviously more convincing when differences between the treatment group and the comparison group are minimal for variables that may be related to the outcome of interest. The designs remain vulnerable to distortion, however, by any unrecognized variables that affect outcomes and are differently distributed in the various groups.

The Multicenter AIDS Cohort Studies (MACS), which were designed to track the natural history of HIV disease among gay and bisexual men, have offered a setting in which the effects of AIDS interventions have been evaluated using matching strategies. One example of retrospective matching is provided by Fox and colleagues (1987), who had the advantage of having collected baseline data. These investigators compared how the knowledge of one's HIV antibody status affects one's sexual activities. Some of the participants in the Baltimore MACS cohort elected to learn their antibody status (the "aware" group) while others elected not to learn their status (the "unaware" group). In a post hoc analysis, investigators matched the aware and unaware men on number of male sex partners, as well as on age, race, perception of illness, manifestation of illness, and proportion who were antibody-positive. The groups were not matched, however, on two other theoretically confounding factors— education and depressive symptoms. Sexual activities were measured at three time points prior to disclosure of test results and at one six-month interval afterward.

Assumptions. Three general assumptions are made when matching without randomization is used, and all three are liable to failure. The first is that matching takes into account all of the variables that are pertinent to selection into a project and to the project's outcome. This assumption is almost certain to fail because unobserved factors are not measured—whether they are individual differences (such as motivation to participate in a program) or community differences (such as decisions to adopt certain AIDS prevention policies). The second assumption is that the biases in the measurement of key variables (e.g., baseline and post-intervention sexual behavior) are equivalent between the treatment group and their matched comparison group. The third assumption, implied by the first two, is that the group constructed as a comparison is fully comparable to the group that receives the treatment.

A simple hypothetical example of the hazards of matching is displayed in Table 6-1. In the top half of this table, five communities hypothetically slated to receive funding for an education project are matched with five other communities on the basis of their population size. The matched communities are approximately the same size, their populations being within three percentage points of one another, based on July 1988 census figures. However, a comparison of annual AIDS rates for the matched communities for 1988 and 1989 shows that disparities exist. For example, Baltimore and Minneapolis–St. Paul both have populations of over 2.3 million, but Baltimore had 20.3 persons with AIDS per 100,000 in 1989, and Minneapolis had 6.6. It can hardly be assumed that local needs for AIDS interventions will be the same for the two communities; likewise, the citizens of these communities should not be assumed to feel similar inducements for changing their behaviors. The same conclusion holds if locales are matched on AIDS rates. The bottom half of the table, for example, shows that Philadelphia and Orlando both had AIDS rates of 16.1 per 100,000 in 1989, but that Philadelphia has a population five times larger than Orlando's, not to mention a different demographic composition. It is thus not safe to assume that their HIV transmission sources are comparable.

Although the panel realizes that few investigators would make matches as simplistic as these, they might attempt to match on both of these variables, and possibly other sociodemographic characteristics. Unfortunately, what the table cannot display is the dearth of community matches possible on even the two observed factors of population size and AIDS rates. Moreover, even the best matching attempts will miss unobserved influential variables. For example, communities slated for sponsorship will probably differ in important respects from communities that have not been chosen to receive funding (they may have more persuasive community leaders, have submitted more sophisticated requests for sponsorship, have less local AIDS funding, and so on).

In addition to the failure of general assumptions, a challenge to matching without randomization is likely whenever the selection of the intervention group is made on the basis that its members are in greater need of treatment. In this case, the treatment group's gain over the comparison group could be explained on the basis of "regression toward the mean." This phenomenon is an improvement that results merely

TABLE 6-1   Hypothetical Matchings of Ten Communities

6-1a.   Comparisons of 1988 and 1989 AIDS Rates Per 100,000
Between Communities Matched on Population Size

City	Population	1988 Rate	1989 Rate	City	Population	1988 Rate	1989 Rate
Baltimore	2,342,500	13.7	20.3	Minnpls-St.Paul	2,387,500	6.3	6.6
Seattle	1,861,700	14.4	19.6	Cleveland	1,845,000	7.0	6.9
Orlando	971,200	18.8	16.1	Louisville	967,000	4.6	4.5
Austin	748,500	13.4	24.5	Tulsa	727,600	6.3	6.3
Las Vegas	631,300	14.4	20.2	Syracuse	650,300	4.6	5.9

6-1b.   Population Comparisons of Ten Communities Matched on
1989 AIDS Rates per 100,000 Population

City	1989 Rate	Population	City	1989 Rate	Population
Washington, D.C.	23.3	3,734,200	New Orleans	22.5	1,306,900
Philadelphia	16.1	4,920,400	Orlando	16.1	971,800
Phoenix	11.1	2,029,500	Wilmington	11.4	573,500
Albany/Schenectady	8.6	850,800	Baton Rouge	8.8	536,500
Salt Lake City	5.2	1,065,000	El Paso	5.6	585,900

NOTE. Source: Population statistics from U.S. Department of Commerce, Bureau of the Census, *News*, September 8, 1989; AIDS case data from U.S. Department of Health and Human Services, Centers for Disease Control, *HIV/AIDS Surveillance Report*, January 1990.

from the group with extreme pretest scores gravitating back toward the population mean score upon retest.

Data Needs. As evident from the example above, it is rarely possible to include measures of "all" the variables that could account for differences in outcomes observed between matched members of treatment and comparison groups. The panel repeats its belief that the state of the art in AIDS prevention research is underdeveloped with respect to predicting how people would behave in the absence of the program (e.g., changes in sexual behavior or needle use), and that it is therefore difficult to specify the types of variables that need to be considered (presumably prior risk behavior and some demographic characteristics are important, but even this is not known with certainty).

Inferences. Several serious problems emerge when inferences are made from matched studies. First, it is not likely that *all* the relevant differences between participants and nonparticipants will be captured by the matching variables. Second, even if the pertinent variables were known, the method becomes difficult to implement if more than a few variables are to be matched, because fewer and fewer close pairs will be found. This practical difficulty may also necessitate reducing the desired sample size; obviously, inferences from reduced samples will be difficult to make. For example, when Chapin (1947) attempted to match on six variables, his original samples of 671 and 523 boys were reduced to samples of size 23 (reported in Cochran, 1965).[39] Finally, the measurement of these matching variables is, itself, subject to considerable error and bias. (See Appendix C for an extended review of the reliability and validity of common measurements of sexual and drug using behaviors.) For all of these reasons, the panel believes that widespread use of matching nonequivalent comparison group designs would be premature in the evaluation of AIDS intervention programs.

Existing Data Sources for Matching Without Randomization

Notwithstanding the inferential problems involved in matching studies, the panel believes that longitudinal cohort studies from which participants in an intervention may be matched with nonparticipants can be rich and useful sources of information for generating hypotheses about project effects. When cohorts are sampled in multiple sites, data collection can be enhanced by coordinating instrumentation across the locations, facilitating cross-site analyses.

Cohorts of Gay Men. Several cohorts of gay men are being studied longitudinally and may serve as sources of matched pairs. For example, the National Institute of Allergy and Infectious Disease supports research on cohorts of men who have sex with men. In the early stages of the epidemic, several MACS cohorts (described earlier) were put together to investigate the epidemiology of AIDS and to draw inferences about the risk factors for acquiring HIV. By administering repeated physical examinations and interviews, the MACS studies have shed light on the natural history of HIV infection and AIDS and the occurrence of behavioral changes made to avoid infection (i.e., reduction of unprotected anal intercourse and number of sexual partners).[40] Although the MACS were not designed to evaluate interventions, they are appealing examples

---

[39] Parametric models might be used when samples are insufficient to obtain exact matches on all variables. The use of such models, however, will introduce an additional degree of uncertainty into the analysis.

[40] Less is known about men in smaller cities where the risk of HIV infection is lower, but it should not be assumed that their behaviors are the same. For example, Kelly and colleagues (1990) surveyed patrons of men's gay bars in three small southern cities (Monroe, Louisiana; Hattiesburg, Mississippi;

because the studies have been coordinated among four sites (Baltimore, Chicago, Los Angeles, and Pittsburgh) to administer the same survey instruments to measure sexual and drug use behaviors and to recruit men who were similar in certain important respects (gay and bisexual men, excluding those diagnosed with AIDS). The generalizability of MACS data is limited, however, because recruitment methods generated a sample of predominately white, middle class, urban men who made a long-term commitment to a research project on men who have same-gender sex.

Several other groups of gay men may serve as additional sources. A cohort similar to the MACS groups is being followed in the San Francisco Men's Health Study (see, e.g., Winkelstein et al., 1987). This study was designed at the same time as the MACS cohorts, but investigators decided during the planning stages to work independently. In addition, CDC sponsors demonstration and education projects among gay and bisexual men in six sites: Albany and New York City; Chicago; Dallas; Denver; Long Beach, California; and Seattle-King County, Washington. CDC also supports, along with the Massachusetts Department of Public Health, a longitudinal study of homosexual men drawn from a Boston community health center (see, for example, McCusker et al., 1988). Additionally, the National Institute of Mental Health is currently supporting longitudinal studies of behavioral change among gay and bisexual men in Chicago (e.g., Joseph et al., 1987), New York City (e.g., Martin and Dean, 1989), and San Francisco (e.g., McKusick et al., 1985).

Cohorts of Intravenous Drug Users. Two cohort studies of drug users provide a potential source of subjects for matching studies within this population. The Treatment Outcome Prospective Study (TOPS) is a longitudinal study of drug users who receive treatment from publicly funded programs. Sponsored by the National Institute on Drug Abuse, the TOPS study seeks to understand the natural history of drug users before, during, and after treatment (see, e.g., Hubbard et al., 1988). The ALIVE group in Baltimore is a cohort of drug users who are being followed to learn more about the natural history of HIV infection in this population. This group of active drug users without AIDS was recruited from street outreach, clinics and hospitals, and drug treatment programs (Nelson et al., 1989). Cohort studies such as these can provide important insights into the factors that lead to behavioral changes and that cause programs to be more (and less) effective. Because of the restricted nature of the samples used in these studies, generalization of findings from such

---

and Biloxi, Mississippi) and found higher rates of risky behavior than those reported in large urban epicenters of the disease. (Note, however, that the source of recruitment—gay bars—may account for some of the differential rates between these cities and the epicenters.)

studies will usually require confirmatory studies using other populations.

In the next section, we examine statistical adjustment and modeling strategies. These strategies constitute the third major approach to nonexperimental evaluation discussed in this chapter.

MODELING AND STATISTICAL ADJUSTMENTS FOR BIAS

We have already looked at two broad answers to the problem of isolating treatment effects: randomization and the deliberate design of nonequivalent comparison groups. Another approach is to search for (or sometimes establish) a comparison group that looks somewhat like the group who received the intervention and then identify, measure, and take into account the many variables that differ between them and that are believed to affect outcome (i.e., "model" the selection bias). Success in this undertaking calls for carrying through three tasks. These tasks are to:

1. Recognize the variables that may influence outcomes,
2. Measure these variables in all participants, and
3. Use the measurements in a way that correctly adjusts outcomes for group differences.

In this section the panel looks at three types of modeling used to eliminate selection bias and to create comparable groups: analysis of covariance, structural equation models, and selection models.

Analysis of Covariance

Analysis of covariance is sometimes used on data from nonrandomized (quasi-experimental) studies to adjust outcome measurements for preexisting differences between groups. In this method, the average outcome in a treatment group comprises two components (plus random error): the effect of the treatment applied in that group, and the effects of relevant confounding variables (for example, age, sexual history, drug use history, and so on). The effects of confounding variables are estimated using some postulated model—perhaps a linear regression—and each treatment group average is thus adjusted. The difference in adjusted average outcomes is then taken as the estimate of the difference in treatment outcomes.

This approach can be very successful in some tightly controlled settings, such as laboratory experiments, where all factors believed to influence the desired outcomes may be measured and included in the model. The success of the method is often equivocal, however, in complex social science investigations because it formally requires identification, measurement, and use of *all* important confounding variables.[41] Unfortunately, it is not generally true that correct adjustment for *some* of the intervening variables will be an improvement over the unadjusted difference. Indeed, one can make projects look far worse or far better than they are by using this approach.

For decades, analysis of covariance has received wide use in behavioral and social investigations. This use is statistically well justified in randomized field experiments. In nonexperiments, however, its use has frequently turned up riddles and complications (Boruch and Riecken, 1975; Boruch, 1986).

Assumptions

Covariance adjustment is dependent on the assumptions of its model, e.g., the assumption of a linear, additive (or other) functional relationship between the covarying independent variables and the outcome measure; this relationship is presumed to be the same in all groups. Moreover, the model assumes that the error term is independent of the treatment and the covariates. Finally, it assumes that no unspecified factors exist that affect both selection and outcome.

Any observational method that attempts to control for selection bias must rely on assumptions that cannot be verified (or can only be imperfectly verified) about the factors that affect the likelihood that individuals will learn of, enroll in, and participate in a project. Examples of several failures of these assumptions and the long debates about appropriate models and inferences can be found in the various evaluations that were performed on the Head Start program. Because Head Start involved several curricular models and three different cohorts of children, various data sets have been analyzed and their results critiqued. The original Head Start evaluation used comparison groups that matched the experimental sample on age, sex, race, and kindergarten attendance. This cohort was not pretested. In the program evaluation, investigators constructed an index of socioeconomic status as the single covariate, and the conclusion from the analysis of covariance was that the program was largely ineffective. This conclusion was roundly criticized because it assumed, incorrectly, that its covariate adequately measured the confounding factors that affected selection and outcome.

---

[41] That is, variables that (1) influence outcomes, and (2) are not equivalently distributed in the treatment and comparison groups.

Subsequent analyses illustrated the danger of assuming that selection factors have been adequately controlled by covariate adjustment. For example, Barnow (1973) reanalyzed the original Head Start data by different racial/ethnic groups and found the program to have positive effects on black and Mexican American children and negative effects on white children, a quite different finding than that of the original study. In addition, Bryk and Weisberg (1976) analyzed the evaluation of another Head Start cohort that adjusted for, among other things, scores on a Preschool Inventory test. The authors criticized the test as being unreliable, and they argued that the covariance model underadjusted for pretest differences between groups and that it overestimated program effects. Later, Magidson (1977) reported small positive effects of the program on white children when he reanalyzed Barnow's data using a model that incorporated allowances for measurement error in the tests and postulated correlations between disturbance terms in a structural equation model (an evaluation method that will be discussed below).

As such 10-year controversies indicate, the process of inference from such nonrandomized designs can be contentious, and closure may be difficult to achieve. This fact was well anticipated by Lord (1967) who observed that "no logical or statistical procedure can be counted on to make proper allowances for uncontrolled pre-existing differences between groups."

Data Needs

Because the selection process influences the ultimate effectiveness of a project, the efforts made by prevention projects to attract and retain participants are of interest. The ability to attract and retain individuals is itself composed of at least two elements: (1) the motivation of the individuals and (2) the ease of access to the program, including its visibility, its convenience in terms of location and hours of operation, and so on. Data on these factors can be collected during the process evaluations, along with other data on program characteristics and program implementation discussed in Chapters 3-5;[42] however, the panel would note that data on motivations is likely to be difficult to collect and fraught with problems (see, for example, Turner and Martin, 1985: Vol.1., Ch.5, 7-9).

---

[42]Data on factors that attract and retain participants can also provide information about important communication links with the population at risk. Such data permit the identification of subgroups that were better attracted to the project, those that were missed, and those who benefited most. This, in turn may help in informing other projects about how to enlist participants, and about which characteristics new projects should avoid or adopt.

Inferences

The success of the analysis of covariance procedure depends on how well its users understand the relationship between underlying variables and the outcomes of interest. For example, if the exact nature of the relationship between age and outcome were known, statistical procedures might be used to model and adjust the estimates of effect to account for differences in the age composition of the treatment and comparison groups. In the evaluation settings we contemplate in AIDS prevention, the state of the art unfortunately does not include knowledge of the important factors determining outcome, let alone measured values for them. It is thus tempting in this situation to measure instead a large collection of all possible variables thought to relate to outcome. If this is done, a decision must be made as to which factors to include in the model and how they should be included. Without strong theory to guide this selection, equivocal answers may result; the approach of measuring as many things as possible and adjusting as best as possible cannot be relied upon to set things right.[43]

Structural Equation and Selection Models

Structural Equation Models

Simply put, a structural equation model is a statistical equation or system of equations that represents a causal linkage among two or more variables.[44] In the context of an evaluation study, this procedure may use complex models of behavior to explain the effects of an intervention on a desired outcome, as mediated through a series of intervening variables and as co-influenced by factors that are exogenous to the intervention. Structural equation models representing these processes may be expressed by path diagrams representing the patterns of influence among these variables. In such diagrams the relationships specified by the equations are represented in a network of causal linkages.

A structural equation model embodies (in a series of equations) an explicit theory about ways in which one variable in a model may (and may

---

[43] The reader may wish, for example, to review the role played by selection and compliance factors in the Clofibrate experience discussed in the section on "Compromised Randomization."

[44] A variety of texts on the topic are available. For example, Goldberger and Duncan (1973) was a seminal effort that brought together theoretical work by econometricians, psychologists, and sociologists. Duncan's (1975) monograph introduced the topic at a simple statistical and logical level. Applications of modeling in the behavioral sciences and education were reviewed by Bentler (1980). In addition, Dwyer (1983) has written a comprehensive technical text on structural equation modeling, which includes discussions of the issues of causal inferences and potential uses of modeling.

not) affect the other variables in the model. Plainly, reliance upon such systems of equations require well-articulated theory or prior empirical knowledge in the present instance of the factors that influence risk-taking behavior and project participation. In particular, this procedure presumes the existence of: (1) explicit theory or empirical evidence about causal relationships among variables and the functional form of these relationships, (2) large samples, especially when the theory is complex, and (3) measurements of the variables specified in the theory.

Where there are sufficient theory and data to use this technique, structural modeling has important advantages. In particular, the structural modeling approach:

- forces the analyst to be explicit in articulating theory,
- facilitates an analytic focus upon how well a particular system of structural equations (a theory) fit the data,
- facilitates comparison of competing models or theories,
- provides an intuitively appealing way of representing complex effects, including direct and mediated chains of causal influence, and
- when successful, such modeling efforts provide some basis for predicting outcomes that may occur as conditions change (e.g., via a policy change that alters the distribution of one or more model variables).

It is nonetheless this panel's judgment that it is unlikely in the near term that structural equation modeling of nonrandomized studies could provide a firmer basis for evaluating the effectiveness of AIDS prevention programs than well-executed randomized experiments. This judgment follows from three considerations:

- theory about causal relations is weak in AIDS settings,
- empirical data that would substitute for theory are sparse,
- the estimates produced by structural models will be subject to considerable uncertainties because competing theories are likely to be plentiful.

For these reasons the panel believes that structural equation modeling would not permit one to make causal inferences (i.e., to declare that a project works) or to measure the magnitude of effects (how well it works) with nearly the same level of confidence that a well-executed experiment does.

Although the panel is not optimistic about our present ability to use structural equation models and data from nonrandomized studies as the *primary strategy* for evaluating the effectiveness of AIDS prevention programs, we do believe that such models will have a role to play and we suspect that this role may grow in the future. In particular, the panel believes that much might be gained by the judicious use of such models as an adjunct to randomized experiments. Modeling efforts might be used, for example, to improve our understanding of the individual and contextual factors that mediate between a treatment and an outcome. Furthermore, as experience accrues in situations where modeling is done *in tandem with experiments,* we anticipate the development of theory and data that may allow modeling approaches to substitute for some experiments in the future.

Selection Models

Another approach to nonexperimental program evaluation comes under the heading of selection modeling. Here the problem of nonequivalent comparison groups is addressed by focusing explicitly on the determinants of project participation. An analysis is conducted of the reasons why some individuals participate and others do not, in the hopes of locating observable variables that can be used to control for, and eliminate, the unmeasured differences between participants and nonparticipants. Such analyses require credible assumptions and sufficient data to explore them. Because this procedure may be new to non-economists, the panel has included a background paper that details selection modeling procedures (Appendix F). A shorter exposition is presented below.

Investigators using selection modeling procedures have generally taken one of two approaches (see, e.g., Heckman and Robb, 1985a and 1985b). The first involves an implicit search for natural experiments (which are expected to present an identifying variable, or set of variables, that theoretically affects project participation but does not directly affect the outcome variable). The second approach involves controlling for the determinants of project participation through the use of longitudinal, cohort, or retrospective data sets containing information on the histories of project participants and nonparticipants.

Selection Models and Natural Experiments. The simplest selection model uses one variable proxy for unobservables. Let us take as an example a natural experiment in which neighborhood A and neighborhood B have equal rates of AIDS incidence and populations with similar demographics and sexual behavior histories. Neighborhood A, however, has more counseling and testing participant slots, purely for political reasons—perhaps the congressional representative from A enjoys seniority over B's representative. Such an identifying variable would explain why participation in neighborhood A is greater, and it would be unrelated to unobservable differences in the preproject levels of the outcome variable.

Once an identifying variable or set of such variables is found,[45] there are several statistical methods that may be used to obtain treatment estimates.[46] The best-known technique is a two-step method called the "Heckman lambda" method in which: (1) an equation is estimated for the determinants of project participation, and (2) from the results of the first step, a "selectivity bias" variable is constructed that is intended to control for the mean levels of the unmeasured differences between participants and nonparticipants. Selection modelers use this second-stage analysis to estimate the effect of program participation on the outcome variable.

Selection Modeling and Historical Controls. The second approach of selection modelers involves identifying determinants of project participation from available data on the histories of project participants and nonparticipants. The philosophy is that the individual histories, taken as a whole, will serve as a proxy for unobservable variables that account for differences in outcomes between groups. The simplest example is one in which unmeasured differences between participants and nonparticipants are explained by preproject measures of the outcome variable. For example, if the difference between those who do and do not participate in a counseling and testing project arises solely because the participants practiced risk reduction behaviors more frequently at some point prior to their entry into a project, having information of their behavior at that point and controlling for it statistically might eliminate the selection bias. This may not always be possible, of course—those who participate may have decided to start practicing less risky behavior between the time their behavior was measured and the time they entered the project.

More generally, if information is available for many different points in the past, a fairly complete history of sexual or drug use behavior can be controlled for. Selection bias will then remain only if participants have the same contemporaneous characteristics (age, location, education, and so on) and the same sexual or drug injection history as nonparticipants, but participants are nevertheless different in some unmeasured way that is not independent of the outcome variable (e.g., their intention to start practicing less risky behavior in the future).

---

[45] Identifying variables can be area characteristics, as in this example, or they can be individual characteristics; they may be discrete variables (city or neighborhood location) or continuous variables (dollar level of funding); or some combination of all of these.

[46] These methods have been explored in depth in the selection modeling literature (e.g., Barnow, Cain, and Goldberger, 1980; Maddala, 1983; Heckman and Robb, 1985a, 1985b).

Assumptions of Modeling

One great merit of both structural equation and selection modeling techniques is that the assumptions needed for these models are made explicit (even though they may be unverifiable). If models are used in an evaluation, their assumptions should be fully reported, so that readers of the research can understand and weigh their plausibility. Moreover, whenever possible, evaluators who use such models need to provide an assessment of whether the study's assumptions were actually met; this assessment can be made with the help of subject-matter experts in HIV disease prevention.

The potential uses of selection modeling in evaluation has generated considerable controversy between economists and statisticians. Examples of that controversy may be found in papers and commentary presented at a 1985 symposium (Heckman and Robb, 1986a, 1986b; Hartigan, 1986; Tukey, 1986a, 1986b), in an exchange recently published by the *Journal of the American Statistical Association* (Heckman and Hotz, 1989a, 1989b; Holland, 1989; Moffitt, 1989), and in the remarks made by participants at the conference held by this panel in January 1990. At present there are divergent and strongly held opinions about the potential uses and misuses of these procedures, and no practical experience applying these procedures to the task of evaluating AIDS prevention programs. In the following pages, the panel briefly reviews some of the key issues that have emerged in the debate over selection models. Given the present state of scientific debate concerning the applicability of these models, it is the panel's belief that it would be unwise to rely upon selection modeling as the mainstay for an AIDS evaluation strategy. Rather the panel believes that careful efforts should be made to learn more about the applicability of these procedures to the task of AIDS evaluation. Such experience may dictate wider use of these procedures in the future.

A critical question in the selection modeling approach is whether selection bias can be eliminated by either of the two methods described above, and whether the analyst can determine when selection bias has been eliminated and when it has not. Critics of this approach have observed that evaluations using selection modeling procedures have often been unsuccessful in replicating the results of randomized controlled experiments (see LaLonde, 1986; Boruch, 1986; and Fraker and Maynard, 1986). Because of the sensitivity of modeling approaches to the assumptions that have to be made, critics claim that selection modeling is unreliable and that it creates substantial uncertainty as to true effects. Some analysts (Fraker and Maynard, 1986; LaLonde, 1986) argue more flatly that the approach does not eliminate selection bias and that the requisite determination cannot be made. Both these analysts find that

TABLE 6-2 Five models of estimated manpower training effects on 1979 earnings

MODEL	Estimate of Effects from Experiment	(s.e.)	Estimated Effects Using Nonexperimental Groups			
			PSID-1	(s.e.)	CPS-SSA-1	(s.e.)
Treatment Earnings Less Comparison Earnings						
Men	886	(476)	-15,578	(913)	-8,870	(562)
Women	851	(307)	-3,357	(403)	-3,363	(320)
One-Stage Econometric Model (Controlling for pre-training earnings and all observed variables including women's AFDC status in 1975)						
Men			-1,228	(896)	-805	(484)
Women			2,097	(491)	1,041	(503)
Two-Stage Econometric Models; Not in earnings equation but included in participation equation:						
Marital status, residency in an SMSA, 1976 employment status, number of children, women's AFDC status in 1975						
Men			-1,133	(820)	-22	(584)
Women			1,129	(385)	1,102	(323)
1976 employment status, number of children						
Men			-1,161	(864)	13	(584)
Women			1,564	(604)	552	(514)
No exclusion restrictions						
Men			-667	(905)	213	(588)
Women			1,747	(620)	805	(523)

NOTES: *s.e.* is standard error of estimate. The estimated training effects are in 1982 dollars. PSID-1 comparison group members were household heads in the Panel Study of Income Dynamics poverty subsample, continuously from 1975 through 1978, who were less than 55 years old and did not classify themselves as retired in 1975. CPS-SSA-1 comparisons were individuals from the Current Population Survey/Social Security Administration matched file, who were in the labor force in March 1976, with nominal income less than $20,000 and household income less than $30,000 (women between ages 20–55 years of age and men less than or equal to 55 years of age).
SOURCE: LaLonde, 1986:Tables 4, 5 and 6. Because LaLonde shows two-stage estimates for only two candidate comparison groups, these are the comparisons reported here. (LaLonde shows eight female candidate comparison groups in Table 4 and six male candidate comparison groups in Table 5.)

estimates of effects are extremely sensitive to the particular "identify-ing" variables chosen (in the first method) and to how much preproject history is controlled for (in the second method). LaLonde, for example, makes side-by-side comparisons of the effects of a manpower training program estimated from a randomized experiment with estimates derived from several nonexperimental models. Table 6-2 reproduces selected es-timates from five of these models in order to compare the results of the randomized control group with estimates from two possible comparison groups.

It will be seen from Table 6-2 that experimentally measured effects are similar for men and women at around $870, as seen in the top two lines of the table. The corresponding estimates using nonexperimental control groups are found in the same top two lines and are *greatly* different: For men the +$886 figure would be replaced by -$15,578 or -$8,870, depending on which comparison group is chosen. For women the observed experimental difference of +$851 would be replaced by -$3,357 or -$3,363. Later lines in the table offer other model-based estimates of the gains for men and for women. One cannot help but be struck by their poor agreement with the experimentally found effects.

On the other side of this argument, Heckman and Hotz (1989a) have argued that many of the different selection models estimated by Fraker and Maynard and by LaLonde can, in fact, be tested and rejected as invalid in the sense that they fit the data poorly. Heckman and Hotz claim that a set of "best" models can be selected by standard statistical methods of hypothesis testing. These authors use nonexperimental data and methods of model selection to argue that the effect estimate obtained in a particular randomized trial can be reproduced with a "best" selection model using nonexperimental data (e.g., the random-growth estimates of effects for high school dropouts and the linear control function estimates of effects for AFDC recipients in Table 6-3).

It will be seen from Table 6-3 that the unrejected linear control function estimate for AFDC recipients closely approximates the estimate derived in a randomized trial (+$267 vs. +$238, with standard errors of 162 and 152 respectively). The random-growth estimates for high-school dropouts, however, were also unrejected—and they would replace an experimentally estimated effect of +$9 by negative effect estimates of -$154 and -$724, respectively. For the latter estimates the inference of effect is also complicated by the larger standard errors that were obtained from the nonexperimental analysis (212 and 502, versus 173 for the experiment).

TABLE 6-3 Experimental and Nonexperimental Estimates of Training Effects for School Dropouts and AFDC Recipients, 1979. (Nonexperimental estimates that were not rejected by Heckman and Hotz's statistical tests are underlined.)

	School Dropouts		AFDC Recipients	
	Est.	(s.e.)	Est.	(s.e.)
Estimates from Experiment	9	(173)	267	(162)
Nonexperimental Estimates				
1: Linear control function estimates*				
Variant 1	-1884	(247)		
Variant 2	-1827	(246)		
Weighted average *(AFDC Model Not Rejected)*			238	(152)
2: Fixed-effect estimates constructed with 1972 pretraining earnings*				
Variant 1	-2172	(277)	508	(193)
Variant 2	-2070	(275)	544	(195)
3: Fixed-effect estimates constructed with 1974 pretraining earnings*				
Variant 1	-1663	(301)	522	(179)
Variant 2	-1636	(269)	500	(184)
4: Random-growth estimates constructed with 1973 pretraining earnings*				
Variant 1			-217	(546)
Variant 2			-263	(557)
Weighted average *(Dropout Model Not Rejected)*	-154	(212)		
5: Random-growth estimates constructed with 1974 pretraining earnings*				
Variant 1			1109	(576)
Variant 2			860	(576)
Weighted average *(Dropout Model Not Rejected)*	-724	(502)		

NOTES: *Est.* is Estimate of effect; *s.e.* is standard error of estimate. Variant 1 assumes that changes in the outcome variable will be the same for nonparticipants as for participants in the absence of treatment. Variant 2 assumes that changes in the outcome variable will vary for people with different characteristics; the average of sample means is shown.

SOURCE: Heckman and Hotz, 1990: Tables 3 and 4. (Heckman and Hotz show additional rejected estimates based on different controlling variables, which the reader may be interested in examining.)

*Controlled for race, sex, marital status, age, education, residency in an SMSA, and participation in NSW (dropouts) or Current Population Survey (AFDC recipients aged 18-64, with dependent children aged 16 and under).

Data Needs of Models

Modelers attempt to control for selection bias by constructing plausible models of selection and then considering the types of data that might be available for fitting a model. In each case, investigators show the assumptions that need to be met in order to obtain *consistent* estimates of the effects of an intervention. Perhaps modelers' major conclusion is that the assumptions necessary to obtain consistent estimates grow less restrictive the richer the data that are available. Multiple comparison groups, multiple independent variables, multiple outcomes, and multiple time points all reduce the number of unverifiable assumptions needed to fit a model. The price paid for this reduction in restrictive assumptions, however, is an increase in error variance, as discussed below.

The minimal data set needed to construct structural and selection models is a single cross-section of post-treatment information (which might be obtained, e.g., from a compromised experiment). The assumptions involved with cross-sectional data have already been described for structural equation models. In addition, use of data from a single cross-section to estimate a selection model requires that the investigator find a plausible identifying variable (that is, a variable that influences participation in the program but not the outcome). If longitudinal data are available from a random sample from periods both prior to and after the treatment, weaker assumptions can be made. For some of the estimation methods, it is more important to have multiple periods of pre-project data than post-project data because the former permit a more adequate control for individual histories prior to the intervention.

To some extent, selection models confront the same inferential problems as natural experiments. How can it be known with certainty that, for example, neighborhood location is indeed independent of the unmeasured differences in the outcome variable between participants and nonparticipants? As discussed in reference to natural experiments, the plausibility of the assumption cannot be tested without gathering additional information. Such information may take the form of institutional knowledge of how the Public Health Service allocates its limited funds or information about the details by which different counseling and testing projects are funded in different neighborhoods and different cities. Alternatively, it may take the form of a search for yet additional sources of natural experimental variations in an attempt to determine whether both neighborhood variation *and* some other type of natural variation give the same, or similar, estimates of effects.

Similarly, one may ask how it can be known with confidence that a single pre-project data point is sufficient to eliminate selection bias?

In this case, the collection of additional data—namely, data from points farther in the past—might be used to make the determination. If the single pre-project data point is sufficient, then controlling for additional pre-project data points will not affect the estimate of effects. One possible consequence of using historical controls, as proposed in Appendix F, is an increase in statistical uncertainty. As in many areas of statistics, a tradeoff must be made between the potential reduction in bias and the potential increase in variance associated with a method that relies on weaker assumptions. The measures proposed for historical controls in selection modeling rely on multiple observations of the outcome variable at different points in time. Estimates based on first, second, and higher order differences involve sums and differences of additional variables, and these estimates can, as a result, have higher variances than simple cross-sectional differences. The actual variance will depend on the structure of the correlations between successive observations.

If the observations are sufficiently correlated (which, of course, is the premise of the approach), the variance of estimates based on historical controls can be lower than those based on cross-sectional data. If, on the other hand, there is no correlation between successive measurements, an estimate based on first differences would have twice the variance as one based on contemporary controls, and one based on third differences would have twenty times the variance. One cannot know, *a priori,* which situation will apply, but "noisy data" (in which the measurement variability is high relative to real changes in the underlying variable) would argue against incorporating multiple observations.[47]

Inferences from Modeling

The panel's concerns about establishing comparability using structural equation or selection models is that they may fail (without detection) because of either flaws in data quality[48] or errors in the assumptions that are made about the relationship of variables that affect selection and outcome. First, at the risk of being redundant, the panel wishes to emphasize that our understanding of the behavioral and other characteristics

---

[47]After the analysis has been completed, of course, it may be possible to estimate the variances and explicitly consider the tradeoffs between bias and variance.

[48]Data quality is an issue for every design. It is a particular concern in the case of modeling efforts (versus experiments) because the device used to produce comparability between groups in a model can be affected by the errors and biases of the measurements, e.g., self-reports of sexual behaviors prior to entry into the program. These measurements are subject to both random errors and to bias in reporting (see Miller, Turner, and Moses, 1990: Ch. 6; included as Appendix C to this report). In a well-executed randomized experiment, the method of producing comparable groups is not subject to such uncertainties.

that are important in changing behaviors that transmit HIV is woefully inadequate. The absence of tested theory or empirical evidence shrinks the basis for the assumptions required by these models.

Second, there are also problems that stem from the quality of the available data. As reported in Miller, Turner, and Moses (1990: Ch.6; reprinted as Appendix C), extant surveys of sexual and drug using practices are riddled with bias. Although the authors are sanguine about the feasibility and replicability of such survey measurement, they note that convincing evidence of measurement validity is sadly lacking for AIDS risk behaviors.

In addition to data problems, the wide variety of estimates possible from both structural and selection models also dampens our enthusiasm. As some critics have pointed out, the model-selection tests are designed to determine if overidentified data fit a model; if the data fit, the test does not reject the model. Moreover, it has been argued that a model that fits the data may not adequately describe the selection function when additional data are considered (see, e.g., Holland, 1989). It is also true that any structural equation model that fits the data is only one of many (Dwyer, 1983). Just because the data *fit* does not mean that the model's effect estimates are valid.

The panel takes a guarded view of the current suitability of modeling approaches to estimate the effects of AIDS prevention programs. The appropriateness of this view may change as experience accumulates in evaluating AIDS programs. In this regard the panel notes that selection models all aim at one desideratum: consistency.[49] But a consistent estimate can have so much variability as to be of no practical value for samples of realistic size. Lacking a theoretical understanding on this matter we can either ignore these methods or get some structured experiences using them, which is the panel's proposed resolution.

The Role of Models

The unresolved debate between modelers and their critics and the available evidence lead us to two conclusions. One, the panel finds little evidence to persuade us that it would be prudent to rely extensively on selection models in the AIDS arena in the near future. Two, we believe that it may be wise to obtain further evidence about the performance and

---

[49]"Consistency" roughly means: a statistic t is a consistent estimate of a parameter T, if with high confidence the differences between t and T approach zero as N goes to infinity. But for N equal to 100 or 1,000 or 1,000,000 that difference need not be serviceably small. (It should be noted that the estimation procedures will, of course, seek efficiency, i.e. minimization of variance between expected and observed values.)

characteristics of these models. Overall, the field of selection modeling is relatively new, having been developed in the 1970s and applied to program evaluation in the 1980s (see, e.g., Heckman, 1979; Barnow, Cain, and Goldberger, 1980), and its full potential has not yet been realized. The panel would like to see its value empirically established, and we believe the federal government should fund the appropriate research.

The panel recommends that the National Science Foundation sponsor research into the empirical accuracy of estimates of program effects derived from selection model methods.

One avenue would be to provide researchers financial support and access to randomized controlled trial data to see if they can reproduce the findings with nonrandomized comparisons. Progress along these lines, if achieved, would be valuable indeed. It would help answer the scientific question about how well nonexperimental approaches work in estimating effects. In addition, this recommendation may help to solve problems not only in the AIDS intervention arena but also in other areas in which it is difficult to implement randomized controlled experiments.[50]

WHEN SHOULD NONRANDOMIZED APPROACHES BE CONSIDERED?

Although the panel believes that randomized controlled experiments ought to form the backbone of CDC's evaluation strategy, we understand that they cannot constitute the exclusive strategy. Under some conditions, randomization is precluded, and an evaluation cannot be conducted unless other methodologies are considered. In this section the panel looks at a set of five conditions under which investigators should seriously consider the use of nonrandomized approaches.[51] Some of the conditions are implicit in the earlier text; for example, where an empirical

---

[50]Another role that models play is to provide a framework for "sensitivity analyses," that is, assessments of the sensitivity of estimates of program effects to departures from the assumptions used in the analysis. When data are not available on selection variables and unverifiable assumptions about the selection process have to be made, researchers can adjust the assumptions in a variety of ways to examine the range of possible estimates of effects (within the contexts of specific models). These results are suggestive of the range of plausible project effects (assuming that a particular model is well specified). This would be useful information to have and it could lead to a more stringent evaluation of the intervention at a later time.

[51]Some scientists argue that there is an additional situation in which nonrandomized approaches should be used, namely when the nonrandomized study is more relevant to the full-scale implementation because the intervention when ultimately implemented on a national scale, will be accompanied by attrition, self-selection, spillovers, etc.

This is a complex issue, but the panel does not, in general, believe that the "messiness" of the real world implementation of a program necessarily argues for a nonexperimental design. The panel believes that the choice of method should be determined by what is feasible, and what will provide an

base needs to be established, alternative observational methods may be quite useful. In addition, positive answers to the following questions invite serious consideration of quasi-experimentation and nonexperimental methods.

1. Can the decision maker tolerate serious ambiguity in estimating the effect of a program or project?

When effects are uncertain and randomization is not feasible, nonrandomized approaches may lead to ambiguous, but tolerable, conclusions. Quasi-experimental evaluations, for example, attempt to estimate an intervention's effect while taking into account plausible competing explanations for its apparent effect, but those competing explanations may involve "causes" that are not fully identifiable or estimable. For example, Kelly and colleagues (1990) were satisfied simply to detect an effect and to tolerate an imprecise measure of effect estimates in their test of a "diffusion-of-innovation" intervention at the community level.[52] By limiting the study to a few sites it was less costly to deliver the intervention. (As discussed under the section on randomized experiments, a sufficient number of units is needed to detect differences in outcome variables, and the cost of delivering an intervention to the necessary number of units—e.g. communities—may be prohibitively expensive when

---

appropriate level of certainty about the answers that are obtained.

In that regard, it should be borne in mind that only some of the "messiness" of a real-world implementation is relevant to assessing the effect of the intervention as implemented. Other aspects have little to do with the intervention, but are of concern to researchers.

For example, in some instances sample attrition will be part of the phenomenon of interest; that is, people will be lost from a treatment (intervention program) itself and that is part of the outcome. (Recall for example the case of Antabuse noted on page 136.) In such cases, as discussed previously, the appropriate analysis should assess the overall outcome (including loss of persons through attrition from the intervention). In other instances, the delivery of an intervention (treatment) may be less than optimal when a program is broadly implemented. In such cases, one might envision an evaluation whose "treatment" was the "intention to deliver the intervention program" and not the optimal delivery of the intervention in a carefully controlled setting. A design for such a study of the joint impact of the treatment and its real-world implementation could be a randomized experiment, or not.

It should be noted, however, that some of the real-world problems one encounters are not germane to the effectiveness of the program although they can make the research task difficult. Sample attrition, for example, may reflect only a poorly implemented data collection plan (and not a treatment outcome). That is, the intervention may have been well delivered to almost all participants, but long-term, post-treatment data gathering may have suffered from a high rate of sample attrition. In this case, there is only a failure of the research effort; it has no necessary consequence to the effectiveness of the intervention. A better executed data collection program might remove this defect; it is not a characteristic of the intervention itself.

[52]Rather than randomize communities, investigators chose three "relatively isolated" communities and measured baseline sexual behaviors at two points prior to the intervention. No intervention was directed at two of the communities, while the third received an intervention that taught risk reduction strategies to men identified as opinion leaders. At two points later, evaluators applied the same behavioral measures and found statistically significant decreases in risky behaviors for the intervention population relative to the comparison community populations.

effects are uncertain.) On the other hand, the lack of randomization into participation categories means that it is not possible to discount the possibility that something other than the planned intervention occurred in the intervention community to cause the change. Thus, this example accepts some ambiguity, but it also may be more feasible than a randomized experiment. In addition, the example reveals the value of quasi-experiments in giving investigators experience with intervention procedures before they are deployed in an experimental study.

2. *Are the competing explanations for the project's effect reasonably assumed to be negligible?*

The number of instances in which competing explanations are negligible will be few. They do exist, however. In testing an algebra course for third graders, for example, it will often be safe to assume that third graders who are not involved in the curriculum will not learn algebra on their own. A before-and-after design would then be sufficient to estimate the effect of the curriculum on children's knowledge.[53] Similarly, a before-and-after design might be acceptable to test the effects on schoolchildren of an intensive CBO project to reduce stigmatization of a prospective seropositive classmate. The media campaign's effects on this population might be assumed to be negligible (given the late hour of most broadcasts of national public service announcements about AIDS and the reading level required for published materials). Any changes in attitudes might then be attributed to the intervention.

3. *Must the program be deployed to all relevant individuals or institutions that are eligible?*

As mentioned earlier, a community-wide intervention project to prevent AIDS may be swiftly implemented and offered to all eligible residents, thus saturating the community and precluding the random assignment of individual residents to experimental and control conditions. Consequently, any evaluation design will have to depend on quasi-experimental or statistical adjustment methods. For example, a time series analysis of trends in condom sales, visits to STD clinics, and sales of safe sex videos or books might be implemented. Note, however, that when multiple sites are involved, the panel suggests that communities themselves might be randomly assigned to an intervention or to a control condition in the interest of estimating the effects of the program.

---

[53]Before-and-after evaluation designs are discussed in Chapter 4.

4. Will a nonrandomized approach meet standards of ethical propriety while a randomized experiment will not?

As discussed in Chapters 4 and 5, random assignment to an intervention or to a control group fails to meet standards of ethical propriety if resources are in ample supply to provide the intervention, it is not otherwise available, and the beneficial effects of the intervention are assumed to outweigh any negative effects. HIV testing, for example, is believed to be an effective medical care procedure, thus making a randomized no-treatment control inappropriate for estimating the effect of CDC's counseling and testing program.[54] In this case, it might be possible to use a time series design to examine the effectiveness of a new counseling and testing setting on the accessibility of services. For example, suppose a small community with HIV test facilities in its public health and family planning clinics wishes to open a new site specifically to attract gay men. Before opening the new site, the community can count the number of test takers using test facilities by their risk exposure group (as identified in Figure 5-1 in Chapter 5). After the new site is open, the number of test takers by risk group can be recounted (actually, a series of before-and-after measurements would be preferred). If the number of gay test takers increases (without a corresponding decrease in the other categories to which they may have assigned themselves), it might be inferred that the new project was effective in attracting gay men.

5. Are theory- or data-based predictions of effectiveness so strong that nonexperimental evidence will suffice?[55]

In some cases, theory may predict dramatic effect sizes. It is often (but not always) true that the larger the expected impact of an intervention, the less accurate an evaluation technique one needs to discern that impact. Extremely persuasive educational and prevention projects might, for example, produce such large effects that the impact would be convincingly evident even with observational designs that are more vulnerable to bias. In other cases, an intervention may have previously been shown to make a difference under a given set of circumstances or within a given subgroup using a randomized experiment. In these cases, suppose the generalizability of this finding is not known, and an investigator wishes to test the intervention in a different setting or among a different target group. Under these circumstances, the inferences from an observational study may be sufficiently convincing as to preclude the

[54] See Appendix D for further discussion of the ethical concerns of evaluating patient care procedures.

[55] Note that it is important to differentiate well-founded predictions of effectiveness from "common knowledge" of what works. Too often hunches or instincts about what works have stood in the way of deciding to conduct a well-controlled randomized study.

need for a full-scale experiment. Consider, for example, the case of a counseling support project that has been tested in a randomized controlled experiment and shown to increase gay men's behavioral skills for refusing sexual coercion (Kelly et al., 1989). The support project's effectiveness among women partners of intravenous drug users, however, is unknown. To test it, a quasi-experiment might be designed.

In a final section, below, the panel considers the investigator's final assessment of the results of his or her study, whether it be a randomized experiment or not.

INTERPRETING EVALUATION RESULTS

The goal of outcome evaluation is to determine how well a project works. Part of this determination, no matter the method chosen for evaluation, involves an investigator's interpretation of results. The degree of certainty that the observed outcomes result from the intervention is a function of, among other things: the reasonableness of the assumptions behind the evaluation strategy, the quality and amount of the data, and the plausibility of counter-hypotheses that could account for the observed data. It is also important for interpretation to address whether results are specific to a given set of circumstances or are generalizable to other populations.

Randomized Experiments

Assuming that randomized controlled trials are used, the assumptions underlying the inference of effects are generally easy to verify, which will facilitate acceptance of a study's interpretation. One still needs, however, to examine the data on project participants and the project itself, to insure the internal validity of the experiment. Such validation is needed to be sure that the project and randomization were implemented as designed and that the degree of attrition is acceptably small. If these conditions are satisfied, differences between units can be analyzed using standard statistical tests.

In the end, even if the results are strongly encouraging for a subgroup of a population, generalizability will often be uncertain. The results from a single experiment may allow strong and rather precise inferences of causality, but because they are likely to be based on small, selective samples, they may be equivocal in terms of how the project will work in other groups, other settings, and other regions of the country. Whatever is known about the experiment should be communicated in the interpretation of results.

Nonrandomized Methods

Nonrandomized methods make greater use of assumptions than randomized trials. In interpreting the results of such studies the plausibility of these assumptions must be considered (and reported) because they will vary from one design to another, and they are crucial to the inferences that will be drawn. Moreover, investigators need to analyze the sensitivity of their inferences to the likely amount of departure from these assumptions.

Accessibility of Assumptions

All of the alternatives to randomization have one thing in common—they rely on assumptions that are not directly verifiable. The nonexperimental alternatives differ, however, in the nature of the assumptions that are necessary.

Observational studies, natural experiments, and matching approaches tend to make assumptions that, although they may not be directly verifiable, can be expressed in accessible everyday terms. Comparison groups must be similar to treatment groups in every respect (other than the treatment) that might influence the outcome; there must be no changes other than the treatment between pretest and posttest; and so on. To the extent that we know the factors that influence the outcome variable, we may be able to assess whether there are differences between comparison and treatment conditions.

Analysis of covariance, selection models, structural equation models and other statistical techniques require assumptions that are generally expressed in formal statistical terms that are somewhat removed from everyday experience. Analysis of covariance, for instance, assumes that the relationship between outcome variables, covariates, and the treatment can be adequately and fully expressed in a particular form of (single-equation) statistical model. Selection models based on historical controls assume that the treatment and comparison groups are similar with respect to the first, second, third, or higher order differences over time in the outcome variable. Structural equation models make complex assumptions about the covariance structure among all of variables in the model. The appropriateness of such assumptions can be quite difficult to assess, even if one is familiar with the statistical language and the subject matter, and external validation data are often unavailable. Although there are some statistical techniques for testing the *inadequacy* of the requisite assumptions for all of these models, there is no general way to determine that the assumptions hold.

In summary, compared to quasi-experimental designs, the complex statistical alternatives to randomization require more elaborate assumptions that can be quite difficult to verify.

Interpretation

Besides plausible assumptions, the interpretation of observational studies is also a function of data quality and competing hypotheses for change in the observed outcomes. The panel has addressed both of these issues in this chapter, but we wish to add a note on how competing hypotheses might be ruled out in a more trustworthy way.

A set of six criteria developed by Hill (1971) to assess observational studies in the field of medicine are of interest. These criteria, which have been modified over the years, point out the need to take into account the whole of the evidence, not just selected studies, in interpreting whether an observed association is causal. A recent report of the Committee on Diet and Health (1989) restated Hill's criteria to include the following:

- the strength of association between the intervention and the observed outcome,
- the "dose-response relationship" in which greater effects are demonstrated from more intense treatments,[56]
- a temporally correct association (i.e., an appropriate time sequence between the intervention and the observed outcome),
- the consistency with which similar associations are found in a variety of evaluations,
- the specificity of the association, and
- plausibility (i.e., the supposed causal association comports with existing knowledge).

Although several of these criteria are applicable to the findings of any one study, the consistency of association and the notion of plausibility argue that a study also be interpreted in the context of other findings.

One of the greatest difficulties for observational studies to surmount is their vulnerability to counter-hypotheses that could account for differences between the comparison and treatment groups (based on factors other than the intervention). Although this problem is inherent to the approach, certainty about a particular causal inference increases as a reservoir of similar findings is accumulated across studies using disparate methods. What is more, even flawed studies can be convincing when a body of evidence is compiled.

When data are drawn from several studies, however, they are sometimes difficult to compare because the studies use different definitions of target audiences, different specifications of causal variables, different

---

[56] A ceiling effect may sometimes appear, thus diluting the dose-response relationship.

outcome measures, different wordings of survey questions, and so on. These differences make it hard to compare results across studies, and detract from their interpretation as a whole. Moreover, differences between studies also make results difficult to generalize, regardless of whether experimental or nonexperimental studies are used. We believe that a way exists to improve their interpretability.

The panel recommends that the Public Health Service and other agencies that sponsor the evaluation of AIDS prevention research require the collection of selected subsets of common data elements across evaluation studies to ensure comparability across sites and to establish and improve data validity and reliability.[57]

Questions about a project's applicability to other populations require information on the populations for which the project succeeded, peculiarities of the region or the population that were important to its success, and the cost of the project and possible areas for cost reduction. The hope is that an evaluation that suggests success for a particular project in one area will lead to a rapid implementation of the project in similar regions and to its gradual implementation in regions less and less similar to the original site evaluated, so that the generalizability of the initial finding is not assumed to stretch too far without empirical verification.

None of this is meant to imply that the panel urges scores of evaluations. The panel believes that more certain and useful knowledge will be gained by a smaller number of well-executed studies than by a precipitous rush to assess the effects of every prevention program that is being mounted. At present, the panel believes the randomized experiment to be the most appropriate design for outcome evaluation, both in terms of clarity and dispatch of results, all else being equal. At the same time, we recognize that the strategy will not always be feasible or appropriate and, for these situations, other designs may have to be deployed until evidence accumulates to make their interpretation dependable or until a randomized experiment can be conducted.

REFERENCES

Barnow, B. S. (1973) The effects of Head Start and socioeconomic status on cognitive development of disadvantaged children. Ph.D. dissertation. University of Wisconsin.

---

[57] Furthermore, methodological research is urgently needed to study the validity and reliability of behavioral measurements. Appendix C is devoted to a discussion of these issues.

Barnow, B. S., Cain, G. G., and Goldberger, A. S. (1980) Issues in the analysis of selectivity bias. In E. W. Stromsdorfer and G. Farkas, eds., *Evaluation Studies Review Annual*, Vol. 5. Beverly Hills, Calif.: Sage Publications.

Bentler, P. M. (1980) Multivariate analysis with latent variables: Causal modeling. *Annual Review of Psychology* 31:419-456.

Bentler, P. M. (1990) Structural equation modeling and AIDS prevention research. Presented at the NRC Conference on Nonexperimental Approaches to Evaluating AIDS Prevention Programs, Washington, D.C., January 12-13.

Berk, R. A., and Rauma, D. (1983) Capitalizing on nonrandom assignment to treatments: A regression-discontinuity evaluation of a crime-control program. *Journal of the American Statistical Association* 78:21-27.

Betsey, C. L., Hollister, R. G., and Papageorgiou, M. R., eds. (1985) *Youth Employment and Training Programs: The YEDPA Years.* Report of the NRC Committee on Youth Employment Programs. Washington, D.C.: National Academy Press.

Boruch, R. F. (1986) Comparative aspects of randomized experiments for planning and evaluation. In M. Bulmer, ed., *Social Science Research and Government.* New York: Cambridge University Press.

Boruch, R. F., and Riecken, H. W., eds. (1975) *Experimental Tests of Public Policy..* Boulder, Colo.: West Press.

Box, G. E. P., and Tiao, G. C. (1965) A change in level of non-stationary time series. *Biometrika* 52:181-192.

Bryk, A. S., and Weisberg, H. I. (1976) Value-added analysis: A dynamic approach to the estimation of treatment effects. *Journal of Educational Statistics* 1:127-155.

Campbell, D. T. (1990) Quasi-experimental design in AIDS prevention research. Presented at the NRC Conference on Nonexperimental Approaches to Evaluating AIDS Prevention Programs, Washington, D.C., January 12-13.

Campbell, D. T., and Stanley, J. C. (1966) *Experimental and Quasi-Experimental Designs for Research.* Chicago: Rand McNally.

Chapin, F. S. (1947) *Experimental Designs in Sociological Research.* New York: Harper.

Coates, T. J., McKusick, L., Kuno, R., and Stites, D. P. (1989) Stress reduction training changed number of sexual partners but not immune function in men with HIV. *American Journal of Public Health* 79:885-887.

Cochran, W. G. (1965) The planning of observational studies of human populations. *Journal of the Royal Statistical Society*, Part 2, 128:234-255.

Cook, T. D., and Campbell, D. T. (1979) *Quasi-Experimentation: Design & Analysis Issues for Field Settings.* Boston: Houghton Mifflin.

Committee on Diet and Health (1989) *Diet and Health: Implications for Reducing Chronic Disease Risk.* Report of the NRC Food and Nutrition Board. Washington, D.C.: National Academy Press.

Coronary Drug Project Research Group (1980) Influence of adherence to treatment and response of cholesterol on mortality in the coronary drug project. *New England Journal of Medicine* 303:1038-1041.

Duncan, O. D. (1975) *Introduction to Structural Equation Models.* New York: Academic Press.

Dwyer, J. H. (1983) *Statistical Models for the Social and Behavioral Sciences.* New York: Oxford University.

Ehrenberg, A. S. C. (1968) The elements of lawlike relationships. *Journal of the Royal Statistical Society*, Series A, 131:280-302.

Emmett, B. P. (1966) The design of investigations into the effects of radio and television programmes and other mass communications. *Journal of the Royal Statistical Society*, Part 1, 129:26-49.

Fehrs, L. J., Fleming, D., Foster, L. R., McAlister, R. O., Fox, V., et al. (1988) Trial of anonymous versus confidential human immunodeficiency virus testing. *Lancet* 2:379-382.

Fisher, B., Redmond, C., Fisher, E. R., Bauer, M., Wolmark, N., et al. (1985) Ten-year results of a randomized clinical trial comparing radical mastectomy and total mastectomy with or without radiation. *New England Journal of Medicine* 312:674-681.

Fleiss, J. L., and Tanur, J. M. (1973) The analysis of covariance in psychopathology. In M. Hammer, K. Salzinger, and S. Sutton, eds., *Psychopathology: Contributions from the Social, Behavioral, and Biological Sciences.* New York: John Wiley & Sons.

Fox, R., Odaka, N. J., Brookmeyer, R., and Polk, B. F. (1987) Effect of HIV antibody disclosure on subsequent sexual activity in homosexual men. *AIDS* 1:241-246.

Fraker, T., and Maynard, R. (1986) *The Adequacy of Comparison Group Design for Evaluations of Employment-Related Programs.* Princeton, N.J.: Mathematica Policy Research.

Friedman, S. R., Rosenblum, A., Goldsmith, D., Des Jarlais, D. C., Sufian, M., et al. (1989) Risk factors for HIV-1 infection among street-recruited intravenous drug users in New York City. Presented at the Fifth International Conference on AIDS, Montreal, June 4-9.

Fuller, R. K., Branchey, L., Brightwell, D. R., Derman, R. M., Emrick, C. D., et al. (1986) Disulfiram treatment of alcoholism: A Veterans Administration cooperative study. *Journal of the American Medical Association* 256:1449-1455.

Goldberger, A. S., and Duncan, O. D., eds. (1973) *Structural Equation Models in the Social Sciences.* New York: Seminar Press.

Gostin, L., and Ziegler, A. (1987) A review of AIDS-related legislative and regulatory policy in the United States. *Law, Medicine & Health Care* 15:5-16.

Hartigan, J. (1986) Discussion 3: Alternative methods for evaluating the impact of intervention. In H. Wainer, ed., *Drawing Inferences from Self-selected Samples.* New York: Springer-Verlag.

Heckman, J. J. (1979) Sample selection bias as a specification error. *Econometrica* 47:153-162.

Heckman, J. J., and Robb, R. (1985a) Alternative methods for evaluating the impact of interventions: An overview. *Journal of Econometrics* 30:239-267.

Heckman, J. J., and Robb, R. (1985b) Alternative methods for evaluating the impact of interventions. In J. Heckman and B. Singer, eds., *Longitudinal Analysis of Labor Market Data.* Cambridge: Cambridge University Press.

Heckman, J. J., and Robb, R. (1986a) Alternative methods for solving the problem of selection bias in evaluating the impact of treatments on outcomes. In H. Wainer, ed., *Drawing Inferences from Self-selected Samples.* New York: Springer-Verlag.

Heckman, J. J., and Robb, R. (1986b) Postscript: A rejoinder to Tukey. In H. Wainer, ed., *Drawing Inferences from Self-selected Samples.* New York: Springer-Verlag.

Heckman, J. J., and Hotz, V. J. (1989a) Choosing among alternative nonexperimental methods for estimating the impact of social programs: The case of manpower training. *Journal of the American Statistical Association* 84:862-874.

Heckman, J. J., and Hotz, V. J. (1989b) Rejoinder. *Journal of the American Statistical Association* 84:878-880.

Hennigan, K. M., Del Rosario, M. L., Heath, L., Cook, T. D., Wharton, J. D., and Calder, B. J. (1982) Impact of the introduction of television on crime in the United States: Empirical findings and theoretical implications. *Journal of Personality and Social Psychology* 42:461-477.

Hill, A. B. (1971) *Principles of Medical Statistics.* 9th ed. New York: Oxford University Press.

Holland, P. W. (1989) Comment: It's very clear. *Journal of the American Statistical Association* 84:875-877.

Hubbard, R. L., Marsden, M. E., Cavanaugh, E., Rachal, J. V., and Ginzburg, H. M. (1988) Role of drug-abuse treatment in limiting the spread of AIDS. *Reviews of Infectious Diseases* 10:377-384.

Joseph, J. G., Montgomery, S. B., Emmons, C. A., Kessler, R. C., Ostrow, D. G., et al. (1987) Magnitude and determinants of behavioral risk reduction: Longitudinal analysis of a cohort at risk for AIDS. *Psychology and Health* 1:73-95.

Kelly, J. A., St. Lawrence, J. S., Hood, H. V., and Brasfield, T. L. (1989) Behavioral intervention to reduce AIDS risk activities. *Journal of Consulting and Clinical Psychology* 57:60-67.

Kelly, J. A., St. Lawrence, J. S., Stevenson, L. Y., Diaz, Y. E., Hauth, A. C., et al. (1990) Population-wide risk behavior reduction through diffusion of innovation following intervention with natural opinion leaders. Presented at the Sixth International Conference on AIDS, San Francisco, June 23.

LaLonde, R. J. (1986) Evaluating the econometric evaluations of training programs with experimental data. *American Economic Review* 76:604-620.

Lohr, W. (1972) An historical view of the research on the behavioral and organizational factors related to the utilization of health services. Social and Economic Analysis Division, Bureau for Health Services Research and Evaluation, Rockville, Md. January.

Lord, F. M. (1967) A paradox in the interpretation of group comparisons. *Psychological Bulletin* 68:304-305.

Maddala, G. S. (1983) *Limited-Dependent Variable and Qualitative Variables in Econometrics.* Cambridge: Cambridge University Press.

Magidson, J. (1977) Toward a causal model approach for adjusting for preexisting differences in the nonequivalent control group situation. *Evaluation Quarterly* 1:399-420.

Martin, J. L., and Dean, L. (1989) Risk factors for AIDS related bereavement in a cohort of homosexual men in New York City. In B. Cooper and T. Helgason, eds., *Epidemiology and the Prevention of Mental Disorders.* London: Routledge & Kegan Paul.

Maxwell, S. E., and Delany, H. D. (1990) *Designing Experiments and Analyzing Data.* Belmont, Calif.: Wadsworth Publishing.

McCusker, J., Stoddard, A. M., Mayer, K. H., Zapka, J., Morrison, C., and Saltzman, S. P. (1988) Effects of HIV antibody test knowledge on subsequent sexual behaviors in a cohort of homosexually active men. *American Journal of Public Health* 78:462-467.

McGlothlin, W. H., and Anglin, M. D. (1981) Shutting off methadone. *Archives of General Psychiatry* 38:885-892.

McKay, H., McKay, A., and Sinisterra, L. (1973) *Stimulation of Intellectual and Social Competence in Colombian Preschool-Age Children Affected by the Multiple Deprivations of Depressed Urban Environments.* Second Progress Report. Cali, Colombia: Human Ecology Research Station, Universidad del Valle. September.

McKusick, L., Horstman, W., and Coates, T. J. (1985) AIDS and sexual behavior reported by gay men in San Francisco. *American Journal of Public Health* 75:493-496.

Miller, H. G., Turner, C. F., and Moses, L. E. (1990) *AIDS: The Second Decade.* Report of the NRC Committee on AIDS Research and the Behavioral, Social, and Statistical Sciences. Washington, D.C.: National Academy Press.

Moffitt, R. A. (1989) Comment. *Journal of the American Statistical Association* 84:877-880.

Moffitt, R. A. (1990) Applying Heckman methods for program evaluation to CDC AIDS prevention programs. Presented at the NRC Conference on Nonexperimental Approaches to Evaluating AIDS Prevention Programs, Washington, D.C., January 12-13.

Mood, A. M. (1950) *Introduction to the Theory of Statistics.* New York: McGraw-Hill.

Nelson, K. E., Vlahov, D., Margolick, J., and Bernal, M. (1989) Blood and plasma donations among a cohort of IV drug users. Presented at the Fifth International Conference on AIDS, Montreal, June 4-9.

Riecken, H. W., and Boruch, R. F., eds. (1974) *Social Experimentation: A Method for Planning and Evaluating Social Intervention.* Report of a Committee of the Social Science Research Council. New York: Academic Press.

Silverman, W. A. (1977) The lesson of retrolental fibroplasia. *Scientific American* 236(6):100-107.

Smith, H. S. (1957) Interpretation of adjusted treatment means and regressions in analysis of covariance. *Biometrics* 13:282-308.

Transportation Research Board (1984) *55: A Decade of Experience.* Special Report 204 of the NRC Committee for the Study of the Benefits and Costs of the 55 MPH National Maximum Speed Limit. Washington, D.C.: National Academy Press.

Tukey, J. W. (1986a) Comments. In H. Wainer, ed., *Drawing Inferences from Self-selected Samples.* New York: Springer-Verlag.

Tukey, J. W. (1986b) Discussion 4: Mixture modeling versus selection modeling with nonignorable nonresponse. In H. Wainer, ed., *Drawing Inferences from Self-selected Samples.* New York: Springer-Verlag.

Turner, C. F. and Martin, E. (1984) *Surveying Subjective Phenomena.* Two volumes. New York: Russell Sage.

Turner, C. F., Miller, H. G., and Moses, L. E., eds. (1989) *AIDS, Sexual Behavior, and Intravenous Drug Use.* Report of the NRC Committee on AIDS Research and the Behavioral, Social, and Statistical Sciences. Washington, D.C.: National Academy Press.

Valdiserri, R. O., Lyter, D. W., Leviton, L. C., Callahan, C. M., Kingsley, L. A., and Rinaldo, C. R. (1989) AIDS prevention in homosexual and bisexual men: Results of a randomized trial evaluating two risk reduction interventions. *AIDS* 3:21-26.

Wilder, C. S. (1972) *Physician Visits, Volume and Interval Since Last Visit, United States-1969.* Vital and Health Statistics, Series 10, No. 75. Rockville, Md.: National Center for Health Statistics.

Winkelstein, W., Samuel, M., Padian, N. S., Wiley, J.A., Lang, W., Anderson, R. E., and Levy, J. A. (1987) The San Francisco Men's Health Study. III. Reduction in human immunodeficiency virus transmission among homosexual/bisexual men, 1982-86. *American Journal of Public Health* 77:685-689.

Ziffer, A., and Ziffer, J. (1989) The need for psychosocial emphasis in academic courses on AIDS. Presented at the Fifth International Conference on AIDS, Montreal, June 4-9.

Appendixes

A

Collaborative Contracting Strategy

In this report, the panel has recommended rigorous evaluation strategies for assessing the projects of community-based organizations (CBOs) and counseling and testing sites. In making these recommendations, we have also noted that some projects may be unable or unwilling to participate in evaluation research because they do not have the funding, time, or appropriately trained personnel to undertake the necessary tasks. In this appendix, the panel lays out a possible strategy that would ensure projects of the necessary resources to conduct evaluation research and that would also lead to separate but mutually informing communities of evaluation experts.

The proposed tactic for evaluating projects located in CBOs and in counseling and testing sites is to use a contract bidding procedure rather than the request-for-proposal process. The contract to be bid on would describe the following:

- demographic characteristics of the target population;
- the scope of the program;
- endpoint objectives—behavioral, psychological, or biological;
- program content objectives;
- policy objectives;
- evaluation objectives for formative and process evaluations and for evaluating whether the project makes a difference and what works better; and
- evaluation methods.

A prospective contractor, in collaboration with a competent evaluation group, would explain in detail its approach to designing a program to meet the contract requirements. The prospective contractor would bid on the contract, relating the bid to program design and to the contract requirement. The evaluation procedure, responsibilities, and budget would be predetermined and included as a contract requirement. The evaluation processes, including random assignment, monitoring, and data collection and analyses, would be dictated primarily by the scope of the program and by whether outcomes are to be assessed internally (as the responsibility of the contractor) or externally (as the responsibility of an outside evaluator to analyze multiple CBO contractors).

The contracting option also engenders further choices. Among these is deciding whether to develop separate contractual arrangements with each project that agrees to evaluation or to develop a single large contract to cover the evaluation of a sample of sites. Developing separate contractual arrangements may involve an independent evaluation team submitting evaluation proposals that show how the CBO would collaborate with such a team and how the evaluation would be carried out. The independence of the evaluation team is justified on grounds of credibility and scientific integrity; however, the collaboration with the CBO is essential.

For CDC to contract separately with six to eight CBO-evaluator groups would be feasible but managerially burdensome. Nevertheless, the strategy arguably is sensible on scientific grounds. In effect, over the long run the approach builds separate but mutually informing communities of experts. The current dependence of AIDS research on only a few universities and research institutes is often sound strategy for massive evaluation but does little to develop local capacity for routinely and locally generated high-quality evaluation. Local evaluative capacity avoids dependence on a single principal investigator who makes decisions about the evaluation of a range of complex projects. Campbell (1987:402) argues that splitting large studies into two or more parallel studies is desirable on grounds that it increases the "size and autonomy of a mutually monitoring scientific community." The latter is essential in building scientific understanding in prevention program research and evaluation.

Contracting with one evaluation group that collaborates with, perhaps, six to eight sites is also feasible, to judge from work by Hubbard and colleagues (1988), among others. This approach is managerially less burdensome than contracting independently with evaluator-project combinations, but has the disadvantages of being vulnerable to the will of a single decision maker (i.e., the principal investigator) and of not building local expertise in the design, implementation, and analysis of what works or what works better.

REFERENCES

Campbell, D. (1987) Guidelines for monitoring the scientific competence of preventive intervention research centers: An exercise in the sociology of scientific validity. *Knowledge: Creation, Diffusion, Utilization* 8:389-430.

Hubbard, R. L., Marsden, M. E., Cavanaugh, E., Rachal, J. V., and Ginzburg, H. M. (1988) Role of drug-abuse treatment in limiting the spread of AIDS. *Reviews of Infectious Diseases* 10:377-384.

B

Oversight and Coordination Strategy

In this appendix, the panel outlines a strategy for overseeing and conducting independent multisite experiments to compare different approaches to reducing the risk of HIV transmission. The strategy described here is illustrated by the cooperative endeavor of six community-based organization (CBO) projects, but it is also relevant for evaluations of the media campaign and the counseling and testing program. We believe that coordinated results from the individual sites, and especially the cross-site results, can lead to the development of sound health education and risk reduction policy.

In the strategy, projects are selected on the basis of their capacity and willingness to engage in randomized tests of two or three interventions that promise better results relative to standard interventions. Each experiment is directed by a different principal investigator and involves CBO practitioners and an independent evaluation group.

As in most community-based endeavors, it is expected that the organization and style of operation of each project will vary despite common goals, as will the character of the local cooperation between the project team and the independent evaluation group. The CBOs and their evaluation associates will vary considerably in experience and in their skill in executing high-quality experiments. The results themselves will vary, and integrating the findings across sites, in the interest of developing health education and risk reduction policy, will then be complex. Given the limited resources available for oversight, the panel suggests a project review team to facilitate the generation of high-quality evidence that is useful both locally and at the aggregate level for determining what works better.

Compared with a conventional advisory board approach, a project review team involves a far deeper commitment and involvement. While this level of involvement and commitment demands more of an oversight body, the panel believes that the potential benefits of such an approach more than justify its use.

THE PROJECT REVIEW TEAM

Three major missions seem appropriate and feasible for the project review team:

- overseeing the progress of each project's evaluation experiments;
- conducting periodic, confirmatory reanalysis of the evaluative data produced by the project experiments; and
- undertaking cross-site analyses of all project evaluations.

The first mission, oversight, is a common function for most advisory boards and is basic to the quality control of projects. For AIDS-related work, however, this oversight must be deeper and more extensive than is customary for advisory boards because the CBOs are engaged in difficult missions that are complicated further by the agreement to cooperate in controlled field tests.

The second mission, periodic confirmatory reanalysis of evaluation data, is not a common function of advisory boards. Following the model used in projects currently sponsored by the National Institute of Justice (NIJ), the team will receive evaluation data and analyses from each site and then conduct reanalyses of those data to confirm the site's original work. Conducted quarterly in the NIJ-sponsored projects, these confirmatory reanalyses have led to improvements in the timeliness of site data production, the quality of site data production systems, the quality of data, and the collective understanding of the operations of the projects (see NIJ, 1989). Use of the project review team approach in AIDS evaluation efforts should offer the same benefits.

The team's third mission, which can be undertaken only after each project evaluation is completed, is to produce cross-site analyses and recommendations that go beyond single-site considerations of experimental results. The product of this aspect of the team's work is an understanding of the variability in project effectiveness—e.g., why projects A, B, and C produced positive effects at various levels while projects D and E produced no detectable effects—and of the policy options suggested by the collective results of the several experiments.

The team might also be responsible for screening the proposals for evaluation submitted by each site. Using the team to both select and oversee the evaluations enhances the continuity of the evaluation process and the uniformity of evaluation designs across sites.

Given these responsibilities, it seems wise to constitute the project review team as a group of five or six experts in various aspects of designing and executing randomized experiments in community-based contexts. The skills required would include those common to experts in the areas of statistics, evaluation, methodology, CBO operations, and public health. Beyond these requirements, membership should be tailored to the special audiences of the projects (e.g., adolescents, women at risk, IV drug users). To centralize team activities, we suggest that one member of the team be directly responsible for a small support group based at a university or research entity that will run the individual site and cross-site analyses.

OPERATIONS

As a practical matter, carrying out the oversight functions will require considerable effort by a number of actors: CBO staffs, the principal investigators responsible for the evaluation experiment at each site, the project review team, and at least one senior CDC staff person with research or evaluation expertise. First, quarterly meetings of the team, the CBO staffs, principal investigators, and the CDC representative are essential to understanding projects and the evaluation experiments. The format of the meetings can be designed to cover sequentially the major problems that are usually encountered in controlled field experiments and the options for their solution. The meetings can also be used to discuss pre-experiment studies, resolve problems in data collection or random assignment that appear during the course of the experiment, and address other issues of concern. The development of an invisible "college" composed of all these actors is part of the potential product of these quarterly meetings. In addition, a quarterly meeting can serve as the venue for presenting evaluative data and analyses produced by personnel at each site. A representative from each site must provide the project review team with updated data files at each meeting to permit the team's subsequent confirmatory reanalyses.

The second team activity relevant to its mission involves repeated site visits to the CBOs participating in the evaluation project. The objective for each visit is to understand local operations, conditions, and problems, and to identify and discuss options (not recommendations) for resolving these problems. The team then reports on these aspects of the projects to CDC.

The site visit reports and the sites' progress reports and provision of data at each quarterly meeting form the basis for the third team activity, reporting to and advising CDC. Such advice includes whether each project's performance justifies another year of funding. The fourth activity is the quarterly reanalysis of data produced by each site. This activity is carried out by a group based in a university or other research environment that is organized to produce the reanalyses and provide them to the project review team. The fifth and final activity is the analysis of data across sites and the production of a report for CDC. This activity can be undertaken using the university-based or research unit-based reanalysis team working under the direction of the team, in combination with the team members' independent work.

The specific products of the project review team process described above are the following:

- reports to CDC on the progress of project evaluations;
- verification or disconfirmation of project evaluations conducted by the sites and reported to CDC;
- advice to CDC on individual project performance and justification and on continuance of each evaluation; and
- cross-site analyses for policy decisions.

The result of a team approach is better evaluative data, more knowledgeable projects, and a greater understanding of what makes a difference and what works better to reduce high-risk behavior.

The discussion above describes the project review team approach for the health education/risk reduction projects of a selected set of CBOs. Yet the approach is also relevant to overseeing and coordinating selected counseling and testing projects and projects supported in the media campaign.

For example, a small number of counseling and testing sites could be invited to participate in comparative experimental tests of new methods for encouraging individuals to return for their test results. The new methods might involve different forms of pretest counseling or more time allotted to such counseling. In agreeing to try out the new approaches, the sites would also agree to randomly assign individuals to the new method and to the standard approach and to cooperate in the multisite evaluation and related activities.

Financial support would be provided to each site for implementing the new approach alongside the standard method and for participating in the cooperative evaluations. Support would also be provided to the local evaluation group with which each site collaborates in implementing the experiment. Finally, support would also be provided to the PRT for project selection, oversight, confirmatory analyses, and so forth.

In the case of counseling and testing sites, as with health education/risk reduction projects, one of the objects is mutual education about implementing the new counseling regimens and executing high-quality randomized tests. Insofar as the project review team activity is intensive, it can offer effective oversight, provide options for resolving problems, and confirm the data analyses produced by each site. The team's cross-site analyses would be dedicated to providing evidence on what works better and addressing policy implications for CDC's consideration in administering the counseling and testing program and developing new initiatives.

For media projects, an evaluation might randomly assign half of a group of communities to a new regimen (set of ads or other materials) or to a control condition, thus creating two groups of communities that do not differ systematically except for the presence of the new regimen in half the group. However, if each community is independently responsible for implementing the regimen and for the collection of evaluation data, an oversight and coordinating body will be essential to producing interpretable results. Here again, the project review team is likely to be a useful option and a more valuable approach than an advisory board, especially if the projects are independent members of a loosely organized cooperative group.

SUMMARY AND DISCUSSION

The project review team approach to evaluation project coordination and oversight is relevant to conducting independent multisite experiments to compare different approaches to reducing the risk of HIV transmission. The team approach, as well as the multisite cooperative endeavor, is innovative in the social sciences, but there are some precedents (see Boruch et al., 1989) and in the medical clinical trials arena (see *Controlled Clinical Trials*).

A distinctive feature and advantage of the team approach is routine periodic reanalysis of data produced by each cooperating site. Although not commonly used in the social and behavioral sciences, the idea comports well with contemporary scientific practice in two respects. First, the feature can be regarded as a data sharing activity because it invites access to the data by a number of scientists beyond the original principal investigators and also allows access among the cooperating sites and the CDC. This kind of data sharing is encouraged by, among others, the National Research Council's Committee on National Statistics (Fienberg, Martin, and Straf, 1985). Given that mistakes and corruption of data may be far more severe a problem in controversial research areas, the purpose of data sharing in this kind of effort is to reduce the likelihood of mistakes in complex data analysis and decrease even further the low likelihood of fraud.

Data sharing may also enhance the usefulness of a scarce resource— in this case, high-quality data on what works better to reduce HIV transmission. The repeated use of the same data set in the interests of confirming the quality of data and analyses and testing new hypotheses is an economic justification for the activity.

A second distinctive feature is that the project review team approach facilitates the coordination of independent project staff and evaluators. Such coordination provides opportunities for the development of local expertise in conducting controlled experiments, an expertise that will, in the long run, enhance local and societal understanding of how to generate sound evidence about what interventions work. An alternative approach—a contract with a single large organization that is employed to develop cooperation and run the experiments locally—generally leads to less local learning (Boruch, Dennis, and Carter-Greer, 1988), although quality control is more certain. Another advantage of the single-contract approach is that the sponsor (CDC) contracts with only one group responsible for executing all experiments in the sites, rather than developing a number of separate contracts with each site that has the capability and willingness to conduct experiments and with the group (i.e., university or research organization) responsible for support of the project review team.

Finally, the team approach is arguably better than conventional advisory boards for coordination and oversight of AIDS prevention project evaluation. The involvement of team members is more extensive and more sustained than is common for advisory board members, leading to a higher quality product. The involvement is such that a "college" of practitioners and researchers develops as a consequence of interactions among various actors, which can lead to more and better mutual education. The team's constitution as, essentially, a blue-ribbon panel, in addition to its level of activity, is likely to lead to high-quality data, especially when coupled with the routine confirmatory reanalyses of site evaluative data. Finally, cross-site analyses are complex enough that conventional advisory boards cannot handle the work; a project review team is designed to handle it well in the interest of providing a timely, policy-relevant product to the sponsoring agency.

REFERENCES

Boruch, R. F., Reiss, A., Garner, J., and Larntz, K. (1989) Coordinating the Spouse Assault Replication Projects: The Project Review Team. Unpublished report. Northwestern University.

Boruch, R. F., Dennis, M., and Carter-Greer, K. (1988) Lessons from the Rockefeller Foundations experiments on the minority female single parent program. *Evaluation Review* 12(4):396-426.

Fienberg, S. E., Martin, M. E., and Straf, M. L., eds. (1985) *Sharing Research Data.* Report of the NRC Committee on National Statistics. Washington, D.C.: National Academy Press.

National Institute of Justice (NIJ) (1989) *Spouse Assault Replication Project Review Team.* Washington, D.C.: U.S. Department of Justice.

C

Methodological Issues in AIDS Surveys

To supplement our discussion of evaluation measurement in Chapter 2, this appendix presents an excerpt on measurement issues in AIDS research from AIDS, The Second Decade *(Miller, Turner, and Moses, 1990:359-471). Readers may also wish to consult the discussion of sampling and related issues in the prior report,* AIDS, Sexual Behavior, and Intravenous Drug Use *(Turner, Miller, and Moses, 1989:147-157, 214-225).*

INTRODUCTION

Surveys or, more generally, the method of asking questions and recording answers, continue to be one of the most important methods for obtaining essential information about the epidemiology of AIDS and HIV, the behaviors that spread HIV, and the effectiveness of AIDS prevention efforts. Previous reports of our committee have included numerous examples of surveys and observations about the methodological difficulties that often attend these measurements.

Because of the central role surveys play in research on AIDS and HIV, this appendix focuses on methodological aspects of this data-gathering method that have important consequences for the usefulness of survey data. This appendix contains much technical material and methodological detail. Our aim in presenting this material is to provide researchers conducting AIDS surveys or analyzing data collected in such surveys with a detailed review of the current state of methodological research in this area. Readers who seek only a synopsis of our conclusions and recommendations may wish to consult pages 27–34 of the summary chapter of the report *AIDS: The Second Decade* (Miller, Turner, and Moses, 1990).

Before turning to specifics, it may be useful to consider data gathering in general and the types of problems that may compromise the collection of accurate and informative data. One may usefully distinguish five aspects of survey data collection: (1) the *definition* of the population to be studied and the drawing of a target sample from that population; (2) the *execution* of the sample design, that is, finding the persons in the target sample and enlisting their cooperation in the survey; (3) the *posing of questions* to elicit the desired information; (4) the *answering of those questions* by the respondent; and (5) the *recording of those answers* (and subsequent data processing and analysis).

To examine these elements, let us consider a hypothetical survey (much like the decennial census) that targeted all households in a particular jurisdiction of the state of Texas. Let us suppose further that the information to be obtained concerned automobile ownership (e.g., how many automobiles were owned by each household, the make and year of the autos, etc.). This survey, although not simple to conduct, would nevertheless be considerably less difficult to conduct than a survey seeking to assess behaviors that transmit HIV; in particular,

- the survey involves matters of fact that are both open to direct observation and matters of public record (e.g., make and year of automobiles owned by household);
- the topic is unlikely to be regarded as sensitive or "private" by respondents, although—as in any survey—some respondents may not wish to take the time to respond;
- developing questions about this topic can draw on a widely shared vocabulary (i.e., there is little ambiguity about what constitutes a "car" or "ownership");
- respondents who are not well informed can consult with other household members or check records (e.g., registration certificates);
- checks of survey accuracy can be made at the group level (by comparing the rates of auto ownership found in the survey and in registration records) and at the individual level (by checking individual registrations[1]); and
- census data on income and statewide auto registration data are available to target the survey efficiently toward segments of the population of particular interest (e.g., current or "potential" owners of Belchfire 500s).

---

[1] The survey may, however, produce detailed information that cannot be verified from public records—for example, the proportion of Belchfire 500s owned by persons with 16+ years of education.

Surveys that inquire about sexual behaviors or IV drug use differ in several ways from the foregoing example, and these differences provide a much greater challenge to the survey (or question-and-answer) method. First, many of the logical "target populations" for drug use and sexual behavior surveys cannot be identified reliably from official statistics. There are few reliable data on the distribution across the nation of persons who engage in behaviors that risk HIV transmission. Furthermore, the behaviors in question occur in private and cannot be verified by direct observation or public records. Many of the behaviors are actively concealed because they are considered illicit (IV drug use is illegal throughout the nation, and many sexual behaviors of interest in preventing HIV transmission are illegal in some states). Thus, the topics these surveys cover are likely to be highly sensitive, which may create difficulties in enlisting the cooperation of persons in a target sample and in obtaining permission from "gatekeepers" (e.g., high school authorities) who control access to particular populations (e.g., high school students).

This appendix considers these problems and reviews the available empirical evidence gathered from surveys of sexual and drug use behaviors. Before beginning this review, however, some cautionary words are in order. The evidence presented here regarding errors in data about sensitive behaviors might lead some readers to unwarranted and wholesale rejection of survey findings on these important topics.[2] Indeed, considering the litany of difficulties presented in this appendix, some readers may ask whether anything at all can be learned from surveys or whether surveys have a useful role to play in research on AIDS and HIV transmission. The following considerations prompt the committee to answer "yes" to these questions.

The most important consideration arises directly from the nature of the disease. HIV infection occurs through the joint operation of the biology of this particular infectious virus and the human behaviors that transmit it. In the absence of vaccines, *all* interventions that seek to retard the spread of HIV infection focus on changing human behaviors to diminish the probability that the virus will be transmitted. Data on these behaviors are needed for a number of important purposes—for example, to understand the factors that motivate and shape the behaviors and to determine whether behaviors that transmit HIV are becoming less frequent in the population.

It might, of course, be argued that merely monitoring changes in the prevalence of HIV would be sufficient to determine whether behavioral

---

[2] The following pages borrow heavily from the discussion of errors in survey measurements in Turner and Martin (1984:Vol. 1, 14–16) and Turner (1989).

change was occurring. Although this argument is true to some extent, there are important deficiencies in any strategy that eschews direct measurement of the behaviors themselves. Reliable data on HIV prevalence and incidence, although of great value for many purposes, are only a final accounting of the number of infected and uninfected persons in the population. From the viewpoint of prevention, such statistics serve best as a catalog of failures. Yet, those who are uninfected are not necessarily successes. For example, the very low rate of HIV infection in states like Wyoming does not necessarily imply that the population has adopted protective behaviors. Instead, the low rate of HIV prevalence could be attributable to an epidemiological happenstance (e.g., isolation—in terms of sexual contacts and injection equipment sharing—from populations with high HIV prevalence.)

Determining whether protective behavioral changes have occurred (in Wyoming or anywhere else) requires asking questions about these risky behaviors. This activity, in turn, raises a host of methodological issues that are germane to survey research of all types plus some questions that are specific to surveys of drug use and sexual behavior. The questions may be quite basic: Are the respondents telling the truth? Do they understand the meaning of the survey questions in the same way the investigator does? Simple or complex, such questions inevitably introduce a degree of uncertainty into the interpretation of all survey data. Grappling with these issues forces an appreciation of the human interactions that produce survey measurements.

Elsewhere it has been argued that fundamental aspects of the survey process

> are quintessentially social psychological in character. They arise from a complex interpersonal exchange, they embody the subjectivities of both interviewer and interviewee, and they present their interpreter with an analytical challenge that requires a multitude of assumptions concerning, among other things, how respondents experience the reality of the interview situation, decode the "meaning" of survey questions, and respond to the social presence of the interviewer and the demand characteristics of the interview. (Turner, 1984:202)

Although this "analytical challenge" may be substantial, researchers are aided in their task by several decades of methodological research (see, for example, Sudman and Bradburn [1974], Bradburn and Sudman [1979], Rossi, Wright, and Anderson [1983], Turner and Martin [1984], and Catania et al. [1990a,b]). A further reason for not abandoning behavioral measurement is that many of the problems encountered in this arena are not unique. Useful lessons may thus be learned from other disciplines that also confront such challenges.

Fallibility of Measurement in Other Sciences

Fallibility and error are not confined to behavioral measurements, as evidenced by the decade-long controversy surrounding the population statistics produced by the decennial censuses.[3] Furthermore, just as fallibility of measurement is not limited to behavioral measurements, neither is it limited to surveys or social statistics. For example, Hunter (1977) and Lide (1981) have noted the variability among measurements of such elementary physical phenomena as the thermal conductivity of copper (Figure C-1). As Hunter observed, "although each analyst measured a physical quality that did not vary with location or time, it is clear that a remarkable variability attended the measurements" (1977:2). He concluded: "The variation in attempting to evaluate the same physical constant is obvious. This example is not unusual. Similar plots of thermal conductivity as a function of temperature for approximately 400 common metals and materials can be found in a supplement to the *Journal* (Ho, Powell, and Liley, 1974). Nor is the observed variation in the measurement of 'thermal conductivity' unique among physical parameters . . . ."

Common biological measurements have shown similar fallibility. Examples include data collected by CDC that show substantial variation in the estimates made by different laboratories of the amount of lead in identical samples of blood. For a sample of blood with a putative lead concentration of 41 milligrams per deciliter (mg/Dl), 100 cooperating laboratories produced measurements that ranged from 33 to 55 mg/Dl; this result prompted the reviewer to observe: "Clearly, whatever the true amount of lead in a sample, the variability demonstrated [in these measurements] guarantees numerous false alarms or—perhaps more important when the true level is high—nonalarms" (Hunter, 1980:870).

Another category of fallibility in the physical sciences involves "discoveries" that are later shown to be experimental artifacts. For example, between 1963 and 1974 more than 500 journal articles (including some in *Science* and *Nature*) discussed a supposed new substance: anomalous water, or polywater. Although it resembled ordinary water, polywater allegedly had a greater density, a reduced freezing point, and an elevated boiling point, among other anomalous properties. In the end, however, it was discovered that this "new substance" was nothing more than an impure solution of ordinary water (Franks, 1981; Eisenberg, 1981).

---

[3]By October 1981, more than 50 lawsuits had been filed challenging the accuracy of the 1980 Census results and their use in legislative apportionment and fund allocation decisions (Citro and Cohen, 1985:9).

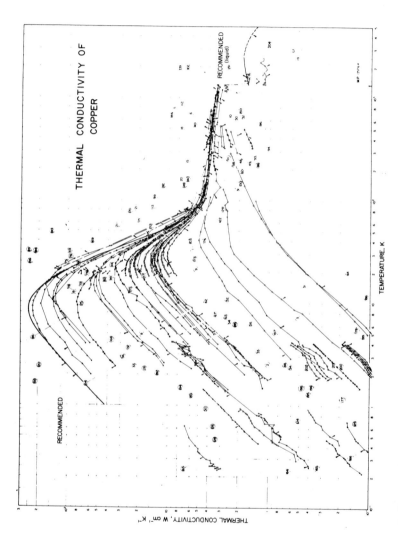

FIGURE C-1 Display of all reported measurements of the thermal conductivity of copper as a function of temperature (reported by Ho, Powell, and Liley, 1974). NOTE: Each set of connected points corresponds to the data given in a single literature source. The recommended curve is based on an evaluation by Ho, Powell, and Liley (1974). SOURCE: Lide (1981).

Such examples indicate that the problems AIDS researchers confront when they seek to assess sexual and drug-using behavior are not unique in the annals of scientific measurement. As Quinn McNemar observed more than 40 years ago, "[a]ll measurement is befuddled with error. About this the scientist can and does do something; he ascertains the possible extent of the error, determines whether it is constant (biasing) or variable, or both, and ever strives to improve his instruments and techniques" (1946:294).

In the following pages the committee reviews what is currently known about the errors that afflict measures of sexual and drug-using behavior and offers some prescriptions for how future measurements might be improved. The first section of the appendix reviews the experience to date in mounting surveys and obtaining responses from the public. The second section considers the reliability and validity of responses obtained in surveys of sexual and drug use behaviors. The final section reviews the use of anthropological research strategies that may provide important complementary information to that obtained in surveys and that may also be crucial in questionnaire development to improve the accuracy and completeness of responses.

RECRUITMENT OF RESPONDENTS IN
SEX AND SEROPREVALENCE SURVEYS

Much of what is now known about the epidemiology of AIDS has come from small-scale, local studies among subgroups thought to be at high risk for infection. Participants in these studies were recruited through various sources and means—from the clientele of local clinics or treatment facilities or the membership rosters of local organizations, through newspaper advertisements and physician referrals, and occasionally from "street sampling." The yield from this research has been remarkably rich. From these studies, researchers have identified the principal mechanisms of HIV infection (i.e., transmission through sexual contact, sharing injection equipment in IV drug use, transfusion of contaminated blood products); verified sexual transmission of HIV from male to male, female to male, and male to female; measured the efficiency of transmission in specific kinds of sexual contacts; and discovered some of the basic features of the long natural history of this devastating disease. As valuable as these studies are, however, the data drawn from them cannot address many other important public health questions that arise because of AIDS, such as: How large is the epidemic? What is the potential for general spread of HIV infection? Can an HIV epidemic be sustained through heterosexual contact alone? To answer questions like these, the knowledge gained from measurements and observations carried out in local studies of special subgroups must be applied in large-scale investigations of populations chosen not because of convenient or ready access but because of their importance in understanding the general course of the epidemic.

This section considers the feasibility of sex and seroprevalence surveys as a means of measuring the distribution of sexual behaviors that risk HIV transmission and the distribution of HIV itself in general populations. Although such surveys may be designed in a variety of ways, all of the studies discussed here employ the same general procedures for participant selection: an unambiguous definition of the population to be studied and a form of sampling from this population that allows the probabilities of selection to be known. The potential advantages of a probability sampling program for selecting survey participants are well known. In principle, probability sampling permits the use of a large body of statistical theory to make inferences from the sample to the larger population and avoids the possible biases inherent in recruitment by other means.

The suggestion to use probability sampling for surveys of sexual behavior was made more than three decades ago in connection with a review of the statistical methods used in Kinsey, Pomeroy, and Martin's *Sexual Behavior in the Human Male* (1948) (Cochran, Mosteller, and Tukey, 1953). The authors of this suggestion were a committee of the Commission on Statistical Standards of the American Statistical Association. At the invitation of Dr. Kinsey and the National Research Council's Committee for Research on Problems of Sex, they were asked to provide counsel on ways to improve the statistical methods used in the Kinsey research. They recommended a step-by-step program of probability sampling, beginning with a small pilot effort. They argued that research of this kind would provide a check on the results obtained with Kinsey's large, nonprobability sample. The committee was aware that problems of cost and potentially high rates of nonparticipation in such surveys would present special challenges. Their comments about the limits of this approach are worth quoting at length because the issues they raised more than 30 years ago in relation to Kinsey's work remain germane in evaluating the potential value of contemporary surveys of sexual behavior.

> In our opinion, no sex study of a broad human population can expect to present incidence data for reported behavior that are known to be correct to within a few percentage points. Even with the best available sampling techniques, there will be a certain percentage of the population who refuse to give histories. If the percentage of refusals is 10 percent or more, then however large the sample, there are no statistical principles which guarantee

that the results are correct to within 2 or 3 percent, . . . but any claim that this is true must be based on the undocumented opinion that the behavior of those who refuse to be interviewed is not very different from that of those who are interviewed. These comments, which are not a criticism of [Kinsey, Pomeroy, and Martin's] research, emphasize the difficulty of answering the question: "How accurate are the results?", which is naturally of great interest to any user of the results of a sex study. (Cochran, Mosteller, and Tukey, 1953:675)

The rationale for using response rates as a "yardstick" to assess the accuracy of survey estimates is twofold: (1) high response rates reduce the influence of selective participation in surveys and hence the potential for bias in the estimates, and (2) for a given target sample size and sample design, the higher the response rate, the larger the actual sample and the smaller the standard error of estimate. In other words, high response rates are better than low rates, provided the procedures used to achieve high response rates do not increase the degree of selectivity or inaccuracy of the responses.

Few contemporary surveys on any topic achieve response rates higher than the 90 percent figure cited in Cochran, Mosteller, and Tukey's review of the Kinsey report; indeed, response rates in most surveys are considerably below that mark. In principle, then, questions about selective participation (i.e., about differences between respondents and nonrespondents) are of concern in judging the accuracy of most survey estimates, not only those that derive from surveys of sexual behavior. Such concerns have generated a substantial literature on the character of nonresponse in surveys and what to do about possibly biased estimation resulting from nonresponse (see, for example, Goyder's 1987 synthesis of nonresponse research and the series of volumes on incomplete data in sample surveys edited by Madow, Nisselson, and Olkin [1983]).

Surveys with response rates that are much lower than 90 percent may still provide useful estimates of population characteristics if it can be established that participation or nonparticipation is unrelated to the characteristic for which an estimate is sought. Furthermore, response rates higher than 90 percent do not guarantee accurate estimation if survey participation is highly selective. Thus, in most cases, the value of the response rate by itself is insufficient justification for claims of accuracy or "representativeness" of survey estimates or for counterclaims that estimates fail in this respect. Such claims should be based on careful study, documentation, and possibly adjustment for bias as a result of refusals and other sources of nonresponse.

In the following review, the committee examines recent efforts to survey sexual behavior and related HIV risk factors that use probability samples from general populations. The review focuses on participation in such surveys and is motivated by the same concerns about nonresponse in probability samples that were expressed in the review of the Kinsey report. It attempts to answer three main questions: (1) What response rates have been achieved in recent surveys of sexual behavior? (2) What survey designs and procedures appear to be associated with higher versus lower levels of participation? and (3) What can be said, at present, about differences between sample persons who participate in sex surveys and sample persons who refuse to participate or do not participate for other reasons? (There is as yet too little information to hazard general statements about differences between participants and nonparticipants in seroprevalence surveys.) Questions about the validity and reliability of survey responses about sexual behavior, which were also noted in reviews of the Kinsey report, will be discussed in the later sections in this appendix.

Scope of the Review

The committee chose 15 surveys for its review, including some that are national in scope and some that target local populations. Most of these studies were initiated after the AIDS epidemic began in response to the need for population-based estimates of sexual behaviors known to be associated with HIV transmission. Both telephone and face-to-face interviewing methods are represented, along with data collection through self-administered questionnaires. There are wide variations among the surveys in the proportion of questions they devote to measuring sexual practices and other risk behaviors. Four surveys were included because of their potential importance for monitoring the prevalence of HIV infection; these surveys attempted to collect a blood specimen for HIV serologic testing from each sample person.

The committee used four criteria for including studies in its review: (1) there was at least a minimal attempt to collect data on personal sexual behavior and, in some cases, other HIV risk factors as well; (2) some form of probability sampling was employed; (3) a response rate of the form (number of survey participants)/(number of sample persons) could be calculated; and (4) enough documentation was available to identify the principal characteristics of the survey design and sampling procedures. Information about the designs, sampling procedures, and participation rates of these surveys appears in Table C-1.

For the most part, the committee collected information about these surveys from published accounts in books, journal articles, and survey field reports. (The source documents are cited in Table C-1.) Occasionally, it was necessary to rely on conversations with survey field managers, especially for surveys that had been completed at the time of this writing. In several other cases, documentation is partial because of incomplete reporting or recordkeeping, or both. For these reasons, and because the total number of surveys is small, the committee has not attempted a statistical analysis of participation rates in relation to survey characteristics. Nevertheless, the review does identify differences in response rates in sex surveys that appear to be associated with procedural and design variations. It also reveals several opportunities for learning more about patterns of participation and nonparticipation.

Participation in Sex Surveys

Data Collection Procedures and Response Rates
Each of the surveys listed in Table C-1 asked respondents to report on certain aspects of their past and present sexual behavior. For the most part, the questions used in recent surveys (i.e., those initiated after the AIDS epidemic began) attempt to measure the occurrence of sexual behaviors associated with HIV infection and transmission and fall into three general categories: sexual orientation (with a focus on homosexuality), selection of sexual partners (number and characteristics of partners, presence of same-sex partnerships), and manner of sexual intercourse (e.g., anal, vaginal, oral). Because of the sensitive and highly personal nature of these questions, virtually all of the surveys made some provision to permit respondents to reveal the details of their sexual behavior without undue embarrassment or fear of disclosure to third parties. Most of the surveys included one or more of the following: special guarantees that responses would be kept confidential; assurance of anonymity—that is, that the person viewing the results would not know the identity of the respondent; privacy during the interview; and placement of the sensitive questions near the end of the interview.

Apart from these similarities, the 15 surveys differ widely with respect to basic methods of data collection and number of questions about sexual behavior. Interviewing was conducted by telephone in four of the surveys (nos. 3, 4, 9, and 10 in Table C-1), by face-to-face interview in five cases (nos. 7, 8, 12, 13, and 14), and by a combination of face-to-face interview and self-administered questionnaire (SAQ) in six (nos. 1, 2, 5, 6, 11, and 15). Virtually all of the surveys that contained long, detailed inventories of sexual questions were conducted through face-to-face or telephone interviews. When SAQs were used, the length of the self-administered forms varied considerably (some did not exceed 1 or 2 pages whereas others [e.g., survey no. 1] were more than 10 pages long).

TABLE C-1 Methods and Execution of Sampling Designs in Recent Surveys of Sexual Behavior and HIV Seroprevalence

Survey	Dates of Fieldwork	Target Population	Sampling Methods	No. of Completed Interviews	Data Collection Methods		Participation Rates	Checks for Nonresponse Bias (in reference document)	Probable Non-Response Bias
					Non-HIV risk items	HIV risk items			
General Population Surveys									
1. Kinsey/ NORC survey	Late in 1970	U.S. residents aged 21+	Multistaged probability sample to block or segment (quotas at person level); interviewed one eligible person per household	3,018	Face-to-face interview in household	SAQ with sealed envelope	None can be calculated; 15% nonresponse on homosexual item among male respondents	Census comparisons; comparisons with 1988 GSS estimates	Probable underrepresentation of "difficult respondents" owing to refusals and lack of callbacks; underrepresentation of older men and black men
2. Danish Institute for Clinical Epidemiology	Feb. to June 1987	Danish men aged 16-55	Random sample from Danish population register (list sample)	1,155	Face-to-face interview in household	SAQ and respondent mailback	Interview RR = 78.3%; sex SAQ RR = 54.8%	Compared age distribution of respondents and non-respondents	Possible higher prevalence of HIV risk factors among nonrespondents
3. Los Angeles Times poll	July 1987	U.S. residents aged 18+ living in households with telephones	RDD with oversampling in Los Angeles, New York City, San Francisco, Miami, and Newark	2,095	Telephone interview	Telephone interview	Interview RR = 33%	Census comparisons	Probable underrepresentation of blacks and persons with less than high school diploma
4. Communication Technologies, Inc./ California Dept. of Health Svcs	Oct. to Dec. 1987	California residents aged 18+ living in households with telephones	Two RDD sampling frames; one RSA per household	2,012	Telephone interview	Telephone interview	RR of identified sample not calculable; interview completion rate = 71%	Comparison with state finance department's demographic estimates	Unknown

5. British National Pilot Survey	Oct. to Nov. 1987	English-speaking residents of Britain aged 16–64	Multistaged probability sample; one RSA per household	785	Face-to-face interview in household	SAQ with sealed envelope	Interview SAQ RR = 47.5%	Comparison with British population projections	Probable underrepresentation of men, persons aged 16–24, and ethnic minorities
6. NORC General Social Survey	Feb. to April 1988	U.S. residents aged 18+	Multistaged probability sample of households; one RSA per household	1,481	Face-to-face interview in household	SAQ with sealed envelope	Interview RR = 77.3%; SAQ RR = 72.6%, item nonresponse = 6%	Comparison with census and current population surveys	Matches census and CPS population estimates
7. National Survey of Family Growth	March to Aug. 1988	U.S. residents, women, aged 15–44	Probability sampling based on HIS enumeration lists	8,450	Face-to-face interview in household	Face-to-face interview in household	Interview RR = 79%; sexual behav. item nonresponse = 4%	Information on non-respondents who were interviewed in HIS	Unknown
8. Sexual Behavior of Young People	1963	Unmarried youth aged 15–19 living in seven London districts	Random sample from lists in NHSAO, supplemented by market research	1,873	Face-to-face interview in local office	Face-to-face interview in local office	RR = 66.2%	None	Unknown
9. Communication Technologies, Inc., San Francisco survey	Aug. to Sept. 1987	Self-identified gay/bisexual men in San Francisco, aged 18+, in households with telephones	Commercial sample of names and telephone numbers; interviewed one eligible person in household	500	Telephone screening for eligibility	Telephone interview	None can be calculated	None	Unknown
10. Seattle pilot study	1985–1986	Selected Seattle area residents, aged 18–45, in households with telephones	Samples from telephone and reverse directories, using RDD	389	Telephone interview	Telephone interview	RR = 55.7%	None	Overrepresentation of persons keeping same telephone number and address over time

Continued

TABLE C-1 *Continued*

Survey	Dates of Fieldwork	Target Population	Sampling Methods	No. of Completed Interviews	Data Collection Methods		Participation Rates	Checks for Nonresponse Bias (in reference document)	Probable Non-Response Bias
					Non-HIV risk items	HIV risk items			
11. Contra Costa County survey, Wave II	Nov. 1988 to June 1989	Persons aged 18+ living in Contra Costa County	Multistaged probability sample; one RSA per household	969	Face-to-face interview in household	SAQ with sealed envelope	Interview RR = 65.8%; SAQ RR = 60.9%	Comparison with census data	Unknown
Local Area Seroprevalence Surveys									
12. San Francisco Men's Health Study, Wave I	May 1984 to April 1985	Currently unmarried men, aged 25–54, living in central San Francisco	Multistaged probability sample of households; all eligible persons in household	1,034	Face-to-face interview in clinic	Face-to-face interview in clinic	Interview RR = 56.2%; blood donation rate = 56.2%, clinic venipuncture	Comparison with census data; analysis of RR and variations over census tracts	Probable underrepresentation of younger and older men, black men, and heterosexual men
13. Belle Glade, Florida survey	Feb. to Oct. 1986	Persons aged 18+ living in 12 neighborhoods of Belle Glade	Probability sample of households; all eligible persons in household	877	Face-to-face interview in household	Face-to-face interview in household	73.1% of contacted households participated; individual RR not reported	None	Unknown

Survey	Date	Population	Sample design	N	Screening	Interview	Response rate	Analysis	Findings
14. San Francisco Home Health Survey	Aug. 1988 to June 1989	Currently unmarried men and women aged 20-44, living in 16 San Francisco census tracts	Multistaged probability sample of households; interviewed any eligible persons in household	1,780	Face-to-face interview in household	Face-to-face interview in household	Interview RR = 59.4%; blood donation rate = 46.2% (venipuncture in home)	Comparison with census data; analysis of data in nonrespondents who were enumerated in screening interview	Not yet available
15. National Household Seroprevalence Survey pilot study	Jan. 1989	Residents of Allegheny County, Pa.; persons aged 18-54	Multistaged probability sample of households; one RSA per household	263	Face-to-face eligibility screening in household	SAQ in sealed envelope	SAQ RR = 81.2%; blood donation rate = 81.2% (venipuncture or finger stick in home)	Analysis of screening RR by sample segment; analysis of sample person RR by enumeration data and interviewer observations	Lower screening RRs outside Pittsburgh and in areas with more married persons (and fewer black persons); lower sample person response rates among married nonblack persons

NOTES: NORC: National Opinion Research Center; SAQ: self-administered questionnaire; GSS: General Social Survey; RR: response rate; RDD: random digit dialing; RSA: randomly selected adult; CPS: Current Population Survey; HIS: Health Interview Survey; NHSAO: National Health and School Attendance Office.

Reference documents for surveys: (1) Fay et al. (1989); (2) Schmidt et al. (1989); (3) Turner, Miller, and Barker (1989); (4) Communication Technologies, Inc. (1988); (5) Johnson et al. (1988); (6) Michael et al. (1988), Smith (1988); (7) Pratt (1989); (8) Schofield (1965); (9) Communication Technologies, Inc. (1987); (10) Borgatta, Blumstein, and Schwartz (1987); (11) K. Trocke, Pacific Medical Center, San Francisco, personal communication, July 14, 1989; (12) Winkelstein et al. (1987); (13) Castro et al. (1988); (14) Wiley (1989); (15) Research Triangle Institute (1989).

The most frequently used data collection procedure was a face-to-face interview followed by a relatively brief SAQ that focused on sexual behavior. In all instances, after the respondent completed the SAQ, it was placed in an envelope (stripped of identifying information except for a serial number, which permitted the questionnaire responses to be linked with interview data), sealed in the presence of the respondent, and collected by the interviewer. In one study (no. 15), the interviewer invited the respondent to accompany him or her to the nearest mailbox from which the questionnaire could be mailed directly to the field office for data entry.

In theory, the SAQ sealed envelope procedure should induce greater cooperation (and perhaps more candid answers) by eliminating the need to verbalize responses to sensitive questions. A potential disadvantage is loss of control over the administration of the questions and recording of responses. Illiteracy or other language problems may prevent the respondent from completing the questionnaire without assistance. In addition, it is easy for a respondent to avoid filling out the questionnaire or to skip questions without refusing directly; on-the-spot checks for item or form nonresponse cannot be conducted without destroying the quasi-anonymous character of the procedure.

Figure C-2 displays response rates for 13 of the surveys[4] classified by type of data collection: face-to-face interview with SAQ, face-to-face interview only, and telephone interview. The response rates for face-to-face and telephone interviewing were calculated by dividing the number of completed interviews by the total number of sample persons. For surveys that used an SAQ, the response rate is the number of completed SAQs divided by the number of sample persons. In three of the surveys (nos. 4, 10, and 13), the reported response rates should be regarded as upper-bound estimates. Item nonresponse rates were generally low or not reported in the available survey documentation.

As noted earlier, the response rate in a study is conventionally used as one yardstick for measuring the potential accuracy of survey estimates. The response rates in Figure C-2 span a wide range, from a low of 33 to a high of 81 percent, with most falling between 50 and 80 percent. Several of the surveys reported levels of participation that compared favorably with rates achieved in surveys dealing with less sensitive issues. The majority of them, however, failed to attain response rates that exceed the usual survey standard of 70 to 80 percent. Given such rates, it is difficult to rule out the possibility of substantial bias from selective participation in

---

[4]Response rates could not be computed for surveys no. 1 and 9.

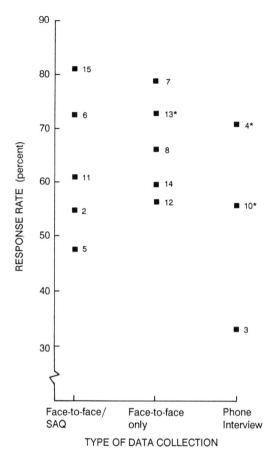

FIGURE C-2 Response rates in selected surveys (from Table C-1) by type of data collection used.

surveys of sexual behavior. It is therefore crucial to document any claims of representativeness by a careful study of patterns of nonresponse.

No obvious association between response rate and the three methods of data collection was found, although response rates in the telephone surveys appear to be somewhat lower than those in surveys using other procedures. (The reader should note that the response rates reported for surveys no. 4 and 10 are probably overestimates; for details, see the section "Use of Telephone Surveys" below.) Similarly, additional comparisons (not shown in Figure C-2) indicate that there is no correlation between response rates and the scope of the sampling (local versus national), the size of the sexual behavior component of the interview, or (surprisingly) whether sample persons were asked to donate blood specimens for serologic testing. Although the variation in response rates appears to be largely unrelated to easily documented characteristics of survey sampling and design in this group of surveys, more specific and detailed comparisons yield some plausible explanations for some of the observed differences. These explanations are discussed below.

Survey Configurations Associated with
High Response Rates

Four of the surveys listed in Table C-1 report response rates higher than 70 percent. The two that are local seroprevalence surveys will be discussed later with other surveys that include a blood component. The focus here is on two large-scale surveys based on national samples of U.S. residents: the 1988 General Social Survey (GSS) and the 1988 National Survey of Family Growth (NSFG).

These two surveys differ in substantive focus, definition of the target population, sampling methodology, and details of survey procedure. Nonetheless, they share certain characteristics that may help to explain why they achieved relatively high rates of participation: they are each part of a series of periodic surveys that have consistently had good response rates; the sexual items consist of a relatively small set of "add-on" questions; the surveys are conducted by the same survey organizations[5] and to some extent by the same supervisory and field staff that have been responsible for previous surveys in the series; and the field procedures include provisions for large numbers of callbacks and special attention to the conversion of refusers.

The 1988 GSS is the fourteenth in a series of annual opinion surveys conducted by the National Opinion Research Center (NORC) under a grant from the National Science Foundation. Since 1977 the GSS sample has been selected using full probability sampling of adults, 18 years and older, living in U.S. households. The GSS interview, which is approximately 90 minutes long, is conducted face to face in the home and is sometimes followed by SAQs dealing with special topics.

In 1988, GSS interviewers gave each respondent a one-page, self-administered questionnaire that included the following questions:

- How many sex partners have you had in the last 12 months?
- Was one of the partners your husband or wife or regular sexual partner?

---

[5]NORC for the General Social Survey and Cycle 1 of the NSFG; Westat for the NSFG cycles 2, 3, 4.

- If you had other partners, please indicate all categories that apply to them

  - close personal friend;
  - neighbor, coworker, or long-term acquaintance;
  - casual date or pick-up;
  - person you paid or person who paid you for sex;
  - other (specify).

- Have your sexual partners in the last 12 months been: exclusively male, both male and female, exclusively female?

The marked questionnaire was placed in an envelope, sealed, and collected by the interviewer.

The conduct of fieldwork was similar to that of previous GSS efforts. One hundred thirty interviewers, most of whom had worked on earlier rounds of the survey, were recruited from NORC's interviewer pool and trained in 1988 GSS procedures by supervisory staff. The target response rate for the survey was 77 percent, with a minimum acceptable response rate per sampled area[6] of 65 percent. NORC employed special procedures to minimize nonresponse. Two hundred preselected respondents living in areas in which recruitment difficulties had been encountered in previous rounds of the GSS were offered $10 to complete the interview and SAQ. In addition, NORC assembled a mobile squad of expert interviewers who were assigned to do refusal conversion interviews. In the later stages of fieldwork, field management authorized interviewers to pay respondent fees from $10 to $50 for completion of interviews after an initial refusal. The field staff completed 1,481 interviews during the 10-week period for a total survey response rate of 77.3 percent. Of those who completed the interview portion of the survey, 93.9 percent returned the SAQ, yielding an SAQ response rate of 72.6 percent. The response rate for fully completed SAQs was somewhat lower (66.7 percent), owing to nonresponse on various items.

The 1988 National Survey of Family Growth (Cycle IV of the series that began in 1973) was conducted for the National Center for Health Statistics by Westat Corporation survey staff from January to August 1988. The target population for this survey consisted of noninstitutionalized civilian women, aged 15 to 44, living in the United States. The target sample for Cycle IV consisted of more than 10,000 eligible and

---

[6]That is, per primary sampling unit (PSU).

randomly selected women who were listed on household rosters[7] from NCHS's National Health Interview Surveys (NHIS)[8] conducted between October 1985 and April 1987. About 80 percent of the sample persons were located through address correction requests and telephone contacts before the beginning of fieldwork.

After a series of screening questions to verify eligibility, interviewers conducted a one-hour face-to-face home interview that dealt with family planning practices, family size expectations and preferences, sources of family planning services, and aspects of maternal and child health. The interview included several questions about personal sexual behavior (e.g., age at first intercourse, frequency of intercourse, lifetime number of male partners, a series of items on beliefs and attitudes about AIDS, and 19 questions about sexually transmitted diseases.

A field staff of 240 interviewers, the majority of whom had at least one year of prior interviewing experience, completed a total of 8,450 interviews by the end of the data collection phase of the survey. This number of completed interviews yielded a total survey response rate of approximately 79 percent (figured by multiplying the 82.1 percent response rate among NSFG sample persons by a 96 percent enumeration response rate[9] in the NHIS). This rate was achieved after considerable investment by reaching sample persons who were not at home during the initial calls and by converting refusals. The response rate (among NSFG sample persons) after the initial interviewer assignments was approximately 69 percent. It increased to 78 percent after nonrespondents were reassigned and contacted by local interviewers; it increased still further (to 82 percent) in a subsequent follow-up of a random half of the remaining nonrespondents who were assigned to a special core of conversion interviewers. Nonresponse to specific questions about sexual behavior averaged about 4 percent.

Judging by the response rates in these surveys, "piggybacking" a small number of questions about sexual behavior onto established surveys appears to be a feasible strategy for obtaining estimates of the prevalence of certain risk factors for sexual transmission of HIV in general populations. Adding sex-related items to the protocols for the 1988 GSS and

---

[7] The NHIS attempted to enumerate all persons living in each household included in its target sample. This was possible for 96 percent of the target households. The names entered on the resulting NHIS "household rosters" provided the basis for the NSFG sampling.

[8] The NHIS is an annual survey of approximately 50,000 households conducted by the Bureau of the Census. The response rate for this survey is more than 95 percent.

[9] The NHIS household rosters were used to sample respondents in the NSFG. Household rosters were missing for approximately 4 percent of the households included in the NHIS target sample.

NSFG[10] had little effect on the response rates normally obtained in those surveys, although item nonresponse may have been slightly higher for the sexual questions than for the nonsexual material. As noted earlier, relatively high rates of participation are typical of these surveys, and the ingredients for such success are well known to survey practitioners: prior experience with similar surveys, continuity of staff, a high "target response rate" combined with a field operation that promotes diligent follow-up of nonresponding sample persons, and an ample budget. Under these conditions, response rates for small subsets of sex-related items can be similar to rates achieved in well-conducted surveys that do not inquire about sensitive personal behaviors.

The above remarks, however, do not necessarily apply to surveys with a greater number of questions about sexual behavior or with questions of a more intimate nature than those in the GSS and NSFG. In both of these surveys, questions about sexual behavior constituted a relatively minor part of the interview and were not emphasized in preinterview contacts with potential respondents. Furthermore, neither survey asked about the details of sexual encounters, such as the full range of types of sexual contact. Surveys dominated by sexual questions, especially those that include long Kinsey-like inventories and sexual histories, may encounter more serious problems of nonresponse than are encountered in piggyback surveys. For example, the demands of prior informed consent in true sex surveys will require more complete advance warning about the nature of the questions to be asked, perhaps increasing respondent concerns about embarrassment and disclosure. Whether the relatively high levels of participation that characterized the 1988 GSS and NSFG can be achieved in more extensive piggyback surveys or in true sex surveys remains an open question.

Use of Telephone Surveys

The collection of survey data through telephone interviews has become an increasingly popular alternative to face-to-face interviewing as a result of the generally lower costs of telephone surveys and developments in sampling and interviewing technology (notably, sampling through random-digit dialing [RDD] and computer-assisted telephone interviewing [CATI]). Comparisons between face-to-face and telephone interviewing in the context of national surveys indicate that the overall response rates for telephone surveys are on the order of 5 percent lower than those expected in personal interviews (Groves and Kahn, 1979). Although

---

[10]The NSFG traditionally had some items on sexual behaviors (e.g., age at first intercourse); in 1988 the number of items was increased.

response rates for the two methodologies tend to converge when unanswered telephone calls are ignored, acceptable standards (e.g., Council of American Survey Research Organizations, 1982) for reporting response rates mandate that a fraction of the numbers not contacted be included in the denominator when calculating response rates for telephone surveys.[11] The generally lower response rates of telephone surveys, along with studies of respondent reactions to the two forms of interviewing, suggest that the rapport and trust between interviewer and respondent attained in face-to-face surveys are harder to achieve in the telephone interview.[12] Thus, it is reasonable to expect somewhat lower rates of participation in telephone surveys that contain explicit sexual content, compared with similar surveys using face-to-face interviewing or a combination of face-to-face interviewing and an SAQ.

Unfortunately, there is only a limited empirical basis for judging the feasibility of conducting interviews about sexual behavior by telephone. Few such surveys have been conducted (four are listed in Table C-1), and only one of the four reviewed by the committee gives an indication of the utility of telephone interviewing for measuring sexual behavior in general populations. Nevertheless, a brief review of response rates in these surveys is warranted, if only to indicate the character of the attempts thus far.

The two local area telephone surveys (nos. 9 and 10)—one of which was conducted in San Francisco, the other in Seattle—are examples of the use of targeted sampling of phone numbers and telephone interviewing to find and interview persons who may be considered to be at higher than average risk of HIV infection. Yet such surveys are not without their drawbacks. Although probability sampling was ostensibly employed, peculiarities in the definition of the target populations and in the execution of the surveys make generalizations about participation in these surveys hazardous.

The 1987 San Francisco survey (conducted by Communication Tech-

---

[11] The ratio of eligible to noneligible contacts found among telephone numbers that *do* answer may be used to deflate the total number included in the denominator. This practice assumes that the proportion of telephone numbers that have no eligible respondents (e.g., business numbers, households without persons meeting screening criteria, etc.) is the same among nonanswers as among those for which responses are obtained.

[12] As part of their comparison of parallel telephone and personal interview surveys, Groves and Kahn (1979:97–99) asked respondents whether they "felt uneasy" discussing various topics that had been included in parallel telephone and personal interview surveys that were conducted in tandem. Survey topics included finances, health, voting, and political attitudes. Groves and Kahn reported finding that larger proportions of respondents interviewed by telephone said they "felt uneasy" about each of these topics. The greatest differences were found for questions on income (17.9 percent "uneasy" in telephone survey versus 15.3 percent in personal interview) and political attitudes (12.1 versus 8.5).

nologies, Inc.) was undertaken to determine levels of high-risk sexual behavior among gay and bisexual men living in San Francisco. It was conceived as a baseline survey, the first in a series that would document changes in risk behavior that might be related to educational campaigns directed at gay and bisexual men. The sampling frame, which consisted of male names and linked telephone numbers, was constructed from commercial lists of households that were stratified by census tract. By oversampling telephone numbers from tracts with a large proportion of unmarried males, the researchers composed 24 replicate samples of 500 names and numbers to be released in sequence to interviewers until 500 interviews had been completed with eligible respondents. Eligibility in this case consisted of being male, 18 years of age or older, and self-identifying in the screening interview as a gay or bisexual man.

Interviewers made as many as four attempts to contact a household and, after initial questioning to determine the presence of a male aged 18 or older, attempted to screen for gay or bisexual behavior. Persons who identified themselves as gay or bisexual were asked a series of questions about their sexual behavior. The report of this survey cited a refusal rate of 19.4 percent. It is not clear, however, whether this rate referred to the initial screening for the presence of an adult male or to the subsequent screening for gay or bisexual behavior. Although there is no mention of the number of households that were not contacted or of the eligibility rate per contacted household, the authors hazard the opinion that "[w]ith a sample size of 500, results were projectable to the universe of self-identifying gay and bisexual men in San Francisco within ±4.5% at the 95% level of confidence" (Communication Technologies, Inc., 1987:25).

The 1985–1986 Seattle survey was a pilot study of the use of telephone interviewing to collect data on sexual behavior in subgroups of the general population who were likely to be at risk of acquiring HIV infection. The target population consisted of persons aged 18 to 45 years living in selected localities of Seattle. Based on census data and "local knowledge," the investigators sampled households in census tracts that were considered likely to include large numbers of homosexual and bisexual men and heterosexually active persons. Households were selected from reverse telephone directories[13] so that names and phone numbers could be recorded prior to the telephone contact with the household. This procedure was necessary because the investigators required that an advance letter be sent to all persons to be contacted indicating the kinds of questions to be asked and the voluntary nature of participation. Of the

[13]Reverse telephone directories are arranged in numerical order by telephone number and give the name and address associated with each listed number.

nearly 3,000 advance letters sent, approximately one-third were returned (as undelivered mail, wrong addressees, or business addresses). Contact was made with seventy-two percent of the remaining households; of these, 46 percent contained no eligible respondents, and 16 percent refused to be interviewed prior to the household enumeration. At the end of fieldwork, 389 interviews had been completed. No interviews were attempted with persons who said they had not received the advance letter. The response rate was estimated to be 55.7 percent, based on the assumption that about one in three of the nonresponding households contained a person who was eligible to be interviewed.

The two telephone surveys targeted to a broader population include a national and a statewide survey. The national survey, conducted by the *Los Angeles Times* in July 1987 (no. 3 in Table C-1), included a short series of questions about sexual behavior at the end of a series of opinion questions. The response rate (reported in a secondary analysis of the poll data) was quite low—about 33 percent—no doubt because fieldwork was completed in five days and only three callbacks were permitted. Low response rates are not unusual in short-term commercial surveys; nevertheless, they provide little indication of what can be achieved in more rigorously executed telephone surveys. Surprisingly, the analysis of reports of one aspect of sexual behavior in this survey appear quite consistent with those obtained in another survey that achieved a much higher response rate (see the discussion below).

The 1987 California survey (no. 4 in Table C-1) was commissioned by the California State Department of Health Services to produce statewide estimates of the distribution of HIV risk factors among adults 18 years of age and older. The investigators generated a sample of telephone numbers by random-digit dialing with deliberate oversampling of prefixes associated with areas containing high proportions of minorities. At first contact, the interviewers attempted to collect information on household composition and to select at random one eligible person to be interviewed. Potential respondents were told in advance about the nature of the questions to be asked. The interviewer then administered a 15-minute series of questions that included screening items pertaining to HIV risk status (e.g., same-gender sexual contact among men, heterosexual contacts with multiple partners or partners in a known HIV risk group, use of recreational drugs). Any respondent who reported one or more of these risk factors was asked additional questions about specific risk behaviors. The interviewers were instructed to make up to 12 attempts to contact each sampled telephone number. Initial refusals were reassigned to other interviewers who made further attempts to complete the interview. At the end of fieldwork, 2,012 persons had been interviewed from a total of 2,834 persons known to be eligible—a completion rate of 71 percent; the 29 percent of incomplete interviews included sample person refusals and interview break-offs. Because noncontacts and enumeration nonresponses were ignored, however, 71 percent must be regarded as a rather generous upper bound on the response rate as conventionally calculated.

The response rates in these few telephone studies appear to be somewhat lower than those obtained in face-to-face interviews of sexual behavior. This conclusion holds true as well for the statewide California survey because the true response rate is undoubtedly lower than the reported completion rate. Experience with sex surveys conducted by telephone is too limited, however, to determine the levels of participation that can be achieved in such surveys and whether the lower response rates in the available cases are a generic feature of telephone surveys or simply the result of early and somewhat idiosyncratic first attempts.

In view of the substantially lower cost of telephone versus face-to-face surveys, as well as the limited scope of current experience, carefully designed experiments should be encouraged to test the feasibility of this methodology for surveys of sexual behavior in general populations. Because noncontacts are a major component of nonresponse in existing surveys, such experiments should include provision for large numbers of callbacks and extended interview periods. Additional increases in response rates may be achieved through research on the best ways to introduce questions about sexual behavior over the phone, improvements in questionnaire design, and more diligent attempts to complete interviews after initial refusals. Another area of possible investigation is to compare—at least at the aggregate and possibly at the individual levels— the results of telephone and personal interview surveys of the same target population.

Participation in Seroprevalence Surveys

If sex surveys are properly executed, they can provide important clues about the potential for sexual transmission of HIV infection in general populations. Survey estimates of the distribution of behaviors associated with HIV transmission, combined with epidemiological findings on the transmission efficiency of HIV in sexual contacts and biological aspects of the natural history of HIV infection, are the raw material for model-based inferences about the future spread of AIDS in known risk groups and in populations not yet considered to be at risk (May and Anderson, 1987; Anderson and May, 1988; May, Anderson, and Blower, 1989; Turner, Miller, and Moses, 1989:Ch. 2). Yet even if the data on sexual behavior in general populations were far more complete than they are at present, the validity of model-based inferences and predictions would be suspect owing to uncertainties about a variety of other forces that govern the epidemic growth of infection. At best, sex surveys of representative samples can indicate degrees of vulnerability to sexual transmission of HIV in individuals and in population subgroups. In this way they can make a significant contribution to prevention and control. Sex surveys cannot, however, substitute for direct assessment of the prevalence of infection.

The most attractive design for direct measurement of the prevalence of infection is the seroprevalence survey.[14] A seroprevalence survey applies well-established principles of probability sampling and survey methodology to the problem of collecting sample blood specimens with the aim of estimating the prevalence of infection in a population. In theory, such surveys could eliminate most of the outstanding uncertainties regarding the size of the AIDS epidemic, the prevalence of infection in major risk groups, and the degree to which HIV has entered populations that are not presently considered to be at significant risk for infection. Yet, the practical difficulties of mounting a seroprevalence survey on a local or national basis are formidable. Not the least of these are the problems of potentially high levels of noncooperation among sample persons and possible correlations between participation and HIV serostatus.

Currently, a national seroprevalence survey is in the planning and development stage under a contract between the National Center for Health Statistics (now a part of CDC) and Research Triangle Institute (RTI). The goal of the first phase of this work, which consists of pilot and pretest surveys, is to select a design that meets several objectives simultaneously: protection of respondent anonymity; attainment of participation rates high enough to justify confidence in prevalence estimates derived from the survey; development of procedures to assess nonresponse bias; and identification of cost-effective fieldwork strategies. Choosing an optimum design requires extensive experimentation with alternative combinations of design characteristics. Among the challenges are determining the best ways: to introduce the study to sample persons and the general public, to maintain anonymity, to collect blood specimens, to ask questions about risk factors, to compensate respondents for the time required for participation, and to minimize fears of disclosure. Survey developers hope that preliminary testing will result in a feasible strategy for a national survey of approximately 50,000 households.

---

[14]Lengthy discussions of the merits of seroprevalence surveys and of the problems of implementing them on a national scale can be found in Turner and Fay (1987/1989) and De Gruttola and Fineberg (1989).

To date, knowledge of what can be accomplished in seroprevalence surveys rests on the results of four local efforts. Only one of these studies, RTI's small-scale pilot seroprevalence survey in Allegheny County, Pennsylvania (which includes the city of Pittsburgh), is part of a program of research to explore alternative designs for a national seroprevalence survey. The other efforts were designed to provide local estimates of the extent of HIV infection in connection with intensive study of the epidemiological factors associated with transmission. In all four surveys, sample persons were selected from local, residentially defined target populations through multistaged probability sampling procedures.

It will be obvious from the descriptions given below that these surveys occupy vastly different positions in the "design space" of potential options for seroprevalence surveys. The RTI Allegheny County (Pittsburgh) pilot survey (no. 15 in Table C-1) is one extreme—a one-time anonymous survey in which blood is collected in the home by venipuncture or finger-stick, accompanied by an SAQ about risk factors. In contrast, the two San Francisco seroprevalence surveys (nos. 12 and 14 in Table C-1) were the first cycles of longitudinal studies that involved periodic collection of blood specimens, extensive personal interviews to obtain risk factor information, and, in one case, routine physical examinations in a clinic setting. Not surprisingly, there is a gradient of response rates in these four studies that corresponds roughly to the intensity and duration of the participation required from each respondent: the response rates for blood samples range from 46 to 81 percent. The highest rates were obtained in the least demanding surveys.

The San Francisco Men's Health Study (no. 12 in Table C-1) is believed to be the first seroprevalence survey of HIV infection conducted in the United States. The baseline survey, which was designed as the recruitment phase of a longitudinal study, began in the spring of 1984 and continued until April 1985. The target population was defined as currently unmarried men, aged 25 to 54 years, living in the 19 census tracts of central San Francisco that in 1984 had the highest cumulative incidence of AIDS for the city. The investigators anticipated that a majority of the eligible men living in the target area, known locally as the Castro District and considered to be a "gay" area, would have had recent homosexual contact. Within the sample strata (census tracts), the sample was drawn by strict probability sampling at the level of households, and all eligible men within each household (with no advance screening for type of sexual activity or sexual orientation) were invited to participate in the study. Interviewers made the initial contact in a visit to each selected household during which they attempted to complete a household enumeration, to identify persons eligible for participation, and to schedule appointments for a visit to a local clinic—where participants were to be interviewed, given a physical examination, and asked to donate blood and other specimens for laboratory assay. Throughout the 12 months of fieldwork for the baseline survey, there were numerous callbacks for hard-to-reach sample persons, frequent rescheduling of missed clinic appointments, and sustained efforts to convert those who initially refused to participate. At the end of the recruitment phase, 1,034 sample persons had completed their first clinic visit, representing a response rate of 56.2 percent (of approximately 1,839 eligible sample persons, including an estimated 157 eligible men in sample households in which the initial household enumeration could not be completed).

In 1986, CDC conducted a seroprevalence survey in Belle Glade, Florida, as part of an investigation of the causes of an AIDS outbreak in that area (see survey no. 13 in Table C-1). The target population comprised persons 18 years of age and older and, with parental consent, children aged 2 to 10 years. Households were selected by stratified random sampling from comprehensive lists for 12 locally defined neighborhoods. Approximately 70 percent of the selected households were located in neighborhoods with the largest numbers of reported AIDS cases in the city. After signing a written informed consent document, sample persons were interviewed at home using a standardized questionnaire; they were then asked for a blood sample (obtained by venipuncture) and examined for signs of HIV infection. The report describing this survey indicates that 557 of the selected households were visited while someone was home, and of these households, 73 percent ($N = 407$ households) agreed to participate in the study, yielding a total of 877 persons who completed the full study protocol. The 557 households do not include those in which no contact was made;[15] thus, 73 percent should be considered an upper bound of the household response rate. The study report did not indicate the response rate for individual sample persons.

A second seroprevalence survey of San Francisco neighborhoods was initiated in 1988-1989, this time to monitor HIV infection in areas thought to be likely candidates for transmission through IV drug use or heterosexual contact, or both. The target population was defined as currently unmarried men and women, aged 20 to 44 years, living in three areas (16 census tracts) characterized by high rates of STDs among women, high rates of admission to drug detoxification programs, and AIDS cases among their residents that were not attributable to male homosexual contacts. Full probability sampling was employed at the

---

[15]Three attempts to contact the household were made at different times of the day (K. G. Castro, Centers for Disease Control, personal communication, May 2, 1990).

household level, and all eligible persons within the selected households were invited to participate in the study. The field protocol included an advance letter to each sample household, signed informed consent, a lengthy personal interview in the home covering HIV risk factors in great detail, and collection of blood (venipuncture in the home or at a local clinic) by interviewers who were certified phlebotomists. Participants were paid $20 as compensation for completing the protocol. Repeated callbacks, rescheduling of home visits, and refusal conversion strategies were employed throughout the 10 months of fieldwork. Based on an estimated 2,983 sample persons living in the selected households, the 1,781 sample persons who completed the interview portion of the protocol constituted an interview response rate of 59.7 percent. The response rate for the blood component of the survey was 46.3 percent because blood specimens were not obtained from 401 of the 1,781 persons interviewed (owing to refusal and, in a few cases, the inability to complete the blood draw).

The initial pilot study to test procedures for a national seroprevalence survey was conducted in January 1989 in Allegheny County, Pennsylvania. As is planned for the national study, the target population for this small-scale pilot consisted of the civilian, noninstitutionalized population aged 18 to 54 years old at the time of the survey. A sample of 539 households was selected by area probability sampling methods, and one eligible adult in each household was randomly chosen as the sample person. The fieldwork protocol called for an enumeration interview (which included questions about the age, sex, race, and marital status of each person in the household), selection of the sample person, signed informed consent (which was left with the respondent at the end of the interview to ensure anonymity), collection of a blood specimen (venipuncture or finger-stick by a phlebotomist who accompanied the interviewer), a $50 incentive payment that was promised before the blood draw, and, finally, completion of a brief SAQ (covering demographic characteristics and basic HIV risk factors) that was subsequently placed in a sealed envelope. Videotapes were shown during the contact with the respondent to explain the survey and motivate participation. Earlier, the existence of the survey and its importance had been stressed on all local television news stations. No names were taken at any time during the visit to the household. At the end of fieldwork, 95.1 percent of the 450 occupied households were successfully screened, and 263 (85.4 percent) of 308 enumerated sample persons completed the survey protocol. The response rate thus was (.951 x .854) 81.2 percent.

The Allegheny County pilot study indicates that relatively high response rates can be obtained in seroprevalence surveys that involve public (e.g., TV news) appeals to participate, that make limited demands on participants' time and that offer substantial monetary incentives. The design of the pilot study stands in sharp contrast to the more epidemiologically oriented surveys that employ lengthy personal interviews covering a much wider range of behavioral risk factors, repeated blood draws (as in the San Francisco longitudinal studies), and invitations to learn antibody status through disclosure counseling. In the Allegheny survey, participation was anonymous: no names were recorded, the risk factor information was obtained by the SAQ/sealed envelope procedure, and there was no feedback of HIV antibody test results to respondents. It is not surprising that response rates in the pilot study were substantially higher than those in more demanding epidemiologically oriented surveys.

These comparisons indicate the trade-off that must often be made between maximizing response rates in a streamlined design and intensive epidemiological investigation with lower response rates. The discussions of the design options for a national seroprevalence survey anticipated the necessity of such a trade-off (Turner and Fay, 1987/1989). Thus, the Allegheny experience suggests that the selection of a survey design that limits the demands on respondents—by making participation relatively easy, anonymous, and nonthreatening—may have been a wise choice. Further testing and refinement of this approach on a larger scale will establish whether it constitutes a feasible design for a national survey.

Nonresponse Bias in Sex and Seroprevalence Surveys

Nonresponse bias[16] occurs when participation in a survey is selective with respect to a characteristic whose distribution is to be estimated from survey responses. A high response rate tends to minimize the effects of such selectivity on survey estimates as long as the procedures used to attain it do not in fact increase the correlation between the characteristic of interest and the act of participation. Response rates in most surveys, however, usually are not high enough to justify ignoring problems of selective participation, and there is in fact, a literature that indicates that certain kinds of persons (notably those of low socioeconomic status) are likely to be underrepresented in most samples in ways that may compromise survey estimates (Turner and Martin, 1984:Vol. 1, Fig. 3-1; Goyder, 1987). The committee's review likewise indicates that the response rates achieved in contemporary sex and seroprevalence surveys

---

[16]Nonresponse bias is the deviation between the distribution of responses obtained from persons who participated in the survey and who responded to the survey question, and the response that would have been obtained if all persons in the target sample had participated in the survey and answered the question.

leave ample opportunity for selective participation to affect the validity of survey estimates of sexual behavior and HIV seroprevalence. (The reader should note that response bias—that is, misleading or inaccurate survey responses—can have similar effects. This issue is addressed later in this appendix; this section deals only with biases that result from selective nonresponse.)

There are three kinds of selective participation that have somewhat different effects on estimates of sexual behavior or HIV infection: (1) selective participation with respect to characteristics that are *independent* of sexual behavior and HIV serostatus; (2) selective participation related to attributes (e.g., marital status) that may be correlated with sexual behavior or HIV infection; and (3) selective participation that is directly related to sexual behavior or serostatus. The first kind of selection can be ignored in the construction of estimates of the sort being considered here because (by definition) this type of nonresponse is unrelated to sexual behavior or infection status. Selection of the second kind does result in biased estimates, but the bias might be remedied if, given the selection factors, the (conditional) distribution of sexual behavior (or serostatus) is known to be the same for respondents and nonrespondents and the distribution of the selection factors among nonrespondents can be ascertained. Let us suppose, for example, that participation in a sex survey is correlated with marital status in such a way that single men are underrepresented. If the marital status of male nonrespondents is known (from, for example, a household enumeration interview) and if there were a good basis[17] for the belief that, for any particular marital status, the sexual behaviors of respondents and nonrespondents were similar, sample estimates of the distribution of sexual behavior might be adjusted, using imputation or maximum likelihood procedures, to adjust for this nonresponse bias. Fay and colleagues (1989) provided a rather sophisticated example of this form of adjustment in connection with estimates of the frequency of male same-gender sexual behaviors from the Kinsey/NORC national survey conducted in 1970.

The most troublesome kind of selectivity is participation that depends directly on sexual behavior or serostatus—for example, when the decision to participate is made in relation to fears about reporting socially proscribed sexual practices or the disclosure of a positive antibody result. In this case, simple imputation from observed data will rarely lead to unbiased estimates of prevalence, although in some cases it may be possible to anticipate the direction of bias. Concerns about this form of selection

---

[17] Such a basis might, for example, have been provided by a methodological study that did more intensive follow-up of a subsample of nonrespondents.

have motivated the development of strategies that make participation in sex and seroprevalence surveys less threatening. Nevertheless, there is likely to be some degree of selection bias attributable to fears about disclosing sexual practices (particularly those considered "deviant") or about revealing one's HIV serostatus in the best executed surveys.

Current knowledge about the structure of nonresponse bias in sex and seroprevalence surveys comes from two kinds of comparisons: comparisons of survey estimates with census data and internal analysis of the correlates of different levels of nonresponse. Roughly half of the 15 surveys reviewed here attempted some form of comparison of survey estimates with census data. There is an apparent positive correlation between years of schooling and participation in several of the surveys but few other regularities in the deviations between survey estimates and census figures could be detected. (See Table C-1 for a summary of the comparisons reported in the source documents.) In any case, a good match between census and sample survey distributions, although encouraging in some respects, does not guarantee that estimates of prevalence rates for sexual behavior or HIV infection are unbiased.

The other major source of information about nonresponse bias comes from analyzing the characteristics associated with nonresponse at different stages of a survey interview. Although such stages vary from study to study, a seroprevalence survey might typically include the following: (1) completing a household enumeration form, which includes basic demographic information about each member of the household; (2) completing the personal interview, which might include an SAQ dealing with sexual behavior and other HIV risk factors; (3) completing every item on the SAQ form; and (4) allowing blood to be drawn for serologic testing. Most of the 15 surveys reviewed here involved some degree of staging of this kind, although not always in this order. In many cases, it is possible to study nonresponse at a given stage in terms of information collected at a previous stage—for example, by comparing (in terms of the responses given by both groups in the personal interview) the characteristics of persons who agreed to give a blood specimen with those who refused.

There were many opportunities for such comparisons in the surveys examined by the committee, but few of those opportunities had been seized. Smith's (1988) study of nonresponse bias in the 1988 GSS is an important exception. Because the GSS consisted of a lengthy personal interview followed by an SAQ covering sexual risk factors, it was possible to examine correlations between the interview responses and two types of nonresponse: nonresponse to the entire SAQ form and nonresponse to specific items. On the basis of this analysis, Smith draws an encouraging conclusion: "In general, the non-response does not appear to be related to differences in sexual behavior. Non-response differentials appear to be absent among those variables most closely related to sexual behavior. Non-response instead is related to general factors such as low education, low political interest, and general uncooperativeness that are not highly related to sexual behavior. As a result, non-response bias to the supplement (i.e., the sex SAQ) appears to be negligible." Smith's conclusion raises an interesting question about the basis for inferring the presence of nonresponse bias. Namely, on what basis can the absence of selection with respect to known or assumed correlates of sexual behavior be taken as evidence of the absence of direct selection (i.e., the third type of selection distinguished above)?

There is clearly a need to encourage further analyses of existing sex and seroprevalence surveys to learn more about the structure of nonresponse. When surveys are organized in a series of stages, which is the case in many instances, analysis can probe more deeply into the potential cause of nonresponse bias than is possible using simple comparisons of survey estimates with external data. Such analyses should provide a firmer basis for estimating population characteristics in the presence of nonresponse, and it would thereby engender increased confidence in the prevalence estimates derived from sex and seroprevalence surveys and surveys of sexual behavior.[18]

NONSAMPLING ISSUES IN AIDS SURVEYS

This section focuses on the survey measurement procedures that yield data for basic and applied studies of the behaviors that transmit HIV. The emphasis here is on nonsampling factors that affect the quality of these data. In this regard, it is important to remember that behind every n–way tabulation, logistic regression, or other analytical model using such data lies a human encounter between two individuals, an interviewer and a respondent. The situational, cognitive, social, and psychological factors that arise within that interpersonal exchange affect the answers that are given and the data that are thereby generated. To understand the sexual and drug-using behaviors that are at issue in survey research on HIV transmission, one must ultimately confront the uncertainties introduced by this question-and-answer process.

Terms and Concepts

In discussing the complex array of factors that can distort survey (and

---

[18] A major aim of the NCHS pilot studies for the national HIV seroprevalence survey is the investigation of the nonresponse bias in surveys that seek to estimate HIV prevalence.

other) measurements, various interrelated terms are used with a reasonably standardized meaning by statisticians and researchers in the behavioral and social sciences. The constellation of sampling and nonsampling factors that influence a particular measurement define the *error structure* of that measurement. Sampling factors can include incompleteness or other errors in the sampling frame used to draw the sample, failure to obtain data from all sampled persons, and so forth. (This type of nonresponse is discussed in the preceding section.) Nonsampling factors that affect measurements include misunderstanding of questions, respondent unwillingness to reveal sensitive information, interviewer mistakes in reading questions, clerical and other errors made during coding and processing of data, and so forth.

Although the factors that affect measurements are diverse, the effects they produce can be divided into two classes: systematic and random. To appreciate this distinction, let us restrict the discussion to phenomena, such as chronological age, for which it seems conceptually simple to sustain the notion of a *true value*.[19] Although any particular measurement procedure might produce inaccurate readings, most people would agree that there does exist a "true" chronological age for all people.

Random errors made in ascertaining age affect the *reproducibility* (widely called "reliability" in this context) of those measurements. Let us imagine, for example, a situation in which interviewers checked one of two boxes: 0-39 years or 40+ years. Assume further that 50 percent of the population were, in fact, 0-39 years old, and 50 percent were 40+. If interviewers accidentally checked the wrong box for 1 in 100 random persons whose true age was less than 40, and there was an equal error rate in coding persons whose true age was 40+, the *aggregate* distribution of ages in the resultant survey data would be identical to the true age distribution for the population. Nevertheless, 1 percent of all individuals in the sample would have been assigned erroneous ages. Random measurement errors of this type produce measurement unreliability, which can be detected in a survey by reinterviewing respondents and asking the relevant questions again. Responses that are inconsistent between the two interviews provide evidence of measurement unreliability.

Systematic errors directly affect the *validity* of a measurement, without altering its reliability. Continuing with the example of chronological age, let us assume that, in some survey, interviewers made neither random

---

[19]In fact, when the argument is pushed far enough, there will always be cases for which the notion of true value becomes difficult to sustain (see Turner and Martin, 1984:97-106). Indeed, even chronological age cannot be known with arbitrarily high levels of precision without careful specification of the precise starting point for life. (The time of birthing, for example, does not readily accommodate specification in milliseconds.)

nor systematic errors but that 10 percent of respondents who were actually 40+ told the interviewer that they were 39. In this case, there would be a systematic error[20] in the aggregate data. The estimates generated from the survey would yield 55 percent who were under 40 and 45 percent who were 40+.[21] This discrepancy between the true distribution and the observed distribution is known as the measurement *bias*. It should be understood that such biases may occur with perfectly reliable measurements. So, for example, the 10 percent of respondents who reported a lower age might well do so again on a reinterview, which would result in perfectly consistent responses in the two interviews: the results would be reproducible, and therefore reliable, but biased nonetheless.

To assess bias in measurements, evidence can often be sought from independent sources. In the case of age, for example, public birth records might be compared with the survey reports to detect bias. (This record check might be performed for a small subsample selected for a validation study rather than for the entire sample.)

Survey Measurement of Sexual Behaviors

Overview

In this section the committee reviews what is currently known about measurement problems that beset surveys of sexual behaviors. Although the survey literature contains much methodological research on nonsampling issues (for reviews, see Bradburn et al., 1979; Rossi, Wright, and Anderson, 1983; Turner and Martin, 1984), there is good reason to suspect that the problems encountered in studying sexual behavior are unique in some respects.[22] There appears to be little that is theoretically unique, however, about the problems of *random* error and the resultant unreliability in survey measurements of sexual behavior, and there is ample evidence in the literature (see below) that respondents do provide reasonably consistent responses to survey questions on sexual behaviors.

When it comes to validation of responses, however, the problems are much more numerous, and they introduce considerable uncertainty into the interpretation of almost all survey data derived from self-reports of sexual behavior and drug use. Moreover, these problems do not appear to be amenable to quick or easy solutions. Indeed, although the committee

---

[20]Systematic error (bias) affects measures of central tendency such as averages and medians, as well as the variability in the distribution of measurements.

[21]This again assumes that the true distribution was 50 percent under age 40 and 50 percent over 40.

[22]For a review see Catania and colleagues (1990a).

later notes a number of reasonably secure inferences that can be drawn from available data and offers several recommendations for improvements in methodology, researchers and other readers of this appendix will find many more questions than answers in the following pages. In addition, these questions will involve the most fundamental matters, such as the issues raised in a question of the sort:

> Given the observation in a survey that X percent of a (probability) sample reported that they had engaged in unprotected anal intercourse during the previous week, and given the possibility that some respondents may knowingly or unknowingly distort their responses, what can be inferred about the actual proportion of the population that engaged in this practice?

A scrupulous answer to this question might well be that it is uncertain how many persons engaged in this behavior.

There are many approaches that might help reduce (but could not eliminate) this uncertainty. Careful investigations of respondents' understanding of a question, for example, could allow an assessment of biases introduced by subjects who did not comprehend the concepts. (There are anecdotal reports, for example, that researchers occasionally find a few heterosexual respondents who confuse rear-entry vaginal intercourse with anal intercourse.) Experiments with alternative question wordings might also be conducted to evaluate the extent to which the wording of a question influenced the responses given. Similarly, investigators could test alternative questioning procedures that afforded the respondent more privacy (e.g., by using self- or computer-administered questionnaires). Simple, probing questions might be used to gauge the extent of misreporting.[23] In addition, the accuracy of summary responses involving, for example, numbers of partners or rates of sexual contact, could be checked by asking a subsample of respondents to keep diaries.

Although each of these tactics provides valuable ancillary information that would reduce some of the uncertainties, none of them provides a completely satisfactory validation of these measurements. There is, for example, good reason (see Table C-4 below) to expect that the sensitivity of the topic is more of an obstacle to accurate measurement than the inherent cognitive complexity of the questions (when the time period being recalled is brief) or the unfamiliarity of the terminology. That is to say, questions such as, "Have you had sexual contact to orgasm with another man in the last week?" may be more prone to bias induced by the sensitivity of the topic than by the respondents' inability to understand the question or remember the event.

---

[23]Newcomer and Udry (1988), for example, had success with the straightforward strategy of asking respondents whether they had given false responses.

Furthermore, although there is ample reason and sufficient empirical evidence to justify experimentation with alternative methods of ensuring respondents' privacy, there is also reason to believe that some respondents may conceal behaviors even in the most private reporting setting and that subsequently they will not admit that they did so. This possibility must be given considerable weight in the face of statutes in many states that classify some sexual behaviors (including oral sex, male-female and male-male anal intercourse) as crimes.[24] Finally, there is the possibility that behaviors in which the respondent engages while under the influence of excessive drugs or alcohol may be poorly recalled, if at all.

Given these considerations, lingering concern about the trustworthiness of such survey estimates is virtually inevitable. Nonetheless, some inferences may be made with relative certainty if one is prepared to make assumptions about the direction of reporting biases.

Inference in the Presence of Bias
It could reasonably be argued that the preponderant source of bias in reports of sexual behaviors or drug use for many (but not all) populations and measurement procedures will be caused by respondents underreporting their behaviors. It might be hypothesized further that this underreporting will follow the norms and taboos of the respondents' society. If this hypothesis were true, one would expect the most extreme underreporting for behaviors that are most disparaged and that carry the most severe penalties for discovery (e.g., adult-child sex, rape, etc.). Similarly, one would expect the least reporting bias for behaviors that are sanctioned or encouraged (e.g., vaginal sex between spouses). (Indeed, in this latter case, one might anticipate an exception to the rule of underreporting. For married couples, it might be reasonable to anticipate some pressure to conceal a low rate or absence of sexual contact between spouses.)

For cases in which underreporting is a reasonable assumption, a safe inference from well-collected survey measurements is that the resultant estimates represent a reasonable lower bound on the true prevalence of the behavior in the population. Such a tack has been explicitly taken in methodological studies of sexual and other sensitive behaviors. For example, investigators who seek to improve the reporting of sexual behaviors such as masturbation (Bradburn et al., 1979) and the reporting of

---

[24]In 1986, the Supreme Court ruled that states could enforce criminal sanctions against consensual homosexual behaviors, even when practiced by adults in the privacy of their own home (*Bowers* v. *Hardwick,* No. 85-140, June 30, 1986). The statute at issue (Georgia Code Annotated at 16-6-2, 1984) held that "(a) A person commits the offense of sodomy when he performs or submits to any sexual act involving the sex organs of one person and the mouth or anus of another . . . ." The argument and opinion in that case implied, however, that although the application of this statute was upheld in the case of male-male sex, it would not be held constitutional if applied to a married male-female couple.

alcohol and drug use (e.g., Waterton and Duffy, 1984) typically assume that the net reporting bias for those behaviors is negative, that is, more persons conceal behaviors in which they have engaged than report behaviors in which they have not engaged. Consequently, these investigators attempt to identify survey procedures (e.g., the use of SAQs) that would increase reporting of these behaviors (in the aggregate). Similarly, a recent attempt to estimate the prevalence of same-gender sex among men in the United States (Fay et al., 1989) argued that the resultant estimates should be treated as lower-bound estimates, on the assumption that the net reporting bias would be negative.

Although this strategy does allow lower bound inferences to be made with relative confidence, it is not an entirely satisfying solution because point estimates (e.g., actual frequencies or means) are, after all, of considerable interest. Indeed, these estimates figure centrally in two of the most important research challenges of the epidemic's second decade: determining whether there are declines over time in the incidence of sexual behaviors that risk transmitting HIV, and assessing the effectiveness of AIDS education and prevention programs by comparing the behaviors of persons who participate in those programs with the behaviors of those who do not. Both of these tasks require comparison of the distribution of behaviors reported by different samples or by the same sample at different points in time to detect differences. Changes in behavior over time or the superior effectiveness of particular interventions in changing behavior could then be inferred. If the only statements about these issues that can be made with certainty must be phrased in terms of lower bounds, these important questions cannot be answered.

Assumption of Constant Bias in Measurements
To answer the questions referred to above, it is neither theoretically necessary to make measurements without bias, nor always required to have accurate assessments of the magnitude and direction of the bias. One can detect change (or intergroup differences) without ever knowing the "true" value, providing it is possible to *assume* that the reporting bias is equivalent at the two points in time (or across the two groups). If the study makes no attempt to validate the self-reports, this assumption is considered to be implicit in studies of time trends or intergroup differences in behavior. This assumption, however, is often problematic.

It is quite possible, for example, that the reporting bias itself will vary over time. Respondents (and the population at large) may become more accustomed to questions about sexual behavior and may be less likely to conceal sensitive behaviors. (For example, condoms, anal intercourse, and other topics that were rarely discussed in the media prior to the AIDS epidemic now appear with greater frequency.) On the other hand, as the result of an educational program or other intervention effort, respondents may become less likely to report unsafe behaviors. Indeed, it might plausibly be argued that the same social and psychological pressures used by intervention programs to encourage behavioral change also make it less likely that respondents will report these same behaviors.[25] Thus, the group receiving an intervention may also have its reporting bias modified in the direction of *less* complete reporting of risky behaviors.)[26]

Approaches to Validation

Measures of sexual behaviors may have much in common with measurements of subjective phenomena (e.g., attitudes, opinions, intentions).[27] Although sexual behavior can, in theory, be observed, there are only a few special circumstances in which the testimony of independent observers could be used to validate respondents' self-reports.[28] Outside these special circumstances, there are no obvious independent measurements that could provide a basis for directly assessing the extent of bias in self-reports of sexual behavior. As discussed below, however, there may be indirect approaches that could be used for such assessments.

---

[25] There is also evidence, however, that in some interventions directed toward IV drug users, increased rapport between clients and program staff over time results in more honest reporting of risky behaviors. D. Worth, Department of Epidemiology and Social Medicine, Montefiore Medical Center, personal communication, June 19, 1989.

[26] Similar arguments apply to efforts to study the "association" between reports of sexual behavior and other variables. Bias in measurements may covary with variables of substantive interest and thus produce spurious correlations. For example, studies of same-gender sexual contact indicate that respondents with college educations report more contacts in childhood and as adults than are reported by those with less than a college education. Although this variation may reflect a true difference between groups with different levels of education, it is also possible that college-educated respondents may be less likely than those with no college education to conceal same-gender sexual behaviors in the context of a survey. To the extent that such differential concealment occurred, a spurious correlation would arise between education and the prevalence of same-gender sexual contacts as a result of the nonequivalent measurement biases in the groups.

[27] In 1984, another NRC panel published a review of concepts and methods for assessing the error structure of survey measurements of subjective phenomena (Turner and Martin, 1984). The report concluded that validation for such measurements might best be sought in demonstrations at an aggregate level that time-series of these measurements were related in a theoretically reasonable fashion to independent time-series that measured objective phenomena to which the subjective phenomena ought to be related. Sufficiently long time-series are not available for most survey measurements of subjective phenomena, but the available data indicate that self-reported attitudes toward the safety of different contraceptives (Beniger, 1984), public perceptions of national "problems" (MacKuen, 1981, 1984), and presidential popularity (MacKuen and Turner, 1984) do show the expected relationships over time.

[28] One such circumstance involves the report of sexual contact by a couple in which each respondent is reporting on the same behavior—for example, the frequency of coitus or the use of a condom; see A.L. Clark and Wallin [1964] and Levinger [1966] for examples.

Validation Using STD Rates. To assess the validity of reports of sexual behavior, the committee's first report recommended consideration of a strategy parallel to that used with subjective measurements. The committee argued:

> It may be possible, for example, to construct a convincing validation by demonstrating that an independent series of measurements of change in the incidence of gonorrhea in a population over time could be predicted from a concurrent time-series monitoring the self-reported incidence of unprotected sexual contacts with new partners in the same population. Although there are many potential pitfalls to executing a successful validation in this way, the committee believes that the feasibility of using such indirect procedures should be given further, careful consideration. (Turner, Miller, and Moses, 1989:150)

The tentativeness of the committee's advice on this validation strategy reflected the practical and theoretical difficulties that attend the use of sexually transmitted disease (STD) statistics for this purpose. The committee noted, for example, that national statistics on STDs may be in need of improvement. It recommended a careful review of these data systems and, if necessary, an increase in resources to improve them (Turner, Miller, and Moses, 1989:167). Furthermore, for any group, the trends in STD rates over time will reflect phenomena such as the changes, if any, in the behaviors of group members that expose them to infection, trends in the rates of STDs among the population from which the group selects its new sexual contacts, and changes in reporting practices. It is thus possible to observe in a particular group a rise in STD rates over time that occurs concurrently with a true decline in the rates of "risky" behaviors. This seemingly paradoxical outcome can result from rising STD rates in the population at large, which mask the protective effect of behavioral change in the smaller subgroup. (That is, although "risky behaviors" are less frequent in number, they are practiced with partners who are more likely to be infected.)[29] Nevertheless, despite the attractiveness of the strategy of conducting validation studies of sexual behavior using STD rates, no assurance currently exists that such a strategy could be made to work.

Psychometric Approaches to Validity. The approaches discussed above follow from measurement traditions in the physical sciences. Yet there is also a robust tradition of measurement in psychology, which has added to the literature both a substantial body of empirical work

---

[29]Numerous other artifacts bedevil this strategy as well. For example, it has been observed that the institution of aggressive STD control programs may inflate the number of cases of STDs that are actually reported. Contact tracing may also serve to bring more STD cases to the attention of public health workers.

and, more important, alternative ways of viewing the error structure of measurements for variables, like intelligence, that are never subject to direct observation. The psychometric literature is vast, and it would be impossible to summarize it here. Excellent texts and reviews are available elsewhere (Gulliksen, 1950; Cronbach and Gleser, 1965; Anastasi, 1976; Wigdor and Garner, 1982). For the purposes of this report, it may suffice to note the approaches to validation offered in this literature. Most important among these are criterion validity, content validity, and construct validity.[30]

- *Criterion validity* for an intelligence test refers to the extent to which a given measurement or test is predictive of the properties it purports to measure. Consider, for example, the Scholastic Aptitude Test, or SAT, which is supposed to measure the test taker's aptitude for college-level coursework. Its criterion validity could be assessed by measuring the correlation between the scores of individuals on the test and some direct indicator of the performance of these individuals in college.[31]

- *Content validity* (sometimes called face validity) is not assessed empirically. Rather, it involves a judgment that the questions being asked are appropriate (or inappropriate) to the characteristic being measured. Thus, it might be judged that questions that tested reading comprehension and written composition had high content validity (i.e., were "appropriate") for a measure that purported to assess the likelihood an individual would succeed in college. In contrast, a measure of the person's athletic prowess might be judged to have low face validity for success in most college programs.

- *Construct validity* refers to the extent to which a set of measurements relate to one another in a coherent way as specified by some (formal or informal) theory. Unlike criterion validity, construct validity cannot be reduced to a single correlation coefficient. Construct validity instead involves a judgment about the extent to which a given measurement fits together with other measurements in a manner that is theoretically meaningful. (In assessing a questionnaire measure

[30] The discussion in this paragraph draws heavily on that in Turner and Martin (1984:Vol. 1, 120–125).

[31] This example simplifies matters somewhat. The criterion validity could be directly assessed by admitting all students to the same college program and then measuring their performance. In reality, practical considerations make such an uncomplicated assessment impossible (e.g., low-scoring students are not admitted to many colleges and universities). These complications require various adjustments and simplifying assumptions.

of psychological depression, for example, psychologists expect to find a coherent pattern of associations between feelings of helplessness and despair, self-destructive fantasy or behavior, somatic complaints such as sleep disturbances, and negative emotions [Hamilton, 1960; Beck et al., 1961; Himmelweit and Turner, 1982].)

While these three psychometric notions of validity can be helpful in approaching the problems involved in validating survey measures of sexual behaviors, their past use has sometimes been less than optimal. One of the most important failings results from overreliance on correlation coefficients in reporting on the validity of measurements. Although ideal self-report measurements of a phenomenon ought to be perfectly correlated with (error-free) direct observations of the same phenomenon, the presence of a very high or even perfect correlation does not, in itself, guarantee that the survey measurement is not contaminated by significant biases. Consider, for example, hypothetical reporting biases that caused the frequency of anal sex to be underreported by 20, 40, and 60 percent from its "true" incidence in three measurements. Such biases would yield three measurements that differed substantially, but that were, nonetheless, perfectly correlated ($r = 1.0$) with one another. These correlations would occur even though the mean frequency of anal sex observed using these three measuring instruments would be quite different.

If one imagines these different reporting biases to be characteristics of different time periods (or different intervention conditions in an evaluation study), one could conceivably report equivalent "validity coefficients" over time (or experimental conditions), although there were, in fact, substantially different and undetected biases in the measurements.[32] It is unfortunately the case that the current literature contains numerous instances in which researchers report only the bivariate correlations as evidence of validity (or reliability). Indeed, readers will note in the following pages numerous instances in which the committee has had to rely exclusively on such coefficients because the published reports of studies do not provide other needed information.

In this regard, the committee also notes that, when examining the validity and reliability of their measurements, researchers would be well advised to avoid a premature rush to rely on statistical procedures that assume (multivariate) normality. Many measurements of epidemiological interest have distributions that are not normal. Indeed, there may be strong reasons to focus special concern on biases that disproportionately

---

[32]These differences *could,* of course, be detected by examining the means or the intercept of the regression of one measurement on the other.

affect extreme segments of the response distribution. For example, persons with very large numbers of sexual and drug-using partners play a disproportionate role in the spread of HIV. It is for this reason that the committee previously recommended that reports of "averages" or tabular displays that hide the long "tails" of the distributions of these variables be avoided whenever possible (Turner, Miller, and Moses, 1989:Ch. 2). For the same reason, researchers who analyze and report on the error structure of their survey measurements should attend not only to the overall performance of their instruments but also to biases and errors that may disproportionately affect the reports of persons who are in the high-activity end of the response distribution.

EMPIRICAL STUDIES OF SEXUAL BEHAVIORS

Validation

There is only a very limited range of evidence that can be collected to provide independent corroboration of the validity of self-reported sexual behaviors. In the past, three broad types of research evidence have been collected:

- partner reports, in which regular sexual partners respond to the same questions as the study respondent;
- "invalidation evidence," which is derived from longitudinal studies in which it is possible to obtain some measure of reporting accuracy by examining the temporal patterns for impossible temporal sequences (e.g., persons who report having engaged in sexual intercourse when interviewed at age 15 but who report at a later age that they have never had intercourse); and
- clinical evidence of sexual activity that can be used to verify the fact that a particular sexual activity has occurred (the committee is aware of only one study in which this sort of evidence has been gathered).

Partner Reports

Kinsey and his colleagues reported the first empirical study of which the committee is aware in which the self-reports of two sexual partners were compared to explore the reports' accuracy. The Kinsey team used 231 pairs of spouses who appear to have been individually interviewed[33]

---

[33]The description of this research (Kinsey et al., 125–128) does not indicate whether the same interviewer questioned both spouses. The text does indicate, however, that "in many instances there were intervals of two to six years or more between the interviews with the two spouses" (p. 127).

TABLE C-2 Findings of Kinsey et al.'s (1948) validation study of sexual behaviors reported by spouses.

COMPARING DATA FROM 231 PAIRS OF SPOUSES

CASES	ITEMS INVOLVED	UNIT OF MEASUREMENT	IDENT. RSPNS. %	WITHIN 1 UNIT OF IDENT. %	COEFFIC. OF CORREL.	MEAN OF HUSBAND'S REPORTS	MEAN OF WIFE'S REPORTS	DIFF. OF MEANS: ♂ − ♀
	Vital Statistics				Pears. r			
229	Years married	1 year	88.6	96.1	0.99	6.35 ± 0.42	6.40 ± 0.42	−0.05
214	Pre-marital acquaint.	12 mon.	57.9	86.9	0.88	42.11 ± 2.83	40.88 ± 2.74	+1.23
156	Engagement	4 mon.	57.1	78.2	0.83	12.64 ± 1.03	12.85 ± 1.07	−0.21
226	Age, ♂ at marr.	1 year	68.6	97.3	0.99	27.27 ± 0.37	27.17 ± 0.37	+0.10
228	Age, ♀ at marr.	1 year	61.8	92.5	0.63	24.88 ± 0.32	24.75 ± 0.32	+0.13
231	No. children	1 child	99.6	100.0	0.99	0.90 ± 0.09	0.90 ± 0.09	0.00
185	No. abortions	1 event	90.3	98.4	0.76	0.32 ± 0.06	0.41 ± 0.08	−0.09
227	Lapse, first coitus—marr.	6 mon.	74.4	89.4	0.85	5.09 ± 0.88	4.72 ± 0.86	+0.37
87	Lapse, marr. —first birth	6 mon.	66.7	89.7	0.96	28.05 ± 1.99	28.19 ± 2.01	−0.14
220	Educ. level, ♂	2 years	84.1	99.1	0.97	16.23 ± 0.26	16.16 ± 0.25	+0.07
223	Educ. level, ♀	2 years	79.4	97.8	0.92	14.41 ± 0.21	14.67 ± 0.21	−0.26
219	Occup. class, ♂	1 of 9	91.8	98.6	0.98	5.32 ± 0.14	5.27 ± 0.14	+0.05
	Coital Freq.							
223	Max. freq., marit. coitus	2/wk.	33.2	68.2	0.54	6.72 ± 0.31	6.74 ± 0.31	−0.02
225	Av. freq., early marr.	1/wk.	34.7	73.3	0.50	2.73 ± 0.13	3.00 ± 0.14	−0.27
226	Av. freq., now	1/wk.	56.6	88.1	0.60	1.91 ± 0.11	2.21 ± 0.13	−0.30
218	% with orgasm, ♀	10%	55.0	71.1	0.75	69.82 ± 2.16	66.83 ± 2.26	+2.99
	Techniques in coital foreplay				Tetra-choric r	% Husbands Reporting Yes	% Wives Reporting Yes	
229	Kiss	Yes, No	97		0.92	95.6 ± 1.35	99.1 ± 0.62	−3.5
228	Deep kiss	Yes, No	85		0.72	85.1 ± 2.36	82.0 ± 2.54	+3.1
228	Hand—♀ breast	Yes, No	95		0.78	95.6 ± 1.36	96.5 ± 1.22	−0.9
228	Mouth—♀ breast	Yes, No	89		0.79	90.4 ± 2.04	86.0 ± 2.43	+4.4
229	Hand—♀ genitalia	Yes, No	90		0.61	92.6 ± 1.73	92.2 ± 1.77	+0.4
226	Hand—♂ genitalia	Yes, No	85		0.70	83.6 ± 2.46	85.8 ± 2.32	− .2
220	Mouth—♀ genitalia	Yes, No	82		0.84	35.9 ± 3.23	37.3 ± 3.26	−1.4
226	Mouth—♂ genitalia	Yes, No	85		0.93	33.6 ± 3.14	35.4 ± 3.18	−1.8
	Coital techniq.							
228	Male above	Yes, No	93		0.75	94.3 ± 1.54	93.5 ± 1.63	+0.8
228	Female above	Yes, No	76		0.74	54.8 ± 3.30	49.1 ± 3.31	+5.7
224	On side	Yes, No	76		0.68	39.3 ± 3.26	37.1 ± 3.23	+2.2
221	Sitting	Yes, No	81		0.63	19.0 ± 2.64	17.6 ± 2.56	+1.4
227	Standing	Yes, No	89		0.64	10.1 ± 2.00	7.9 ± 1.79	+2.2
224	Rear entrance	Yes, No	83		0.77	24.6 ± 2.88	17.4 ± 2.53	+7.2
186	Coitus nude	Yes, No	90		0.82	87.1 ± 2.46	89.2 ± 2.28	−2.1
223	Multiple orgasm, ♂	Yes, No	95		0.74	4.9 ± 1.45	4.1 ± 1.33	+0.8

following the normal procedures used in the Kinsey studies (see Gebhard and Johnson, 1979; Turner, Miller, Moses, 1989:80–83). The results obtained from comparing the reports of each spouse regarding coital frequency and technique are summarized in Table C-2. The table shows— as Kinsey, Pomeroy, and Martin (1948:125) themselves remark—"[a]n amazing agreement between the statements of the husbands and of the wives in each marriage . . . " Given the relatively small sample size, few instances of bias in this study would reach conventional standards of significance. There is, however, a modest trend for females to report less frequently than their male partners the practice of female superior and rear-entry coitus; females also tended to report a higher average frequency of coitus both in their early marriage and at the time of the interview. In assessing the rather high degree of congruence between the reports of spouses in Kinsey's study, one is also well advised to note the interpretive caveat that Kinsey, Pomeroy, and Martin (1948:125) offered, namely, that "allowance must be made for the possibility that there may have been collusion between some of the partners, and a conscious or unconscious agreement to distort the fact[s]."

Following the example set by Kinsey, subsequent sexual behavior researchers have on occasion gathered data from spouses and other partners to gauge the accuracy of self-reported data. With some exceptions, these studies do not cover as comprehensive a range of sexual behaviors as Kinsey explored. They are, nonetheless, perhaps of more relevance for understanding the qualities of the behavioral data that are routinely used in AIDS research. This is so not only because the social norms regarding sexual activity have changed since the 1940s but also because the methodologies employed in recent studies tend to involve standardized interviews or self-administered questionnaires rather than the Kinsey-type interviews that last many hours.

Table C-3 summarizes the results of selected recent studies that use spousal reports to gauge the accuracy of reporting of sexual behaviors. One of the first things regarding this tabulation that will be noted—and lamented—is the relative dearth of information on response congruence that is typically supplied. Kinsey and colleagues presented the proportions of spousal pairs who were in perfect agreement and who agreed within ±1 unit; in addition, they supplied correlation coefficients and means and standard deviations for reports by husbands and wives. In contrast, recent studies typically present only correlation coefficients. As noted previously, these coefficients do not provide some of the information that is most crucial in understanding the error structure of measurements. They do not, for example, allow any statement about bias—for example, for heterosexual couples, the extent to which husbands' reports

TABLE C-3 Post-Kinsey Validation Studies of Self-Reported Sexual Behaviors Comparing Reports of Sexual Partners

Study	Sample	Method	Findings
Clark and Wallin (1964)	428 male-female couples (married)[a]	SAQ; frequency of coitus[b]	Correlations of .57 to .61 between husbands' and wives' reports; roughly equal means for husbands and wives
Levinger (1966)	60 male-female couples (married)[c]	Interview question; frequency of coitus (average in relationship)[d]	Mean frequency reported: 7.78 (wives) and 6.96 (husbands); correlation not reported
Seage et al. (1989)	170 male-male couples	Interview	Spearman correlations between number of occurrences reported by two partners: .63 to .76 for oral sex without ejaculation;[e] .63 to .80 for oral sex with ejaculation; .60 to .92 for anal sex without ejaculation; .75 to .79 for anal sex with ejaculation; .73 to .87 for rimming; .48 to .99 for fisting
Jacobson & Moore (1981)	36 male-female couples (married) including 16 "distressed" & 20 non-distressed	Daily checklists of various sexual behaviors[f]	60 percent agreement[g] between spouses in "distressed" couples; 67 percent agreement between spouses in nondistressed couples; (difference was not significant)
Blumstein & Schwartz (1983, 1989)[h]	3,600 male-female couples (married); 650 male-female couples (unmarried); 965 male-male couples; and 770 female-female couples	SAQ	Correlations of .78 to .86 for frequency of intercourse over last year;[i] .66 to .70 for how frequently cunnilingus is part of sex;[j] .71 (heterosexuals) and .38 (gay men) for how frequently fellatio is part of sex;[j] .65 (gay men) for how frequently anal intercourse is part of sex[j]
Coates et al. (1988)	75 male-male couples (one partner with AIDS)	Interview	Correlations between frequency reported by index case and by partner: .82 to .88 for mouth-penis contact;[k] .72 to .75 for ejaculation in partner's mouth;[l] .90 to .91 for insertion of penis in rectum; .85 to .89 for ejaculation in rectum; .57 for insertion of finger in partner's anus;[m] .53 to .71 for tongue-anus contact;[n] .68 to .81 for insertion of object in anus;[o] .49 to .69 for insertion of hand in anus[p]

NOTES: SAQ: Self-Administered Questionnaire.

[a]"White, native born, and when first studied were predominantly residents of Chicago. Only a fifth of the men and a third of the women lacked some college education" (Clark and Wallin, 1964:168).

[b]Question: "About how many times a month have you had sexual relations with your wife [husband] in the past 12 months? (Give the number that tells the average number of times per month.)"

[c]"60 middle class couples, all of whom had children, had been married four to twenty-two years, and who lived in the Greater Cleveland area. The average couple was in its late thirties, had been married 13.6 years, had three children ..."

[d]Question: "Ordinarily, how many times a month do you have sexual relations with your wife [husband]? (Except during periods of pregnancy or physical illness)."

[e]The range reflects correlations reported for three groups: concordant HIV-negative couples (both partners are HIV negative), concordant HIV-positive couples (both partners are HIV positive), and discordant couples (one partner is HIV positive, the other is HIV negative).

[f]Spouse Observation Checklist (SOC): "The SOC, consisting of 409 items, is a comprehensive list of potential events that can occur in a marital relationship" (Jacobsen and Moore, 1981:271). Self-Monitoring Checklist (SMC): The SMC was a parallel checklist that required the spouse of the respondent also to track his or her own behaviors. "Sex" behaviors included items such as: "we engaged in sexual intercourse; spouse petted me; spouse caressed me with his mouth."

[g]Results were calculated as the total number of individual behaviors checked by both spouses divided by the number checked by both plus the number checked by one spouse but not the other. Unfortunately, the report of the study does not break down the results by different behaviors. It is reasonable to suspect that there might be more agreement about intercourse than about ambiguous and possibly less memorable events such as "spouse caressed me with his mouth."

[h]Original research reported in Blumstein and Schwartz (1983); reliabilities reported by Blumstein (personal communication, June 21, 1989).

[i]Eight-point scale: (1) daily or almost daily, (2) 3–4 times a week, (3) 1–2 times a week, (4) 2–3 times a month, (5) once a month, (6) once every few months, (7) a few times in last year, (8) never.

[j]Five-point scale: (1) always, (2) usually, (3) sometimes, (4) rarely, (5) never.

[k]Note that two correlations are reported: one for insertion by the index case and one for insertion by the partner. They are not, however, markedly different.

[l]Note that two correlations are reported: one for ejaculation by the index case and one for ejaculation by the partner. They are not, however, markedly different.

[m]Reliabilities were identical for case-partner and partner-case contacts.

[n].53 is reliability reported for index case having tongue contact with partner's anus; .71 is correlation for partner having tongue contact with index case's anus.

[o].68 for index case inserting object in partner's anus; .81 for the reverse case.

[p].49 for index case inserting hand in partner's anus; .69 for the reverse case.

systematically differ from those provided by wives.

Overall, the results in Table C-3 together with the Kinsey results suggest that there is substantial but not complete agreement between sexual partners in describing the behaviors in which a couple has engaged. Indeed, in some of the instances reported in Table C-3, the nature of the questions makes the levels of agreement that were obtained somewhat surprising. Coates and coworkers (1988), for example, requested that the gay men in their study report the total number of sexual encounters they had with a particular partner and the total number of times (or percentage of encounters) during which they engaged in specific sexual behaviors. Given that these men reported a mean of more than 250 encounters with their partners occurring over an average of more than two years, accurate reporting from memory was clearly beyond the ability of most respondents. Nonetheless, the correlational evidence suggests that sexual partners provided quite similar reports of their behaviors.

Similarly, Levinger (1966) asked heterosexual married couples to estimate the mean frequency of intercourse during their marriage. (The couples were married an average of approximately 14 years.) Although one would prefer some report of the joint distribution of spouses' reports, it is impressive nonetheless that the mean monthly frequency of intercourse reported by husbands and wives in this study varied by less than one act per month. Blumstein and Schwartz (1983) report parallel evidence from male-male, male-female, and female-female couples indicating that reports of the frequency of intercourse over the preceding year were quite consistent between partners ($r = .78$ to $.86$), although somewhat lower levels of consistency were found for questions about other sexual behaviors.

Other Validation Techniques

Although partner validation provides the most obvious source of independent information on sexual behavior, it is not the only validation method that has been used.[34] In 1966 J.P. Clark and Tifft reported the use of a polygraph (lie detector) to motivate respondents to correct misreports

---

[34] Occasionally, the literature reports studies that use expert judgments to validate behavioral measurements. For example, Koss and Gidycz (1985) reported the use of a self-administered questionnaire to identify "hidden" rapes (i.e., those not reported to police) in samples of college students (242 female and 144 male). Validity was subsequently assessed by comparing questionnaire responses with the results of interviews with a "post-master's level psychologist." Twenty-five percent of survey respondents consented to the interview, and the author reported correlations of .73 (female) and .61 (male) when questionnaire data and judgments made by psychologists were aggregated in categories (no victimization, sexual coercion, sexual abuse, and sexual assault). The interpretation of these results is problematic, however, because there is no assurance that the judgments made by the "psychologist" were more accurate than those obtained from the survey questionnaire.

they may have made in a previously completed questionnaire. By monitoring the changes made by the respondents, Clark and Tifft obtained a measure of the magnitude and direction of reporting biases that may occur in surveys of sexual behavior. Clark and Tifft's subjects were 45 college males who reported on (lifetime) experiences with prostitutes, sexual coercion, homosexual contacts, masturbation, and nonmarital sex. (It should be emphasized that the criterion measure was not the polygraph judgment but rather the subjects' behavior in "correcting" their answers to the questionnaire when confronted with the polygraph.)[35]

Table C-4 presents selected results from this study. It will be seen that for every measurement a substantial fraction of the sexual behaviors that were finally reported were reported only after the possibility of lie detection was introduced. Thus, although virtually every male (95 percent), when confronted with the polygraph, indicated that he had masturbated, 30 percent of the men in the sample denied masturbating on the initial questionnaire and subsequently changed their response. Similarly, although 22.5 percent of these college men ultimately reported some male-male sexual contact, 15 percent of the men initially denied such contact and subsequently changed their answers.

As these results indicate, the response bias in questionnaire measures can be substantial. Furthermore, the net bias (i.e., the difference between the percentages overreporting and underreporting) is typically weighted in the direction of underreporting. Empirical evidence such as this underlies the common assumption that survey measurements of sexual and drug use behaviors may set lower bounds on the actual frequency of these behaviors in the population.

Udry and Morris (1967) used a different strategy to study a behavior that may have been less sensitive to report—that is, intercourse for married women. These investigators collected daily urine specimens for a period of 90 days and tested the specimens for the presence of

[35] Subjects were given multiple opportunities to change their initial answers. In postsurvey interviews, researchers would ask a respondent for his "utmost cooperation in making his response accurate and [the researchers] strongly alluded to the likelihood of inaccurate responses being given on questionnaires administered in group situations" (J.P. Clark and Tifft, 1966:519). The respondent was then asked to retrieve his questionnaire using the identification number that had been assigned and "to make whatever modifications (in private) that were necessary to bring it to 100 percent accuracy."

Subsequently, subjects were told that the researchers would like them to submit voluntarily to a polygraph examination. (No subjects refused the polygraph.) During the polygraph examination, the researchers reported that "when an indication of deception occurred with one of our respondents, the examiner asked the respondent if he wanted to make a change in his response." The responses supplied by respondents after all "corrections" had been made are taken to be more accurate than those originally supplied in the survey. Although this assumption seems fair, there is, nonetheless, some possibility that respondents may have altered their answers for reasons that would not result in increased accuracy (e.g., to comply with covert social pressure).

TABLE C-4 Selected Results Reported in Clark and Tifft's Study of Bias in Questionnaire Measurements of "Deviant" Behavior: Percentage of college men ($N = 45$) who: (a) report selected sexual behaviors when confronted with lie detector, (b) deny behavior in questionnaire but report it when confronted with lie detector (underreporting), and (c) report behavior in questionnaire but deny it when confronted with lie detector (overreporting)

	Percent Reporting Behavior With Lie Detector (a)	Estimate of Bias	
Behavior		Under-reporting (b)	Over-reporting (c)
Had sex relations with a person of the same sex	22.5	15.0	5.0
Masturbated	95.0	30.0	5.0
Attempted to force or forced a female to have sexual intercourse with me	15.0	7.5	2.5
Had sex relations with a person of the opposite sex (other than my wife)	55.0	17.5	15.0
Gotten a female other than my wife pregnant	7.5	2.5	2.5
Visited a house of prostitution	17.5	2.5	2.5
Had in my possession pictures, books, or other materials which were obviously obscene and prepared to arouse someone sexually	50.0	12.5	7.5

SOURCE: J.P. Clark and Tifft (1986).

sperm to validate the women's self-reports of intercourse (which were also obtained daily). Although the absence of sperm does not provide definitive evidence that intercourse had *not* occurred, the presence of sperm can be taken as evidence that intercourse had occurred at some point in the recent past.[36] Fifteen (of 58) women in this study showed evidence of sperm in their urine on one or more occasions. For 12 of the women, all 32 reports of the presence of sperm in their daily urines corresponded with *prior* reports of coitus. Among the other 3 women, there were 5 (of 9) instances in which sperm were present but the subject had not reported intercourse during the preceding 48 hours.

Independent evidence validating self-reports is precious. Yet for

[36]There is some uncertainty about how long sperm may be found after intercourse. Udry and Morris adopted the standard that the sighting of three or more intact sperm was consistent with a report of coitus during the previous 48-hour period. (In making these judgments, the authors centrifuged the urine specimens and analyzed one drop of the sediment for 10 minutes.)

many studies, obtaining such evidence is impossible (owing to the "private" nature of the behavior) or so difficult as to become infeasible. Consequently, other evidence is required to sustain the claim that a particular data collection method is useful for research.

Replication of Surveys on Samples of the Same Population

In lodging a claim that measurement in a particular domain is "scientific," one may legitimately pose the question: Do independent attempts to measure the same phenomenon produce consistent results? Given the litany of possible contaminants that can corrupt the measurement process, there is substantial interest in knowing whether similar answers about characteristics of the same population can be obtained by different survey organizations using roughly comparable techniques. Because of the dearth of basic research on sexual behavior in particular and the lack of investment in methodological research in general, there is no ample stock of material from which to make such comparisons. There are, however, two examples that demonstrate the important point that survey measurements of sexual behaviors can produce reliable measures of behavior in well-defined populations.

Proportion of Teenagers Who Are Sexually Active

The most thorough demonstration is offered in the literature on teenage sexual activity (an area that fortunately received some investment prior to AIDS to pursue studies to understand patterns of sexual behavior). Kahn, Kalsbeek, and Hofferth (1988) recently published a comparison of rates of teenage sexual activity reported by the 1959-1963 birth cohort in three independent surveys:

- the 1979 national survey of young women undertaken by Zelnik and Kantner (1980) and the Institute for Survey Research of Temple University (KZ79 in Figure C-3);
- the 1982 National Survey of Family Growth conducted by Westat for the National Center for Health Statistics (NSFG in Figure C-3); and
- the 1983 wave of the National Longitudinal Survey of Youth conducted by the National Opinion Research Center (NORC, University of Chicago) for a consortium of federal agencies (NLSY in Figure C-3).

The comparison undertaken by Kahn, Kalsbeek, and Hofferth involved surveys that had several systematic differences in methodology. The three studies differed, for example, in the precise wording of the

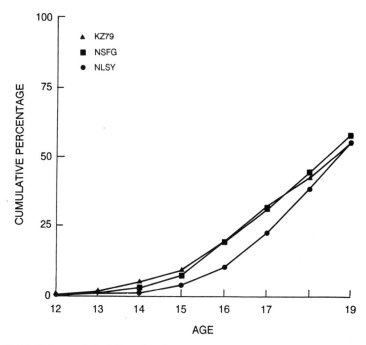

FIGURE C-3 Estimates derived from three independent surveys of the cumulative percentage of teenagers sexually active, by exact ages. NOTE: Survey estimates have been adjusted to make surveys as comparable as possible by, for example, eliminating population segments that are not included in all three surveys. SOURCE: J. R. Kahn, Kalsbeek, and Hofferth (1988).

question, the age of the respondents at the time they were asked to recall their early sexual experiences, and study design. Adjustments were made (e.g., eliminating population segments that were not included in all surveys) to make the studies as comparable as possible; the adjusted proportions of women reporting sexual activity by each age are shown in Figure C-3.[37] This plot shows that there is a very close correspondence between two of the three surveys and that the third survey (the National Longitudinal Survey of Youth) produces estimates that are quite similar for ages 12 to 15 and 18 to 19; however, it provides substantially lower estimates of sexual activity for this cohort of women at ages 16 and 17. Although these observed discrepancies are not trivial and are

[37]Respondents in the 1979 survey by Zelnik and Kantner (1980) were asked: When was the first time you had intercourse? That is, in what month and year? How old were you at the time? Respondents in the National Survey of Family Growth were asked: Thinking back after your first menstrual period, when did you have sexual intercourse for the first time—what month and year was that? (If date was not known): How old were you at that time? Was it before your n-th birthday, or after? Respondents in the National Longitudinal Survey were asked: At what age did you first have sexual intercourse? (Source: Kahn, Kalsbeek, and Hofferth, 1988:193, Table 3).

much larger than would be expected to occur as a result of sampling error alone, one cannot lose sight of the very substantial similarity of the findings obtained by the three surveys. Furthermore, Kahn, Kalsbeek, and Hofferth (1988) go on to demonstrate that the three surveys produce statistically equivalent estimates of the net *association*[38] between sexual activity (i.e., having engaged in intercourse at a given age) and various background variables. The background variables used in this analysis included the exact year of birth, mother's education, whether the respondent was Catholic, and whether the respondent lived with both natural parents at age 14. Of 93 tests for survey-specific differences in the net association between the background variable and sexual activity, in only one case was the estimated discrepancy judged to be different from zero with a *p* less than 0.05.[39]

The discrepancies observed among young women aged 16 to 17 are large enough to suggest that naive comparisons of results obtained in different surveys can be misleading if the basis for inference is sampling error alone. It has come to be a well-accepted notion in the literature on survey measurements (as it long has been in analytical measurements in other disciplines) that variability in measurements among procedures, investigators, and laboratories cannot be determined by a simple extrapolation of the variances observed in measurements from a single experiment. Rather, different procedures, investigators, and laboratories typically produce measurements that converge on values over repeated measurements that are nevertheless not the grand mean of all measurements. Thus it is not unusual to find that the effects of minor variabilities in the particular procedures used by different investigators and research organizations may contaminate individual measurements to some degree. In the case of the three surveys discussed above, however, the overall impact of this effect, although large enough to be statistically detectable, is not so large as to lead to markedly different inferences about the patterns of teenage sexual behavior in this cohort of young women. Indeed, it is somewhat comforting to note that the two cross-sectional surveys (by Zelnik and Kantner and the NSFG) produced very similar results at all ages.

As for the discrepant results of the longitudinal survey, surveys that perform repeated measurements of the same respondent may have many

---

[38]The net association was tested by entering as dummy variables the product of the dichotomous variable reflecting the characteristic of interest (e.g., Catholic or not) and dummy variables for the surveys.

[39]Note that with 100 independent comparisons, one expects random fluctuations to produce five discrepancies of this magnitude when the true discrepancy across all tests is zero (and the significance level is set at .05).

characteristics that can affect typical survey measurements. At a minimum, the design of the longitudinal survey must not only accommodate nonresponse at the initial interview stage but is also subject to attrition of respondents from the sample over time. Furthermore, the experience of repeated interviewing can create a different interview climate which may influence the results that are obtained.[40]

Number of Sexual Partners Reported by Adults

A second example is provided by surveys performed in 1987 by the *Los Angeles Times* and by the 1988 NORC General Social Survey (GSS). Both surveys asked respondents about the total number of sexual partners they had had during the past year.[41] The responses to this question yielded a number of interesting results. Of most interest for methodological purposes was the substantial similarity of results obtained in the two surveys. This similarity is surprising owing to the following:

- The quality of survey execution varied markedly. As noted in Table C-1 the GSS obtained one of the highest response rates of the surveys reviewed by the committee and the *Los Angeles Times* survey obtained the lowest.
- The surveys differed in the wording of questions, survey content, and mode of administration (phone survey versus self-administered questionnaire in a face-to-face survey).
- The 12-month time period did not cover the same dates. (The time periods were approximately July 1986 to June 1987 for the *Los Angeles Times* survey versus March 1987 to February 1988 for the NORC survey.)

Nonetheless, analysis[42] of a five-way crosstabulation of the two surveys by using five age groups, gender (male, female), marital status (married, not married), and number of partners (0, 1, 2, 3+) provided surprising evidence of consistency in the survey findings. (This table is presented in the Appendix.) In this five-way tabulation, once the demographic marginals of the two surveys were made comparable,[43] it

---

[40]Careful studies of the responses of persons interviewed in the Bureau of the Census Current Population Survey indicated that employment experience reporting was subject to artifacts resulting from repeated interviewing (Bailar, 1975; Brooks and Bailar, 1978).

[41]The following questions were posed to respondents: About how many sexual partners would you say you have had in the last year? (*Los Angeles Times*); and, How many sex partners have you had in the last 12 months? (NORC).

[42]See Turner, Miller, and Moses, 1989:104-108.

[43]The four-way demographic marginals (age by marital status by gender by survey) differed owing to divergences in the populations included in telephone versus personal interview surveys and to substantial differences in the quality of the execution of the sampling plans.

was virtually impossible to discriminate statistically among the results obtained in the two surveys with regard to the number of sexual partners in the last year or in the patterns of association found between this variable and marital status, gender, or age.[44]

Replication of Measurements Using Same Respondents

A parallel approach to the replication of entire surveys on new samples from a population is the repeated measurement of a (stable) characteristic of the same respondent, a method that effectively reduces some of the sources of "noise" in comparisons (e.g., differences that arise from variations in the methods of survey measurement). Indeed, for characteristics that are unchangeable during the interval between repeated measurements, such as age of first intercourse (for nonvirgin respondents), a survey measurement that was perfectly reliable might be expected to produce 100 percent consistency of response between two separate interviews. In reality, however, errors of recall, misunderstanding of questions, miscoding of responses, and a host of other factors may cause two survey measurements made at two different times to be less than perfectly consistent. This lack of consistency is true not only for questions that might be "sensitive" (e.g., those about sexuality), but also for seemingly innocuous inquiries about demographic characteristics.

As a standard component of careful survey practice, it is common for surveyors to recontact a (random) subsample of respondents and to repeat questions that provide crucial measurements. The tabulation of these repeated measurements against the original survey responses provides an index of the reliability of the survey measurements. That is, it provides a way of assessing the consistency of survey response. As

---

[44]Using a stratified jackknife procedure to fit a hierarchical series of log-linear models to the five-way table (Turner, Miller, and Moses, 1989:104-108), it was found that a model that fit the {PAGM} and {AGMS} marginals (where P = partners, A = age, M = marital status, G = gender, and S = survey) could be improved slightly by also constraining the model to fit the {PS} marginal (jackknifed likelihood-ratio chi-square for comparison of two alternate models: $J^2 = 1.49$, d.f. = 3, p = .051). This improvement is of borderline statistical "significance." An examination of estimates of the $\lambda^{\{PS\}}$ parameters for this "improved" model indicates that the observed intersurvey discrepancy was largely attributable to minor variations between the surveys in the numbers of persons with no sexual partners and with one partner. Estimates of the $\lambda^{\{PS\}}$ parameters (and standard errors) for a log-linear model constrained to fit {PAGM} {SAGM} {PS} marginals were .127 (s.e. =.070) for zero partners; -.123 (.063) for one partner; .035 (.073) for two partners; and -.040 (.072) for the category three or more partners. (Model parameters are [arbitrarily] coded so that positive values indicate an "excess" of NORC cases in the specified category.) With the effects of weighting and the complex sample design in the range of $deff$ = 1.6, significant effects were not found for other multivariate parameters involving P and S (e.g., {PAS}, {PGS}, {PMS}, etc.). It should be noted that all model comparisons fit the {SAGM} marginals, which allows for intersurvey differences in the demographic composition of the samples drawn by the two surveys.

noted earlier, consistency alone is no guarantee that the measurements are meaningful or valuable. However, survey measures that have zero (or very low consistency) between repeated measurements are inherently suspect (if the trait being measured is stable over time).

Because repeated measurements can be performed within the context of a single survey, there is opportunity for amassing these measurements, and the published literature (as well as unpublished technical documents) provides greater detail than is available on replicated surveys. Table C-5 summarizes some of the relevant results, which indicate substantial levels of consistency between answers to questions about sexual behavior obtained at two different points in time.

The observed consistency, however, is not as great as the consistency obtained for some other topics. Saltzman and colleagues (1987), for example, report test-retest reliabilities for two administrations of a questionnaire asking about sexual orientation, sexual behaviors, and change in sexual behaviors. Respondents were 116 gay men participating in an HIV study being conducted at the Fenway Community Health Center in Boston.[45] Compared with the test-retest reliabilities of .94 obtained for questions about smoking behavior and .79 for dietary habits, the reliabilities for reports on sexual behaviors were in the range of .40 to .99. The lowest reliabilities were found for number of nonsteady partners during last six months (.53) and number of partners for insertive anal intercourse without a condom (.61).

Other studies summarized in Table C-5 found test-retest reliabilities in the range of approximately .5 to .9. The retests in several studies assessed behaviors in a different time period than the first measurements (e.g., this past week). As a result, temporal instability in actual behaviors masquerades as "unreliability" in some of these studies.

Although the reliability analyses reported in Table C-5 encourage the belief that respondents can report consistently on their sexual behaviors, they do not, in themselves, tell anything directly about the systematic distortions that may occur in reporting. In an enlightening analysis of similar test-retest data, Rodgers, Billy, and Udry (1982) used data from successive waves of a longitudinal survey of adolescents (ages 11 to 16) to deduce evidence of invalidity. In this study, 408 adolescents completed two parallel sexual behavior questionnaires at an interval of 12 months. Rodgers and colleagues reported reliability analyses using items for which different responses at the two points in time are logically impossible. For example, teens who said they had had intercourse one or more times in their life in the first survey should give the same answer in

---

[45] Respondents with AIDS or AIDS-related complex were excluded.

all subsequent surveys. However, 43 percent of adolescents who reported "ever masturbating" in the first survey reported no such experience in the second survey; for intercourse the comparable figure was 19 percent. As a comparison, a similar analysis was conducted for reports of using alcohol; this effort yielded an inconsistency rate of 6 percent. The authors also reported results for an extremely vague question ("Have you ever grown several inches in height very quickly?"), which produced a 34 percent inconsistent response rate.

Across a series of 11 behavior measurements, the authors reported that adolescent respondents were most likely to rescind reports (between times 1 and 2) of touching of sex organs and, to a lesser extent, sexual intercourse. Less intimate behaviors (hand-holding, kissing) were less likely to be rescinded. For masturbation (in wave 1) and sexual intercourse (in waves 1 and 2), reliability was also assessed within each interview by asking questions at the beginning and end of the session. Inconsistent responses within interviews averaged 7.8 percent for intercourse and 8.3 percent for reports of masturbation in the first survey,[46] but there was substantial variation by race and sex. For both intercourse and masturbation, the greatest inconsistency in reporting was observed among black males.[47]

EMPIRICAL STUDIES OF DRUG-USING BEHAVIORS

Many of the methodological issues investigators face in studying drug use behaviors are identical to those found in studying sexual or other sensitive or illegal behaviors (see, for example, Siegel and Bauman, 1986; Kaplan et al., 1987; Zich and Temoshok, 1987; Kaplan, 1989). Yet some of the difficulties encountered in studying drug use behaviors are unique to this area of inquiry. Some of the most difficult research challenges arise from the fact that patterns of drug availability and injection behaviors may change rapidly. In the last several years, for example, considerable evidence has accumulated that drug-using populations in some communities have changed their needle use practices to avoid HIV infection (Chaisson et al., 1987; Friedman et al., 1987b; Des Jarlais, Friedman, and Stoneburner, 1988; Des Jarlais et al., 1988; Robertson, Skidmore, and Roberts, 1988). These changes have included both decreased needle-sharing and increased use of disinfection regimens for injecting equipment.

---

[46] Results for the second survey are reported for intercourse alone, for which 4.3 percent of respondents gave inconsistent responses within the interview.

[47] In the first survey, 23.7 percent of black male respondents gave inconsistent responses within the interview to the question on sexual intercourse, and 26 percent gave inconsistent responses to the questions on masturbation. In the second survey, 13 percent of black male respondents gave inconsistent responses to the question on sexual intercourse; no results were reported for masturbation.

TABLE C-5 Reliability Studies of Self-Reported Sexual Behaviors

Study	Sample	Method	Findings
Saltzman et al. (1987)	116 asymptomatic gay men, volunteers from community health center in Boston, who were homosexually active in 6 months prior to study	SAQ[h] with retest at 6 weeks (retest ranged from 2 to 18 weeks later): frequency of sexual acts and numbers of partners	Kappa statistic (measure of agreement relative to that expected by chance): For frequency of practice in last 6 months: .52 for insertive oral sex; .45 for receptive oral sex; .53 for insertive anal sex without condom; .50 for insertive anal sex with condom; .56 for receptive anal sex; .47 for kissing. For number of partners in last 6 months: .60 for insertive oral sex; .52 for receptive oral sex; .46 for insertive anal sex without condom; .60 for insertive anal sex with condom; .50 for receptive anal sex; .53 for kissing.
Koss and Gidycz (1985)	386 college students (242 women, 144 men)	SAQ[a] test with QI retest; sexual victimization and aggression	Pearson correlation between SAQ test and QI retest: .73 between women's levels of victimization and .61 between men's levels of aggression.
DeLamater (1974)	237 unmarried undergraduates at University of Wisconsin	Interviews varying the order of measures: (1) Current partners—depth of relationship and sexual behaviors; (2) Ideology (sexual attitudes)—personal ideology and peers' ideology	Analysis of variance showed no significant differences among respondents of either sex in measures of current partners' sexual behaviors or in measures of depth of relationship when the item order was varied. Among female respondents only, analysis of variance showed more liberal ideology when personal ideology was measured prior to peers' ideology.
DeLamater and MacCorquodale (1975)	432 single male undergraduates, 429 single female undergraduates, 220 single male nonstudents, and 293 single female nonstudents from Madison, Wisconsin	Three measures were compared: (1) SAQ and QI[b]; (2) location (middle or end of list about sexual experience), and (3) order of measures on current behaviors, partner characteristics, and partner ideology	Analysis of variance showed no significant differences by type of questionnaire administration, location of questions, or order of measures.
Anderson and Broffitt (1988)	57 healthy and 66 women with gynecological disorders	Face-to-face interviews; test with retest at three 4-month intervals using the SES, which assesses the range of current activities	Pearson correlation statistics showed a range in stability in SES responses from .55 to .85 for healthy women and from .62 to .85 for women with gynecological disorders.[c]

Study	Sample	Method	Results
Catania et al. (1986)	193 college students (66 males, 127 females)	Test with retest at 2 weeks using SAQs[d]; additional retest at second 2-week interval by face-to-face interview using the SSD to study sexual experiences and activities	Pearson correlation of SSD showed high internal consistency (.92); no significant order effects were found within the SAQs.
Zuckerman et al. (1976)	221 male and 331 female college students enrolled in personality psychology (control group) or human sexuality courses (experimental group)	Test at beginning and retest at end of 15-week course; SES	For the four sex-course groups, correlations on the 14-item heterosexual experience scale ranged from .80 to .95. The range for the 4-item homosexual experience scale was from .49 to .84. The range for the item on masturbation was from .63 to .90.
Allen and Haupt (1966)	56 male and 28 female college students at University of Miami	Test with retest at 3 months; sex inventory of 200 true-false items forming 10 scales of sexual behaviors and attitudes	Intraclass correlation coefficients on the scales ranged from .67 to .89.
Marks and Sartorius (1968)	17 psychiatric hospital patients with sex deviations	Test with retest at 24 hours; 260-item questionnaire forming 13 scales on attitudes toward sexual and nonsexual concepts	Pearson correlation coefficients for the 13 sexual scales ranges from .44 to .80, with only 2 scores below .64.
LoPiccolo and Steger (1974)	15 heterosexual couples recruited through ads placed on university bulletin boards	Test with retest at 2 weeks; 11-item scale of sexual adjustment and satisfaction	Pearson correlation coefficients for the 11 scales ranged from .53 to .90.
Harbison et al. (1974)	15 subjects	Test with retest at 3 to 5 months; 140-item sexual interest questionnaire forming 5 subscales and 1 overall scale	Pearson correlation coefficients for the 6 scales ranged from .68 to .92.
Derogatis and Melisaratos (1979), Derogatis (1980)	Normal and sexually dysfunctional individuals[e]	Test with retest at 2 weeks; sexual functioning inventory of 258 items forming 10 subtests on sexual behavior and attitudes	Correlations for the subtests ranged from .42 to .96.
Coates et al. (1986)	26 gay men in Toronto, recruited through local gay organizations	Face-to-face interviews with retest at least 72 hours after initial interview: volume of sexual partners, percentage frequency of certain sexual activities	Pearson correlation coefficients for the variables regarding number of sexual partners ranged from .71 to .99, with one exception.[f] The range for the percentage frequency of specific sexual activities was from .40 to .99, with most .70 or higher.

Continued

266

TABLE C-5 *Continued*

Study	Sample	Method	Findings
Catania et al. (1990a)	Sample of sexually active adolescent women	Questions asked at two different points within a SAQ: sexual activity in prior 2 months	The reliability coefficient for frequency of total intercourse (unprotected and protected across partners) was .98, and for frequency of condom use was .97. Reliability was slightly lower for those with three or more partners versus those with one partner.
Catania et al. (1990a)	Sample of heterosexual college undergraduates	SAQ test with retest at 2 weeks: frequency of intercourse for varying retrospective periods	Longer retrospective intervals were associated with lower test-retest reliability (one month = .89, six months = .65, one year = .36).
Millstein and Irwin (1983)	108 adolescent female patients recruited from three university hospital clinics	Comparison of: (1) SAQ, (2) computer-assisted SAQ, and (3) face-to-face interview in obtaining sexual histories	Girls assigned to the face-to-face interview reported lower levels of sexual activity than girls assigned to either of the SAQ types. (Roughly 74% of the girls responding to SAQs reported ever having sexual intercourse, compared with 63% of the other girls.)
Rolnick et al. (1989)	268 females at Midwestern University, identified through health service visits for STD treatment or to obtain contraceptives	Comparison of: (1) face-to-face interview with multiple questions on heterosexual history, (2) mail SAQ with multiple questions, and (3) mail SAQ with only 2 sexual history questions	Contingency table comparisons showed little difference by method in tendency to give "socially acceptable" responses.

NOTE: SAQ: self-administered questionnaire; QI: questionnaire interview; SES: sexual experience scale; SSD: sexual self-disclosure scale.

Table includes only studies reporting test-retest analysis of measurements or analysis of measurements made under different conditions (e.g., variations in question order, mode of administration). Studies reporting on scalability or internal consistency of sets of items that were not intended to measure the same behaviors have not been included (e.g., Podell and Perkins, 1957; Brady and Levitt, 1965; Bentler, 1968a,b; Zuckerman, 1973).

[a]SAQ administered in university class. [b]QI was face-to-face and SAQ was given as part of face-to-face interview. [c]The authors expected lower correlations for the women with gynecological disorders than for the healthy group, but the correlations for the two groups were similar. [d]SAQs administered to sample in classroom with alternate seating. [e]Information in Schiavi et al. (1979) suggests that these studies are reporting on 200 normal and slightly fewer than 200 dysfunctional individuals. [f]The exception was a coefficient of .24 for the variable "percentage of male partners since 1978 with whom sexual contact has occurred more than 5 times." [g]Checks on validity of responses (comparing answers with medical histories) showed no differences by methods. [h]Study coordinator reviewed completed SAQ with respondent for missing or inconsistent information.

As noted in Chapter 1 of the committee's most recent report (Miller, Turner, Moses, 1990), changing patterns of cocaine use complicate this picture. The 1980s saw a dramatic increase in the use of cocaine (Drug Enforcement Administration [DEA], 1988); in a related development, trade in "crack" (smokable) cocaine burgeoned from initial reports in 1981 of its availability in 3 cities, to its availability in 47 states and the District of Columbia during 1987 (DEA, 1988). Similarly, some observers[48] believe that "ice," a synthetic amphetamine that is smoked, may play a major role in drug use in the United States in coming years.

Changes in the illicit drugs in most common use can have important implications for HIV transmission. Studies presented in 1988 and 1989, for example, indicated that the injection of cocaine was associated with elevated rates of HIV infection (Chaisson et al., 1988, 1989; Des Jarlais and Friedman, 1988b; Friedman et al., 1989; Novick et al., 1989). This association is thought to be the result of high frequencies of injection and decreased needle hygiene over the course of an injection session (Friedman et al., 1989). Further studies in New York (Friedman et al., 1988) and San Francisco (Fullilove et al., 1989, 1990) have found that smoking crack cocaine, which in itself presents no direct risk of HIV transmission, is nonetheless associated with risky sexual behavior. Indeed, cocaine use has been associated with a higher incidence of syphilis (Minkoff et al., 1989). Such findings suggest that an outbreak of HIV infection among cocaine-using adolescents and adults is a possibility.

Accuracy of Self-Reports of Drug Use Behaviors

Huang, Watters, and Case (1988) point out that the lack of standardized measures, combined with the heterogeneity of the population of drug users and the impaired cognitive functioning that may result from extensive drug use, tends to make survey research in this population a difficult task. A drug user who is inebriated, for example, cannot be expected to recall needle-sharing episodes accurately. Furthermore, the wording of key questions in past AIDS research has sometimes been ambiguous. Consider, for example, the following hypothetical experience of an injection drug user:[49]

> Bill selected the syringe that looked least-used from among four in a half-filled water glass. Its action was a little stiff, so he took it apart. He swished the plunger around in the foil packet of a lubricated condom and then dipped the metal needle into a small vial of bleach. Putting the "works"

---

[48]L. Thompson, "Ice: New smokable form of speed," *Washington Post*, November 21, 1989, A-11.

[49]The term *injection user* is used to include both those who inject drugs, like heroin, intravenously and those who insert drugs intramuscularly.

back together, he tested it by drawing up water from the glass. Very smooth now. Then he, his wife, and their friend cooked up the heroin. Bill used the syringe first, then his wife used it, but they wouldn't share with the friend, who had his own set. The next morning at the detoxification clinic Bill agreed to be interviewed for a research project. The AIDS researcher asked how often does he use condoms, clean his needles with bleach, what percent of the time does he share needles?

The drug user in this vignette could report that he uses condoms frequently (to lubricate his syringes), that he "never" shares needles (only doing so with his wife), and that he cleans his needles "every time" (even though he may subsequently contaminate a clean needle with water shared with other syringes). Furthermore, a survey question about how often Bill shared needles could be answered accurately only if it clarified that "sharing" included using needles with his wife.

Similarly, most questionnaires about the use of needle-cleaning regimens are not sensitive enough to distinguish between disinfection that is thought to provide some protection and disinfection that is clearly ineffective. (Wermuth and Ham [1989], for example, report that some drug users disinfect their syringes by using bleach before and after sessions of sharing them with others but not between use by different persons.) Clarifying some of the ambiguities in survey measurements of these behaviors may eventually explain why longitudinal studies have failed to demonstrate a relationship between needle cleaning and rates of seroconversion among injection drug users (see, for example, Moss et al., 1989).

Measurement Bias

As with sexual behaviors, a major problem in measuring the risk behaviors of injection drug users is that researchers usually cannot observe the behaviors of interest directly. Occasionally, outreach workers may unobtrusively observe behaviors in such sites as "shooting galleries" (places in which drug users inject drugs together), but in general, drug use is not open to observation by research workers. Consequently, most AIDS research on drug use behaviors has relied heavily on the self-reports of persons who use IV drugs. Response bias, however, is a serious problem in such research.

Because of such potential biases, there has been ongoing concern among drug use researchers about the accuracy of injection drug users' self-reports. The most frequently asked validity question has been whether subjects underreport their drug use. Several studies have investigated the accuracy of injection drug users' self-reports of their drug use. The results of these studies are quite varied. Amsel and colleagues (1976), for example, followed 865 criminally involved drug users and employed various methods to assess the reliability and validity of self-reports of criminal and drug-taking behavior. Overall, their results indicated that, although the self-reports tended to have a downward bias, 74 percent of respondents accurately reported their drug use during the previous four weeks. That is, their self-reports were consistent with urinalysis findings. (In another 9 percent of cases, a validity check could not be made owing to incomplete data.) In 14 percent of cases, however, respondents reported no drug use, whereas tests of their urine indicated the presence of drugs.

Although these findings are encouraging, it should be noted that urine specimens were provided by only 267 (of a total of 865) respondents. The rates of drug use reported by those who did and did not provide specimens showed little difference,[50] but it is possible that, in many cases a respondent's prior inaccurate reporting on the questionnaire may have prompted him or her to refuse to provide a urine sample. If this were, indeed, true, the high rates of consistency observed in this study would not be a good indicator of the overall validity of the self-report data.

In addition to using urinalysis as a validity check, Amsel and coworkers obtained evidence of reliability in two ways. First, they examined questionnaire responses to detect inconsistent reporting of patterns of drug use. In only 7 percent of cases were inconsistencies detected in reports of the frequency of drug use and the reported cost of the habit. Inconsistency in the reporting of illegal activities was found in somewhat more cases (13 percent). The investigators also assessed the reliability of their measurements by readministering a small number of questions in a separate questionnaire two to six weeks later. They found that 97 percent of respondents gave consistent responses over time to the two questions asked about drug use in this second measurement. In a similarly designed study, Bale and colleagues (1981) interviewed 272 male veterans who were heroin users about their heroin use and compared their statements with a urine sample. The investigators found self-reports to be reasonably accurate in that 84 percent of those denying heroin use in the previous three months and 78 percent of those claiming no use in the previous week had urine samples that were negative for opiates.

Table C-6 summarizes the results of 17 other studies reviewed by Magura and colleagues (1987) in which self-reports of drug use were validated by urinalysis. Several studies obtained reports of drug use that were as consistent with urinalysis findings as the studies of the Amsel

---

[50]Of those providing urine specimens, 41 percent reported no drug use, versus 45 percent of those who did not provide specimens for testing.

(1976) and Bale (1981) research teams. Yet the findings summarized in Table C-6 also show great variability in the results achieved by different investigators and in the results achieved by the same investigator when obtaining reports of the use of different drugs. Use of heroin and other opiates, for example, is consistently reported with greater accuracy than is the use of other illicit drugs. Yet even for heroin use, the range of validity results is quite broad ($.26 \leq K \leq .78$),[51] and the median level of agreement between urinalysis results and self-reports is relatively modest ($K \approx .5$). The range of results improves, however, if the comparison is restricted to studies that assessed heroin or opiate use within seven days of the urinalysis ($.59 \leq K \leq .78$).

Although the direction of the reporting bias in most studies is toward underreporting of drug use, the results are not entirely consistent with that interpretation. Focusing on those surveys (marked with an asterisk in Table C-6) that asked about drug use within the period (seven days) for which urinalysis can reliably detect it, one finds instances of major studies in which underreporting biases of up to 13 percentage points were found (McGlothlin, Anglin, and Wilson, 1977; $N = 497$). On the other hand, one major study (W. F. Page et al., 1977; $N = 896$) and one small-scale study (Wish et al., 1983, $N = 26$) found small biases in the opposite direction (i.e., more respondents reported drug use than were detected in urinalysis). (Such divergences might be attributable to the fallibility of the urinalysis itself.)[52]

Although the results shown in Table C-6 are "usually interpreted as supporting the validity of addicts' self-reports,"[53] they also provide clear evidence of the errors that can affect these measurements. Furthermore, although the studies are not unanimous in their findings, it does appear

---

[51] Coefficient reported is kappa (see Bishop et al., 1975:395).

[52] It should be recognized that the validity criterion in these studies is also subject to error. In blinded testing of the proficiencies of 50 laboratories performing urinalysis for opiates, cocaine, and other illicit drugs, Davis, Hawks, and Blanke (1988) found that, of 389 urine specimens known to be negative for particular drugs, the laboratories reported five false-positive readings (a false-positive error rate of 1.3 percent). The majority of these false-positive results involved identification of the wrong drug in urine specimens that were positive for some drug; however, two false-positives were given for cannabis and for methadone in samples that were actually drug free. In 350 tests involving urine specimens known to be positive for particular drugs, the laboratory tests had a 31 percent false-negative rate (109 of 350). The substances most often missed were phenylcyclidine (51 percent), morphine (47 percent), cocaine (38 percent), and methamphetamine (28 percent). The false-positive and false-negative rates obtained in such testing are, of course, a function of analytic method and the cutoff values that are used. Although the above findings provide some indication of the error rates obtained by standard practices in contemporary drug testing by commercial laboratories, it is possible that the procedures used in the validity studies reported in Table C-6 may be different.

[53] This characterization is offered by Magura and colleagues (1987), who cite the writings of Aiken and LoSciuto (1985) and Harrell (1985) as examples of such interpretations.

TABLE C-6 Summary of Studies on Validity of Self-Reported Drug Use in High-Risk Populations[a] (from Magura et al., 1987 and other sources)

Investigators	Subjects	Drugs	N	Percent Using Drugs by		Kappa
				Self-report	Criterion[b]	
*Ball (1967)[n]	Noninstitutionalized narcotics addicts	Opiates	25	20	28	.78
*W.F. Page et al. (1977)[o]	Arrestees	Opiates	896	16	15	.69
		Stimulants	896	9	7	.29
		Sedatives	896	16	18	.38
*McGlothlin, Anglin, and Wilson (1977)[h]	Drug treatment admissions	Opiates Last 5 days	497	27	40[i]	.59
*Bale et al. (1981)[p]	Former VA detox and drug treatment clients	Heroin All subjects	272	35	45	.61
*Wish et al. (1983)[q]	Drug users criminals	Heroin	26	58	50	.69
		Cocaine	26	58	46	.77
		Methadone	31	52	52	.61
Eckerman et al. (1971)[c]	Arrestees	Heroin	1,693	19	15	.48
		Barbiturates	1,693	7	11	.12
		Amphetamines	878	6	3	.10
		Methadone	1,693	3	2	.16

continued

TABLE C-6 Continued

Investigators	Subjects	Drugs	N	Percent Using Drugs by		
				Self-report	Criterion[b]	Kappa
Cisin and Parry (1979)[d]	Drug treatment clients	Heroin	85	13	27	.29
		Barbiturates	85	35	41	.23
		Tranquilizers	85	25	31	-.08
		Amphetamines	85	39	34	.04
		Cocaine	85	39	32	.23
Cox and Longwell (1974)[e]	Methadone patients	Heroin[f]	175	23	20	.57
Amsel et al. (1976)[g]	Civil commitment applicants	12 drugs	267	59	70	.60
McGlothlin, Anglin, and Wilson (1977)[h]	Drug treatment admissions	Opiates Last 4 weeks	497	38	40[i]	.56
Bale (1979)[j]	Former VA detox and drug treatment patients	Heroin By questionnaire	55	51	38	.53
		By interview	55	36	38	.65
Ben-Yehuda (1980)[k]	Methadone patients	All illicit drugs	47	47	72	.34
Hubbard, Marsden, and Allison (1984)[l]	Drug treatment clients	Heroin	767	10	20	.26
		Other opiates	767	29	22	-.08
		Cocaine	767	10	5	.18
		Minor tranquilizers	767	30	7	.10
		Barbiturates	767	13	3	.07
		Amphetamines	767	21	2	.03

	Heroin	Other opiates	Cocaine	Barbiturates	Sedatives/tranquilizers	Marijuana
	291	287	282	281	274	75
	21	4	11	8	20	15
	23	14	7	8	14	24
	.54	.22	.31	.33	.17	.62

Aiken and LoSciuto (1985)[m] — Methadone and drug-free outpatients: Heroin, Other opiates, Cocaine, Barbiturates, Sedatives/tranquilizers, Marijuana

Zuckerman et al. (1985)[r] — Pregnant women: Marijuana

NOTES: TLC: thin-layer chromatography; EMIT: enzyme multiplied immunoassay technique.

[a] Excludes general population and student surveys. [b] Urinalysis, clinic records, counselors, etc. [c] Subjects: Arrestees at central booking; Los Angeles, Chicago, New York City, San Antonio, St. Louis, New Orleans. Procedures: Drug use within last month from interview vs. single research TLC urinalysis. [d] Subjects: Drug treatment clients in 1974; San Francisco Bay area. Procedures: Self-administered questionnaire vs. clinic records; data grouped as "ever used" and "never used." [e] Subjects: Methadone patients (N = 106) admitted for at least 3 months; Tucson clinic. Procedures: Drug use over 3 months by period interviews vs. clinic's weekly TLC urinalysis over same 3 months; data grouped as "low" and "high use." [f] N and % refer to interviews. [g] Subjects: Applicants to NIMH civil commitment between 1967 and 1971 (follow-up); PHS hospital at Lexington and Ft. Worth. Procedures: Drug use over 4-week period by interview vs. single research TLC urinalysis. [h] Subjects: Admissions to civil commitment in 1962-63, 1964, 1970 (follow-up of nonincarcerated sample); California, statewide. Procedures: Drug use by interview (last 5 days and last 4 weeks) vs. single research urinalysis (quantitative immunoassay). [i] "Positive" and "probable positive" classed as positive. [j] Subjects: Former VA detox and drug treatment patients (1-year follow-up); Palo Alto/Stanford area. Procedures: Mailed questionnaire (drug use during past month) and subsequent interview (drug use during past week) vs. single research urinalysis (TLC confirmed by radioimmunoassay). [k] Subjects: Methadone patients; Chicago clinic. Procedures: Self-administered questionnaire (drugs taken "now") vs. clinic's TLC urinalysis over 6 months (grouped as 0-3 and 4+ urine positives). [l] Subjects: Drug treatment clients admitted 1 month (outpatient detox; drug-free and methadone outpatient; and residential); numerous programs in 10 cities in 1979, 1980, 1981. Procedures: Interview (drug use during last month) vs. clinic's TLC urinalysis during that month. [m] Subjects: Methadone and drug-free outpatient; 16 programs in New York, Washington, Chicago, Los Angeles, San Francisco in 1977. Procedures: Client (N=300) vs. counselor (N = 85) interviews (drug use in past 30 days). [n] Subjects: Noninstitutionalized narcotics addicts; former federal inmates at Lexington and Ft. Worth. Procedures: Current drug use by interview vs. single research analysis (apparently TLC). [o] Subjects: Arrestees booked for felony in 1973; Dade County, Florida. Procedures: Drug use in last 48 hours by interview vs. single research urinalysis by spectrofluorometry and/or EMIT and/or TLC. [p] Subjects: Former VA detox and drug treatment clients (2-year follow-up); Palo Alto/Stanford area. Procedures: Interview (drug use during past week) vs. single research urinalysis (TLC confirmed by radioimmunoassay). [q] Subjects: Drug users recruited off street; New York City. Procedures: Interview (drug use during past 36 hours) vs. single research urinalysis (TLC and EMIT). [r] Subjects: Women registering at prenatal clinic; Boston. Procedures: Personal interview (marijuana use in previous week) vs. urinalysis (EMIT). (This study was not discussed in Magura et al. [1987].)
* Study measured drug use during time period of 7 days or less prior to urinalysis.

that a bias toward underreporting of drug use is quite common.

In considering the implications of these results for AIDS research, there are further reasons to constrain one's optimism about the overall validity of drug use measurements. First, the committee notes that one statistic of considerable interest is the *prevalence* of drug use in broadly defined populations. Chapter 3 of the committees's most recent report (Miller, Turner, and Moses, 1990), for example, discussed surveys that attempted to assess the prevalence of drug use among high school students using the students' self-reports. It is quite possible that surveys of such general populations may be subject to a rather different pattern of bias and errors than that afflicting the surveys included in Table C-6.[54] The populations sampled in Table C-6 were all drawn from groups who were publicly identified as drug users. Because these respondents were already labeled as users of illicit drugs, not only by researchers but by treatment personnel and the criminal justice system, they may have been less motivated to conceal drug use. Furthermore, the routine use of urinalysis in research and in monitoring of treatment may further discourage attempts by this population to hide drug use.

Generalizations from these findings to AIDS research are further limited by the subject matter covered in the survey questions. As Rounsaville and coworkers pointed out in 1981, investigators in the drug use field traditionally examined a relatively restricted range of factual data. In AIDS research, however, the knowledge required is somewhat more extensive. Questions of particular interest include not just whether subjects use drugs but how they use them. How often do they use needles? share needles? clean needles? Little is known about the accuracy of responses to more fine-grained questions such as these, although the accuracy of self-reports of drug use has been studied extensively. A recent study by McLaws and coworkers (1988) found rates of infection with hepatitis B virus that suggested that respondents were actually sharing needles at a rate higher than that reported to researchers.

As with self-reports of sexual behaviors, differential reporting bias is a danger in the use of self-reports of drug use behaviors. In evaluation studies, for example, subjects assigned to an intervention (versus a control) group might tend to underreport such behaviors as needle sharing after having gone through an intervention that stressed the importance of

---

[54]Some surveys of adolescents have attempted to test for overreporting of drug use by asking teenage respondents how often they had used a fictitious drug (e.g., bindro, adrenochromes/wagon wheels, etc.). Negligible percentages (0 to 4 percent) of respondents in these surveys reported using these fictitious drugs (see Haberman et al., 1972; Whitehead and Smart, 1972; Petzel, Johnson, and McKillip, 1973; Single, Kandel, and Johnson, 1975; Needle et al., 1983). Yet although this result is encouraging, it does not speak to the more likely bias, that is, underreporting of drug use.

stopping these risky behaviors.[55] There is some evidence that reporting biases may sometimes work in the opposite direction. Worth and colleagues (1989), for example, found that women drug users tried to be "good survey takers." After participating in an AIDS prevention group they tended to give responses indicating more frequent risk taking. The authors attribute this finding to the subjects' greater degree of honesty, reflecting increased comfort with the questions and the interviewers. Such a differential reporting bias would tend to mask the effects of interventions.

SUMMARY OF FINDINGS

Although there is ample evidence of error and bias in extant surveys of AIDS risk behaviors, and such evidence should be of concern to investigators, some important conclusions can nevertheless be drawn from this body of work.

Feasibility

First, based on the empirical evidence presented in the first section of this appendix, there appears to be little question that such surveys can enlist the cooperation of the vast majority of the American public. Carefully designed surveys inquiring about sexual matters, for example, appear to be capable of obtaining response rates that rival those of commercial and academic surveys on less sensitive topics. Of course, special efforts may be needed to ensure high levels of cooperation, and, as always, careful collection of evidence of response bias is necessary. There appears to be little question, however, that such surveys are feasible as scientific enterprises.

Replicability

Second, the recent literature contains two demonstrations that independently conducted national surveys of aspects of sexual behavior (age at first intercourse and number of sexual partners in past year) produced reassuringly similar estimates. This similarity was achieved despite variations in survey methodology. These results, if repeated across a wider range of measurements, provide salutary evidence that surveys of AIDS risk behaviors can, indeed, provide replicable measurements—that is, different investigators using roughly similar methods to survey the same population can obtain equivalent results.

---

[55] Some of the potential for bias might be eliminated by using research interviewers who are independent of the staff who deliver the intervention. This tactic, however, should not be expected to eliminate completely the potential for bias.

Validity

In most sex surveys, it will be difficult (if not impossible) to obtain convincing evidence of measurement validity. The committee finds nonetheless that the research literature contains several important demonstrations of the validity of sexual and drug use behavior measures. When couples report independently on factual aspects of their own sexual interactions, for example, there is considerable agreement between the survey reports that are obtained. Similarly, in one instance in which physical evidence could be obtained, it was found that, when questioned in an interview, a very high proportion of married women for whom there was physical evidence of intercourse reported that they had, indeed, had intercourse. Furthermore, studies that have validated self-reported drug use with urinalysis have found moderate levels of agreement. These results are certainly encouraging, but there is also a variety of other evidence that suggests that some sexual and drug-using behaviors may be considerably underreported in surveys. Although the evidence is limited, it appears that male-male sexual contacts may be massively underreported (at least by college student populations).

Reliability

There is a fairly large body of research reporting on the consistency of responses over short periods of time in survey reports on various AIDS risk behaviors. These studies have generally demonstrated moderate levels of response consistency over time. It is possible, however, that some of the inconsistencies observed in these studies reflect true changes in behavior over time rather than errors in reporting on behavior.

IMPROVING VALIDITY AND RELIABILITY

The above evidence leads naturally to questions concerning how the reliability and validity of self-report data on these behaviors might be improved. In this regard there are a number of tactics that should be considered.

Literacy

Literacy is an obvious concern when self-administered forms or other written materials are to be used to collect data. In designing surveys, researchers should be sure that their survey questionnaires (as well as their consent forms, information sheets, etc.) are readable and, in particular, that the difficulty of the materials does not exceed the reading level of their subjects. In cases in which there is a possibility that some of the respondents recruited for a study may be illiterate, provisions must be made for detecting this problem and providing an alternate data collection method.

In this regard the committee notes that Hochhauser analyzed the readability of AIDS educational materials in 1987 and found that, on average, they required a 14th grade (i.e., college) reading level.[56] Such a mismatch in the reading level of educational materials intended for the general public suggests that sensitivity to literacy problems is not widespread. The literacy problem may be even more complex when it is extended to include the research consent forms and information sheets required by institutional review boards. It may in fact be very difficult to make these quasi-legal documents truly readable. One study of the reading level of patient information at a psychiatric institute revealed that all brochures were written below the educational level of 85 percent of their readers but that the patient's consent form was written above the educational level of 77 percent of the patients (Sorensen and Leder, 1978).

Alternatives to Self-Reports

In addition to adopting procedures that ensure that respondents can understand the questions they are being asked, it is desirable to supplement self-reports with alternative measures whenever possible. Such measures, which include ethnographic observations, physical evidence, skills demonstrations, and reports of "significant others," can provide important data on the biases that may affect key measurements. Ethnographic observations, which are discussed at length in the next section, can be a particularly valuable tool in understanding responses to quantitative self-report measures. Lange and colleagues (1988), for example, recently reported that, according to self-reports collected in survey interviews, only 70 percent of IV drug users in New York City had shared needles at some time in their life. Ethnographic studies provided a quick corrective to this inaccurate conclusion. These studies indicated that *essentially all* IV drug users in New York had used someone else's injection equipment at least one time in their life—when they first began to inject drugs (Des Jarlais and Friedman, 1988c). In this case, ethnographic observations helped clarify a limitation of data gathered through interview methods. Other alternative measures are discussed briefly below.

---

[56]Wells and coworkers (1989) found somewhat lower reading levels in a random sample of brochures, cards, inserts ($N = 104$), and pamphlets, books, and monographs ($N = 41$) selected from the 1988 *AIDS Information Resources Directory*. Wells et al. reported that a preliminary analysis of 57 brochures found that 72 percent were written at the equivalent of tenth grade or above and 10 percent at a grade level beyond high school.

Physical Evidence

A variety of other data can supplement self-reports of drug use. Skin examinations for puncture marks and urine drug screens can be used as cross-checks against self-reports (Sorensen et al., 1989c), and low-frequency physiological surrogate markers can sometimes be useful if the population is large enough. For example, Bardoux and colleagues (1989) interpreted a declining incidence of hepatitis B among injection drug users in Amsterdam as a reflection of decreases in needle-sharing and related risk behaviors among that population. Similarly, as noted previously, some researchers have monitored prevalence rates of hepatitis B virus and used these rates as a cross-check on self-reports of needle-sharing among their respondents.

Skills Demonstrations

A further supplement to self-reports are skills demonstrations in which subjects show their ability to practice preventive behaviors. For example, a test of a prevention program with injection drug users has used demonstrations of the ability to clean needles and use condoms properly as outcome measures (Heitzman et al., 1989). Such demonstrations can provide useful cross-checks against self-reports. For example, even if a subject reported cleaning needles 100 percent of the time, the preventive value of this "cleaning" would be questionable if the subject's demonstration of needle cleaning skills revealed unfamiliarity with the basic procedures needed to prevent transmission of HIV.

Other Safeguards for Surveys

Although firm guarantees cannot be made as to the beneficial effects of any particular tactic noted here, the committee believes that there is strong presumptive evidence to indicate that a considerably larger investment of resources needs to be made in exploratory work prior to the fielding of major survey investigations.[57] (This problem is not confined

---

[57] Also needed are careful methodological investigations of the relative merits of different methods of survey administration, including use of self-administered questionnaires versus interviewer questioning in surveys of sexual behavior and telephone versus face-to-face surveys. The effects of different data collection methods have not been extensively studied by drug researchers. Magura and colleagues (1987) found with their 248 methadone patients that the age of clients and the type of interviewer directly affected the rate of underreporting. On the other hand, Skinner and Allen (1983) randomly assigned 150 drug treatment clients either to a computerized interview, face-to-face interview, or self-report format and found no important differences in reliability, level of problems, or consumption patterns of alcohol, drug, and tobacco use. Similar results were found by Needle, Jou, and Su (1989), who compared adolescents' reports of drug use when randomly assigned to report with mailed questionnaires or in-person survey interviews.

to studies of sexual or drug use behaviors; inadequate investment in such exploratory work is common to surveys of other topics according to knowledgeable observers. See, for example, comments by Cannell and coworkers [1989:3].) For surveys of behaviors that risk HIV transmission, this lack of exploratory work is particularly troubling, given the underdeveloped state of research in this field. In this regard, the committee notes that some of the questionnaires it reviewed made impossible demands on the cognitive capacities of respondents, an unfortunate error that would have been detected if the questionnaires had received more thorough pilot testing. For example, one previously cited survey asked respondents to report the total number of sexual encounters they had had with particular partners during the entire length of relationships whose *median* duration was 24 months. The survey further asked respondents to report the total number of times (or percentage of encounters) during which they engaged in one or more of 13 different sexual practices.[58]

As is discussed below, there may be good reasons for collecting such data despite the frailties of respondents' recall. Empirical studies of memory for other events, however, suggest that a respondent's ability to recall such events is limited, and random and systematic errors intrude on the responses. Such studies argue for careful research conducted as ancillary efforts to the epidemiological undertaking that would characterize these errors. Indeed, it might be argued that (in some instances) there would be good cause for restricting recall to time periods in which accurate recall might be assumed with greater certainty. So, for example, reports on sexual encounters during the preceding one to three days place more manageable demands on respondents' memory (although, even here, perfect recall should not be assumed).

Although the arguments for use of different time frames are complicated (see below), there is little doubt that researchers' appreciation of the problems that attend key measurements can be sharpened by greater use of exploratory studies prior to the launching of major surveys. Among the techniques that can be profitably employed are ethnographic studies and focus groups whose aim is to explore the frames of reference and language that respondents use in approaching a given topic area; pretests and pilot studies that explore the respondents' understanding of preliminary versions of questionnaires; and cognitive research strategies that detail the limits of recall and the strategies respondents use in answering questions that demand recall of events that are not directly accessible (e.g., how many sexual encounters have you had with John in the past

---

[58] For example, masturbation, insertive and receptive oral sex, insertive and receptive anal sex, and so forth.

two years?). Furthermore, major surveys can embed experimental studies in their designs to assess the effects of key aspects of the research process (e.g., the nature and perceptions of confidentiality guarantees, question wording and context, and the measurement variance and bias introduced by interviewers themselves). Examples of such techniques are provided below.

Randomized Response Techniques

A widely known set of tactics for increasing cooperation and accurate reporting of sensitive information in surveys are the randomized response techniques. These techniques are intended to provide an estimate of the distribution of a sensitive characteristic in the population without requiring that individuals reveal sensitive information about themselves. They introduce a random element into the response process so that no individual respondent is *definitely* identified as admitting to the sensitive trait. One variant of this technique instructs a random half of the sample to answer "yes" regardless of the question while the other half of the sample is asked to give an accurate answer to the sensitive question. (The randomization might be performed by having the respondent flip a coin without letting the interviewer know the result of the coin toss.) Because one-half of the sample would be expected to answer "yes" as a result of the coin toss, the proportion who answered "yes" to the sensitive question can be estimated. (Variations on this basic strategy include one that requests respondents to answer one of two questions—one sensitive and one not—based upon a coin toss or other randomizing device.)

Although these techniques are attractive in theory, they do have some drawbacks (Campbell, 1987). Accordingly, researchers applying randomized response methods should recognize the need for careful pilot testing prior to embarking on a major research effort using them. One drawback is that larger sample sizes are required to obtain estimates of equal precision because the randomization procedure substantially increases the sampling error.[59] Second, although these techniques permit estimation of the univariate distribution of discrete population characteristics (e.g., proportion having same-gender sex in last year); they are not easily adapted for use in estimating continuous variables (e.g., number of sexual partners).[60] Finally, respondents may not understand or follow

---

[59] Even where the total sample size is large, use of randomized response techniques may yield estimates for subpopulations (e.g., unmarried males, ages 21–30) that have unacceptably large standard errors.

[60] See Fox and Tracy (1986:44–48) for a discussion of the randomizing devices that have been used and the estimation procedures. See Tracy and Fox (1981) for a successful application to estimating arrest rates.

the instructions used in these techniques, or they may distort their responses despite the theoretical safeguards afforded by the randomization technique. Empirical evidence on the success of these techniques is mixed. Although there have been convincing demonstrations of their ability to increase response rates and to reduce bias in some instances (Goodstadt and Gruson, 1975), the evidence from other studies has been equivocal (e.g., Bradburn et al., 1979:8-13). Boruch (1989), in reviewing the results of 23 studies using randomized response techniques, concluded that these methods appeared to increase cooperation and decrease bias in about one-half of the cases in which they had been used. Unfortunately, the available evidence does not provide clear guidance as to the conditions under which these techniques will work.

Pilot Studies
Survey researchers typically distinguish between two types of exploratory studies. Pilot studies are commonly semistructured inquiries conducted prior to the design of the final (or penultimate) version of a survey questionnaire. These studies are used to gather information that is helpful in drafting the instrument. Pretests, on the other hand, are structured tests of a survey questionnaire, one or more of which may be conducted prior to the fielding of a typical survey. Pretests provide information on the range of difficulties that may be encountered in administering a questionnaire–for example, respondent difficulty in understanding the questions, respondent resistance to providing sensitive information, interviewer difficulty in following "skip patterns,"[61] and so forth.

Although examination of survey questionnaires used in past research on AIDS reveals some deficiencies resulting from the rush to gather data, there have also been some laudable examples of careful preparatory work. The committee notes, for example, that Britain's Social and Community Planning Research unit[62] has included provisions for a three-stage development effort prior to fielding the British survey of sexual attitudes and behavior. This program (see L. Spencer, Faulkner, and Keegan, 1988:3) includes a pilot study[63] (consisting of a series of unstructured in-depth

---

[61] Skip patterns are instructions to skip blocks of questions that depend on responses to prior questions. For example, a series of questions on *first* sexual experiences would be skipped for respondents who indicated that they were inexperienced.

[62] Under contract to the British Health Education Authority.

[63] The work by L. Spencer, Faulkner, and Keegan (1988) testifies to the inconsistent use of the terms *pilot study* and *pretest* among survey researchers. In their publication, *pilot study* includes testing of structured questionnaires, and the large-scale test of the final questionnaire is called a large-scale pilot study or feasibility test. The preliminary unstructured research is termed an "investigative study" (p. 3).

interviews), the development of structured questionnaires and small-scale pretests, and a large-scale pretest of the final questionnaire. The pilot phase of the research included among its aims exploration of the dimensions of the topics that were to be included in the survey, clarification of appropriate language to be used in posing questions, identification of sensitive issues and ways of gathering data on these topics, and preliminary examination of the impact of interviewer characteristics (e.g., gender, sexual orientation) on the willingness of respondents to discuss their sexual behaviors.

These British investigators learned several valuable lessons from their pilot work, which used semistructured interviews with 40 respondents. Three of these lessons are reported here, not because they will necessarily generalize to other samples but rather to indicate the important design considerations that can be missed without careful preparatory work. As a result of debriefing respondents about their reactions to the interviewers to whom they were assigned, the investigators learned the following:

- Women expressed a strong preference for women interviewers;[64] some women indicated that they would not consent to an interview with a male interviewer, whereas other women said that "they would not have been as open and might have refused to answer some of the more personal questions" (L. Spencer, Faulkner, and Keegan, 1988:10).

- Masturbation, surprisingly, seemed to cause respondents more embarrassment than oral or anal sex. Furthermore, there was considerable variability in the use of this term depending on the respondent's sexual orientation. Among respondents with predominantly heterosexual histories, masturbation was usually understood to refer to self-stimulation to orgasm in the absence of a partner. Among gay-identified men, mutual masturbation was a readily acknowledged behavior. For women who identified themselves as lesbians, masturbation referred exclusively to self-stimulation; stimulation by a partner's hands or fingers was "making love" or "having sex."

- There was a strong preference among respondents for use of formal rather than street language in discussing sexual behaviors. Furthermore, although terms such as penis and vagina were well understood, some of the terminology that

---

[64]The evidence reported in this study was based entirely on respondents' statements to female interviewers. In the pilot study, male interviewers were never assigned to female respondents.

has become standard in the epidemiological literature was quite foreign to respondents (e.g., vaginal sex), and there was considerable variation in what was inferred from the terms homosexual and bisexual.[65] Other terms (e.g., anal sex, oral sex) were widely understood.

One cannot, of course, assume that such findings with 40 British adults will generalize to other samples—or, indeed, that one such study fully canvasses the problems involved in surveying the British population. The study does, however, alert researchers to important aspects of the way in which these individuals perceive and talk about their sexual lives and the factors that may impede collection of accurate survey data.

Pretests

Usually, pretests are dress rehearsals for the final survey. As such, they can have great value in allowing field staff and investigators to identify any procedural problems inherent in a questionnaire. Similarly, selective debriefing of interviewers and a subset of survey respondents can help identify aspects of the survey that were difficult to administer or understand. Indeed, simple tactics, such as asking respondents to restate in their own words what was meant by an individual survey question, can be tremendously useful in identifying survey questions that do not have equivalent meanings for all respondents (or, equally important, do not have the same meaning for respondents and the investigator).

Although much can be done using these procedures, some investigators have introduced more systematic data gathering into the pretest process. Cannell and colleagues (1989), for example, implemented ancillary data-gathering activities during pretests to provide additional information on interviewer problems with asking the questions as worded, respondent problems of comprehension, and respondent problems with knowing or providing the required information. In brief, three types of supplemental data were collected during the pretests:

---

[65]Thus, the authors (L. Spencer, Faulkner, and Keegan, 1988:24-25) write: "Some people are clear that [homosexual] refers to both men and women who are attracted to and have sex with their own sex. There are, however, a number of people of different ages and social classes who associate the word exclusively with men: *'Homo equals men.' (Woman, 37 years, married)* For these people, women who have sex with each other are lesbians, not homosexuals."

The Spencer group also reported that although most respondents identified bisexuals as persons who had sex with both sexes and heterosexuals as persons who had sex with persons of the opposite sex, there were a few notable confusions. One 31-year-old single man, for example, thought bisexual meant "kinky sex, 3 in bed, that sort of thing" (p. 25); some respondents seemed confused by "ordinary people" being labeled at all with regard to sexual orientation and defined heterosexuals as persons who "liked either sex" or their own sex.

- Coding of behaviors of interviewer and respondent: survey interviews were recorded, and relevant aspects of the survey interview were coded to indicate whether the interviewer asked the question as written, whether the respondent asked for clarification, and so forth. Systematic coding of the pretest interviews provides useful data for identifying questions that pose special difficulties for the interviewer or the respondent, or both, and that may need to be redesigned.

- Probes: follow-up questions are used to determine whether the respondents understood the question in the manner that the investigator intended.

- Rating of questions by interviewers: after completing their interviews (and after completing training on the nature of questionnaire problems), interviewers were asked to rate individual questions and to identify the different types of problems they encountered in asking the question.

These data, which go beyond those usually collected in pretests, can provide important ancillary information on the extent to which the survey interview is "standardized": that is, whether questions are asked in identical fashion and have the same meaning across respondents.

Cognitive Research Strategies

A further preliminary strategy to be considered involves the use of the findings and techniques of cognitive research. These strategies are particularly appropriate when the task at hand is likely to make substantial demands on a respondent's memory.

In that regard the committee notes that two examples used previously may be atypical of the types of information in which AIDS researchers are most interested. Questions regarding chronological age and sexual activity during the past day (or week) solicit information that is easily remembered. Most individuals can readily recall their sexual experiences of the previous day, and chronological age is such an important variable in this culture that the inability to recall it is considered an almost certain sign of dementia.

In contrast, many survey researchers ask for information involving matters to which respondents do not have direct and immediate access— for example, the average number of times per week they have had intercourse over the past six months or year. A mistaken estimate in this case may not be the result of "distortion"—either conscious or unconscious—but may simply be due to the relative unavailability to immediate memory of the information that has been requested.

When such information cannot be directly and easily recalled, two factors must be considered. The first factor is the recall strategy used by the respondent. For example, in estimating frequency of sexual activity over a prolonged period, the respondent may concentrate on a particular short time interval (e.g., the last week or two) and then multiply. Alternatively, the subject may rely on a recent conversation with someone else about the issue or even on some external benchmark (e.g., "I have always had intercourse at a rate twice the averages I've heard reported so therefore my rate must be . . . "). There are a number of such strategies, and each results in different types of systematic biases. A "free scan" may yield events or a period that is particularly memorable—for reasons unrelated to the purposes of the question. For example, researchers working on other topics have found that events (e.g., victimization) that have led to some subsequent actions on the part of the respondent (reporting to the police, collecting insurance) are recalled more clearly than those that have not (Wagennar, 1986). (See Bradburn, Rips, and Shevell [1987] for a more detailed discussion of such strategies.)

The second factor, as noted by Bartlett in 1932, is that memory is basically a reconstructive process and hence is amenable to influences that are described in the memory literature by such terms as "schemata," "scripts," "good stories," and so on. The reason such effects occur is simply that respondents carry out recall on the basis of the information currently available to them, and just as current expectations and preconceptions can affect perception, they can also affect memory—only often more so (see Neisser, 1981; Pearson, Ross, and Dawes, 1989).

The effects of these recall factors may not always constitute a disadvantage from the perspective of the researcher, but they certainly present problems often enough that they must be considered in designing research protocols and questionnaires. Two studies illustrate this conclusion. In the first, by Smith, Jobe, and Mingay (in press), subjects kept a diary of what they ate over a four-week period and were then asked to recall their food intake from the most recent two weeks and from the more remote two weeks. The recall for the most recent two-week period more closely matched the actual items eaten during those two weeks (i.e., those in the diary) than the recall for the items eaten during the more remote two weeks. In contrast, the recall for the more remote period matched the previous two weeks and the remote two weeks equally well. The authors concluded that recall for food intake prior to the previous two weeks produced a "generic" result (based on foods that were commonly eaten by the person recalling) whereas people had a more direct recall of the previous two weeks. Even though personal recall may be subject to social scripts and schemata, such distortions may be unimportant to the researcher. Indeed, for many purposes, the "generic" result may be of equal or greater interest.[66]

During the last decade, a number of promising examples of the use of cognitive research techniques in survey development have been proposed (Biderman and Moore, 1980; Jabine et al., 1985). The last year in particular has witnessed publication of several studies that used such techniques to evaluate and improve survey measurements of health-related and other events (Brewer, Dull, and Jobe, 1989; Lessler, Tourangeau, and Salter, 1989; Means et al., 1989; Tucker et al., 1989). Yet, although these techniques offer researchers new possibilities to "take account" of the effect of the recall strategy and belief factors in assessing responses, such a task is difficult and may present problems for which there are no easy solutions. Clearly, if the phenomena of interest can be restricted to time frames that do not make impossible demands on the accuracy of the respondent's memory, then there is much to be gained by ensuring that the phrasing of questions appropriately restricts the time frame, although this kind of restriction may be impossible in some situations. In other situations, there may be no alternative. Some epidemiological research, for example, requires information on patterns of behavior that are sufficiently removed in time to make severe demands on memory. If the information is needed for distant time periods, then researchers have no alternative but to buttress their survey measurements with carefully conducted studies that probe the character of the memory processes that underlie subjects' reports (and misreports).

A final strategy that can be used profitably in developing more accurate survey instruments involves the use of ethnographic research techniques. Not only can these techniques be helpful in preliminary investigations to develop better questionnaires and research designs, but they also provide an important research strategy in their own right for studying questions and populations that may be inaccessible using other research techniques. This appendix concludes with a brief overview of current AIDS research using these techniques.

ETHNOGRAPHIC STUDIES

Anthropologists often deal with phenomena for which other scientific methods are unsuitable. For example, a description of the day's events in a drug shooting gallery or the attempt to understand the meaning of condom use for certain individuals and groups are problems of quite different

---

[66]Neisser (1981), for example, found (by comparing John Dean's testimony before the discovery of Nixon's White House tapes to the evidence of the tapes) that the "gist" of what happened was maintained, even though the recall was wrong in almost every detail.

dimensions than determining the HIV status of those same individuals and populations. The anthropologist's task is one of observation and interpretation rather than statistical evaluation or prediction and thus depends more on human powers to learn, understand, and communicate. Although anthropologists consider an understanding and interpretation of the unique aspects of social life to be an important part of their research, they also analyze their data for patterns and systematic relationships that can lead to generalizations and theory building.

Ethnographic data gathered in the course of fieldwork requires intimate participation in a community and observation of ways of life that often differ from one's own. Long-term participation in the everyday events of a community, neighborhood, or group provides access to detailed information on behaviors, the contexts in which they are enacted, and the vocabulary used to describe them. Participant observation can thus help to identify contradictions between what people say they do and what they actually do. The recording and interpretation of another people's way of life (ethnography) is a process that reveals alternative conceptual frameworks, modes of being, forms of property, and ways of organizing domestic, religious, or political affairs. An appreciation of the diversity of social and cultural forms challenges the aura of naturalness that surrounds the institutions and conventions of life at home and allows one to rethink the basic categories and assumptions of one's own society.

Ethnographic research methods provide particularly useful tools for gathering information about hard-to-reach populations, for acquainting investigators with the diversity of conceptual frameworks and social forms used to organize and interpret events, and for refining and assessing the appropriateness of questionnaires and other research instruments.

Examples of Studies Related to HIV Transmission

Male-Male Sexual Contacts

Anthropological research among Mexicans and Mexican Americans in southern California[67] provides a telling example of the benefits of an ethnographic approach to data gathering. Studies of sexual behavior in Mexico indicate that Mexican men who engage in same-gender sex have

---

[67]By August 1989, 1,151 cases of AIDS had been recorded in Orange County, mainly among homosexual (67.8 percent) or bisexual (18.3 percent) men. Although most cases so far have occurred in the Anglo community, in the past two years the number of Latino cases has grown more rapidly than the number of cases in the Anglo community. Mexicans (sojourners who move back and forth across the border) and Mexican Americans (those born in the United States) constitute the largest proportion of the Latino male population in California (Carrier and Magana, n.d.).

a strong preference for anal intercourse over fellatio. Conceptually, the male playing the receptive role is considered homosexual (by societal standards), but the one playing the insertive role is not, a view that is not shared by men in the Anglo community. Because many Mexicans who engage in same-gender sex may not consider themselves to be homosexual or bisexual, AIDS education programs designed for Anglo gay men may not seem relevant to them (Carrier, 1989; Carrier and Magana, n.d.). Alonso and Koreck (1989) confirmed these findings among rural workers in northern Mexico, adding that similar patterns of sexual behavior may be found among other Latino groups, such as Cubans, in the United States. These researchers caution, however, that other important differences will become apparent once such variables as class and geographic location are considered.

Carrier and Magana (n.d.) similarly note the variability of same-gender sexual behaviors among immigrant Mexican men. Although most immigrant Mexican men continue to engage in behaviors patterned on their prior sexual experiences in Mexico, some adopt mainstream Anglo behaviors. The major determinant of the change appears to be the extent to which their socialization in adolescence was with Mexican or Anglo-American sex partners. The development of appropriate AIDS intervention strategies thus depends on an appreciation of the range, context, meaning, and distribution of sexual practices among different ethnic groups within the United States. Targeted educational interventions may also be required for people who are less educated or for those who are preliterate (Carrier, 1989; Carrier and Magana, n.d.).

Variation in Drug Use Patterns

A second example of how ethnographic research may broaden and enhance the knowledge base on hard-to-reach populations concerns stereotypical views of IV drug users. Anthropological descriptions of the diversity of behaviors, social networks, and self-distinctions that exist in different drug-using communities discount the widely held image of the "dope fiend" as a person who devotes his life to acquiring and using drugs. Although IV drug users in a black community in Baltimore (Mason, 1988) can certainly identify "dope fiends among their numbers," they also recognize and distinguish several other types of drug users:

- "addicts" who pursue drugs constantly but who often have families and jobs and thus participate to some extent in the "straight" world;
- "hope fiends" who are either unable or unwilling to pursue money to support their habit but who hang around drug

areas waiting for an opportunity to get drugs by hustling or through cunning;

- casual users or "chippers" who use IV drugs recreationally on the weekends; and

- people who at various points in their drug-using careers move between these categories.

Seen in this light, IV drug users are a diverse and shifting population, and consequently, prevention and outreach services must be tailored to meet a variety of needs and objectives (Mason, 1988).[68]

Ethnographic Methods

Anthropologists thus investigate, interpret, and attempt to explain cultural difference and its changing nature. By emphasizing the diversity of beliefs, practices, and social conditions in different communities, anthropologists counter the tendency to see Hispanics, blacks, whites, Asians, Native Americans, men, women, or adolescents in the United States as undifferentiated monocultures. Such an appreciation, however, requires a foundation of quantitative data for better interpretation of the illustrative case. Demographic data, usually gathered by the ethnographer using techniques of mapping and census-taking in the study of small-scale societies, are supplemented by census or epidemiological survey data in larger, more complex settings.

In recent years, anthropologists have become more sensitive to sampling issues as greater theoretical attention has been given to variations in the ideologies and beliefs of different individuals in tribal societies. The question of sampling becomes more acute in large populations in which cultural diversity, social stratification, and rapid change raise greater concern regarding methodological precision and the validity and reliability of ethnographic data (see Pelto and Pelto, 1978; Bernard, 1988). The task of ethnographic analysis is further complicated by an awareness that, like data in all the sciences, anthropological data are not acquired through a pristine encounter with the world. Rather, observation, recording, and measurement are directed by concepts and theories, and these concepts and ideas are subject to modification and change. Unless ethnographers take what they suppose to be a purely empirical approach to the world, they often have a "double sense" of the way they go about their work: they assume that their ideas are suitable for interpreting other peoples'

---

[68] Koester's (1989b) study of black IV drug users in Denver also challenges the common stereotype of the drug addict. In Denver, Koester found heroin habits that rarely required more than a $50 a day to sustain, and the petty thefts that supported the drug user's habits were often directed at other addicts.

beliefs but that these ideas, like the beliefs they are intended to interpret, are also the products of particular historical and social circumstances.[69]

The methods used to gather ethnographic data fall into five main categories:

- direct observation of daily life on mundane and ceremonial occasions, description of the observed environment (sometimes with detailed accounts of commerce or household economies), and the recording of spontaneous conversations in which the ethnographer may or may not be a participant (careful records of speech events provide important material for linguistic analysis);

- relatively open-ended interviews and discussions with key informants, as well as the recording of life histories;

- gathering of information from existing records, "native" texts, songs, visual material, government records, and historical archives;

- surveys using structured interviews and involving large numbers of respondents; and

- an important type of learning that receives little attention and involves knowledge not reported in notebooks or on filecards comes from long-term residence in the study community. Memories of experiences, as well as perhaps unconscious recollections and understandings (associated with certain sights, sounds, and smells) often form the backdrop for the patterns and connections that are made during interpretations and analysis of field data.

Much ethnographic data collection depends on developing relationships of trust with those whose lives are the subject of study. Such relationships may develop over an extended period of time, and to some degree they determine the accuracy, sensitivity, and complexity of the data. The researcher has an ethical responsibility to ensure that identities are protected and that the study causes no harm, an objective that the subjects of the study often monitor and probe.

AIDS research presents a special methodological challenge as anthropologists investigate the worlds of men and women who have bisexual and same-gender sexual relations or who may be IV drug users and their sex partners, prostitutes and their clients, male hustlers, prison inmates,

---

[69] Analysis of anthropological data is tempered by an awareness that knowledge in various societies is distributed and controlled in different ways. Anthropologists thus see cultures not as fixed entities but rather as the products of continual processes of creation and contest.

and undocumented laborers. Some ethnographic studies have looked at health care workers, insurance companies, or students and staff in schools, but most research concerns populations that are seen as "marginalized"— outside the mainstream, often impoverished, and involved in activities that are illegal or that are seen as deviant. Methods of ethnographic or anthropological fieldwork developed in other contexts may not be well suited to studies of sexual behaviors and IV drug use, the behaviors that need to be understood and changed in order to stem the epidemic. Both of these areas of study thus present a challenge to accepted notions of participant observation.

Ethnographic Methods in AIDS Research

The difficulties encountered in AIDS research have elicited a variety of methodological responses from the anthropological community. Some ethnographers continue to undertake something close to what is thought of as classical fieldwork. Working alone, they establish rapport and trust with the subjects of study and observe incidents in natural settings. Outside the United States, in Haiti and Brazil, for example, the researcher "lives" in the field, participating extensively in community affairs (Parker, 1987; Farmer and Kleinman, 1989; Farmer, 1990). In the United States, on the other hand, investigators tend to follow an approach often used in urban fieldwork, that is, "visiting the field" more or less on a daily basis (Leonard, 1990; Connors, 1989; Sterk, 1989).

To overcome the difficulties of research with contemporary drug users, for example, the ethnographer may belong to a team that includes former drug users as outreach workers. As a participant observer, the ethnographer documents the kinds of questions, attitudes, and theories the former drug users express, training them to do the same in their own daily reports. In turn, the ethnographer learns about drug use from these outreach workers, and their presence facilitates his or her acceptance as an outsider asking questions on sensitive issues (Mason, 1988; Weibel, 1988). The use of a field station storefront appears to provide a context in which surprisingly sensitive information can be gathered. The protocol of an AIDS intervention project for the sex partners of IV drug users in the predominantly black south side of Chicago, for example, began with a preliminary questionnaire (to gather sociodemographic and epidemiological data), followed by a longer, open-ended conversation that reconstructed the routines of everyday life and some aspects of the respondent's life history. This latter session was designed to alert the sexual partners to the dangers of their day-to-day behavior and offered the chance for a discussion of more subtle issues and personal concerns that were not elicited by the questionnaire (Kane, 1989a,b).

292 | APPENDIX C

"Captive" populations are also the subject of anthropological study. Hospital clinics, county health departments, and bars provide settings for personal interviews, focus group discussions, or the distribution of questionnaires to be filled in and returned to the investigator (McCombie, 1986, 1990; Marshall et al., 1990; K. Kennedy, personal communication).[70] Although this approach is constrained by its inability to compare self-reported and observed behaviors, it can provide information on sexual behavior and drug use that is otherwise difficult to obtain.

Adaptation of the traditional methods of kinship charting to construct a visual image of concrete social relations is an ethnographic method that has been used to elicit information from male and female black and Puerto Rican patients at a methadone clinic in the Bronx. Patients and an anthropologist worked together to create a visual chart of the patient's kin and friends, to which were added color-coded records of his or her drug-using and non-drug-using associates, the particular drugs chosen, sexual and social intimates, those who were aware of the patient's HIV status, those who were informed about their own HIV status, and the patient's household composition as well as that of his or her children (who often lived separately). From an anthropological point of view, the chart is only a starting point for more extended enquiries about various aspects of social life. For an epidemiologist, however, the chart provides an index of the number of people at risk for HIV infection because it records the frequency of sexual intercourse, the categories of sexual partners (those who live together, those who are lovers or more casual partners, and those involved in prostitution), and whether contraceptives are used.[71]

Regional comparisons, which are commonly used in ethnographic research, have been rare in the anthropology of HIV infection. A comparison of two ethnically distinct neighborhoods in Baltimore, however, provides some insight into the different drug choices and the motivations for and meanings of multiple drug use among African Americans and European Americans, as well as the relative risks of HIV infection (Mason, 1989). Similarly, an ethnographic study of the social contexts of injection equipment sharing conducted in New York City and San Francisco revealed that, in the "shooting galleries" of New York, several sets

---

[70] K. Kennedy, Montefiore Family Health Center, Bronx, N.Y., personal communication, August 1989.

[71] A. Pivnik, Montefiore Hospital, Bronx, N.Y., personal communication, October 1989. A different kind of creative mapping plots the distribution of circumcision practices in Africa with areas of high and low AIDS prevalence, an association that has provided significant results, as it suggests that uncircumcised men run a greater risk of becoming infected during sexual intercourse than do those who are circumcised (Reining, 1989). In response to the uncritical use of ethnographic data that marked the early years of the AIDS epidemic, a computer-assisted data base is also being designed to collate cultural information from a variety of sources to complement local, national, and international data bases on HIV seroprevalence (Conant, 1989).

of injection equipment might be shared by more than 100 individuals in a single day. In San Francisco, however, smaller circles of friends shared injection equipment. Given New York's much higher seroprevalence among IV drug users, documentation of these widely varying conditions of injection equipment use provides some contextual understanding of the spread of the virus and the differing character of the epidemic in each location (Watters, 1989).

Although most social research on AIDS has concerned the behaviors that put people at risk for HIV infection, a recent review of the ethnographic literature on sexual behaviors (Cassidy and Porter, 1989) attempted to identify "safer" (nonpenetrative) sexual practices that might form a core of culturally sensitive interventions to control the spread of the virus (keeping in mind that the concept of "safer" sex is a peculiarly Western medical notion). As the review shows, low-risk nonpenetrative behaviors (interfemoral intercourse, masturbation, mutual grooming, sexual joking, and so on) occur commonly throughout the world. A mere listing of sexual behaviors that appear to be universal—including coitus, other forms of intercourse, masturbation, same-sex relations—is not very informative, however, and may even be misleading because the contexts in which the behaviors occur, the attitudes people express about these behaviors, and the meanings of the behaviors vary enormously from locale to locale. Sexual behavior cannot be understood apart from its cultural context, which includes historical, economic, and political aspects. As the example of Mexican American and Anglo sexual behavior in Orange County illustrates, "homosexual" and "bisexual" relations may have a different meaning and expression for different ethnic groups living in the same community. Thus, to communicate effectively with people at risk, AIDS research and interventions must be sensitive to the variability of sexual meaning and experience within and among cultural groups (Cassidy and Porter, 1989).

Findings of Ethnographic Research on AIDS

Ethnographic research on the spread of HIV infection is still in the preliminary phases of data gathering. Nevertheless, some suggestive patterns appear to be emerging. First, prostitutes' use of condoms for professional but not personal sex has been widely observed in Europe and in some parts of the United States (Kane, 1989b; Worth, 1989), the West Indies (McCombie, 1990), and Africa (Bledsoe, 1990). That a similar pattern does not currently exist among prostitutes in Orange County, southern California (Carrier, 1989; Carrier and Magana, n.d.) or among church women in Zaire (Schoepf et al., in press) is a salutary reminder that cultural data should always be examined for its internal variability and in appropriate historical context.

Second, studies of the perceptions of some segments of the scientific community in the United States suggest that scientists—like people everywhere—may hold local views of the world that are at variance with statistical or scientific understanding. Thus health care professionals sometimes fail to adopt precautions when they are at risk, although they show excessive caution in less risky situations. The perception of whether an individual is considered "safe" or "unsafe," for example, depends on a combination of social, economic, and visual criteria (McCombie, 1989).

Third, despite the hazards of attempting to compare heterogeneous data from several countries, some consistent cultural themes can be identified. A comparison of data from Central and East Africa (Zaire, Zambia, Tanzania, and Uganda) and West Africa (Nigeria and Sierra Leone), for example, indicates that condom use poses problems for populations that stress fertility in heterosexual relations; in addition, condoms are associated with promiscuity. Moreover, polygyny is an accepted cultural behavior among men in all three regions, and women may also have multiple sexual partners, often as a result of economic pressures (Bledsoe, 1990).

Finally, several studies indicate that educational messages concerning the dangers of unprotected sex reach some audiences but have actually increased the dangers of HIV infection for other segments of the population. In response to public education about AIDS, men in some parts of Africa continue to pursue an active sexual life but have turned from high-risk groups (e.g., prostitutes) to low-risk pools (e.g., schoolgirls, who may be willing to exchange sex for money to finance their education) (Bledsoe, 1990). Similarly, as a result of educational campaigns in the United States, the clients of street prostitutes in New Jersey report choosing novices and apparently inexperienced young girls in hopes of avoiding long-term drug users who may be infected with HIV (Leonard, 1990).

Gaps and Deficiencies in Current Ethnographic Research

The current flurry of anthropological research on sexual behavior and drug use suffers from the absence of a sustained scholarly tradition in both fields. Although there is more research on sexual behavior than on drug use, the study of sexuality has focused for several decades on sexual meanings and beliefs and has tended to ignore sexual behaviors. The usefulness of such data for HIV research thus is limited. When sexual behaviors were reported, normative behaviors were highlighted rather than the varied ways in which people often choose to lead their sexual lives. Moreover, this earlier literature provides little information concerning the substantial changes that have now altered behaviors in once-isolated regions.

Studies of drug use have provided information on patterns of behavior in homes and shooting galleries (Koester, 1989a,b; Watters, 1989; B.P. Page et al., 1990), on the meaning and practices of injection equipment use (Connors, 1989), and on different patterns of multiple drug use and high-risk behaviors in different ethnic communities (Mason, 1989). Attention is now beginning to turn to the broader determinants of high-risk drug behaviors—such as the history and political economy of drug use and drug marketing (Hamid, 1990; Mason, 1989) and the way in which laws that make carrying a syringe a crime increase the probability that drug users will adopt risky behaviors (Koester, 1989a,b). Much more information is needed, however, on such social determinants, as well as on individual perceptions of the risky behaviors associated with drug use.

Anthropologists and epidemiologists have had some success in identifying and investigating "risky" behaviors in many locations. Yet intervention strategies have sometimes been directed too narrowly at behaviors rather than at people in context. Effective intervention may require a broader understanding of both the personal and social determinants of risk behaviors (cf. O'Reilly, 1989). A further area in which much ethnographic work deserves to be conducted involves the relationship between belief and behavior. In this regard, there is a distinction to be drawn between constructs that constitute a public language and constructs that guide individual choices in specific situations. Recent studies point to the way in which individuals personalize the rules of behavior to fit their own wishes and the limited options from which they might choose (Eyre, 1989; Kane, 1989a,b; Cassidy and Porter, 1989). The ability of impoverished women to practice "safer" sexual behaviors, for example, may be particularly circumscribed. Furthermore, very little is known about the interaction between private worlds of erotic behavior and the public domain of shared meanings recently explored by Parker (1989). It has been suggested that rules regulating sexual behavior may be particularly prone to individual negotiation and improvisation (Cassidy and Porter, 1989). All of these factors emphasize the continuing valuable role to be played by ethnographic research and the discipline of anthropology.

RECOMMENDATIONS

Given the evidence reviewed in the foregoing pages, the committee concludes that there is good reason to believe that accurate measurements of AIDS risk behaviors can be obtained. The committee notes, however, that there is substantial room for improvement in current efforts. This potential is not surprising given the immaturity of many of the relevant research fields.

The committee believes that appropriate investments to create a better foundation of relevant methodological knowledge can lead to more certain scientific understanding about the behaviors that transmit HIV and the factors that motivate and shape these behaviors. Toward this end the committee makes the following recommendations.

The committee recommends that the Public Health Service and other organizations supporting AIDS research provide increased support for methodological research on the measurement of behaviors that transmit HIV. Such research should consider inferential problems introduced by nonresponse and by nonsampling factors, including (but not limited to) the effects of question wording and question context, the time periods and events that respondents are asked to recall, and the effects of anonymity guarantees on survey responses.

The committee recommends that researchers who conduct behavioral surveys on HIV transmission make increased use of ethnographic studies, pretests, pilot studies, cognitive laboratory investigations, and other similar developmental strategies to aid in the design of large-scale surveys.

The committee recommends that, where appropriate, researchers embed experimental studies within behavioral surveys on HIV transmission to assess the effects of key aspects of the survey measurement process.

The committee recommends that, whenever feasible, researchers supplement self-reports in behavioral surveys on HIV transmission with other indicators of these behaviors that do not rely on respondent reports.

REFERENCES

Aiken, L. S. (1986) Retrospective self-reports by clients differ from original reports: Implications for the evaluation of drug treatment programs. *International Journal of the Addictions* 21:767–788.

Aiken, L. S., and LoSciuto, L. A. (1985) Ex-addict versus nonaddict counselors' knowledge of clients' drug use. *International Journal of the Addictions* 20:417–433.

Allen, R. M., and Haupt, T. D. (1966) The sex inventory: Test-retest reliability of scale scores and items. *Journal of Clinical Psychology* 22:375–378.

Alonso, A. M., and Koreck, M. T. (1989) Silences: Hispanics, AIDS, and sexual practices. *Differences* 1:101–124.

Amsel, Z., Mandell, W., Matthias, L., Mason, C., and Hocherman, I. (1976) Reliability and validity of self-reported illegal activities and drug use collected from narcotic addicts. *International Journal of the Addictions* 11:325–336.

Anastasi, A. (1976) *Psychological Testing*. 4th ed. New York: Macmillan.

Andersen, B. L., and Broffitt, B. (1988) Is there a reliable and valid self-report measure of sexual behavior? *Archives of Sexual Behavior* 17:509–525.

Andersen, R., Kasper, J., Frankel, M. R., and Associates. (1979) *Total Survey Error.* San Francisco: Jossey-Bass.

Anderson, R. M., and May, R. M. (1988) Epidemiological parameters of HIV transmission. *Nature* 333:514–519.

Aral, S. O., Magder, L. S., and Bowen, G. S. (1989) HIV risk behavior screening: Concordance between assessments through interviews and questionnaires. Presented at the Fifth International Conference on AIDS, Montreal, June 4–9.

Axinn, W. G. (n.d.) The influence of interviewer gender on responses to sensitive questions in less developed settings: Evidence from Nepal. Population Studies Center, Institute for Social Research and Department of Sociology, University of Michigan, Ann Arbor, Mich.

Baddeley, A. D. (1979) The limitations of human memory: Implications for the design of retrospective surveys. In L. Moss and H. Goldstein, eds., *The Recall Method in Social Surveys.* London: University of London Institute of Education.

Bailar, B. (1975) The effects of rotation group bias on estimates from panel surveys. *Journal of the American Statistical Association* 70:23–30.

Bailar, B., Bailey, L., and Stevens, J. (1977) Measures of interviewer bias and variance. *Journal of Marketing Research* 14:337–343.

Bailey, L., Moore, T., and Bailar, B. (1978) An interviewer variance study for the eight impact cities of the National Crime Survey cities sample. *Journal of the American Statistical Association* 73:16–23.

Bale, R. N. (1979) The validity and reliability of self-reported data from heroin addicts: Mailed questionnaires compared with face-to-face interviews. *International Journal of the Addictions* 14:993–1000.

Bale, R. N., Van Stone, W. W., Engelsing, T. M. J., Zarcone, V. P., and Kuldau, J. M. (1981) The validity of self-reported heroin use. *International Journal of the Addictions* 16:1387–1398.

Ball, J. C. (1967) The reliability and validity of interview data obtained from 59 narcotic drug addicts. *American Journal of Sociology* 72:650–654.

Ball, J. C., Lange, W. R., Myers, C. P., and Friedman, S. R. (1988) Reducing the risk of AIDS through methadone maintenance treatment. *Journal of Health and Social Behavior* 29:214–226.

Bardoux, C., Buning, E., Leentvaar-Kuijpers, A., Verster, A., and Coutinho, R. A. (1989) Declining incidence of acute hepatitis B among drug users in Amsterdam may indicate a change in risk behavior. Presented at the Fifth International Conference on AIDS, Montreal, June 4–9.

Bartlett, F. C. (1932) *Remembering: A Study in Experimental Social Psychology.* Cambridge University Press: Cambridge, Great Britain.

Batki, S. L., Sorensen, J. L., Coates, C., and Gibson, D. R. (1989) Methadone maintenance for AIDS-affected IV drug users: Psychiatric factors and outcome three months into treatment (abstract). In L. S. Harris, ed., *Problems of Drug Dependence 1988: Proceedings of the Committee on the Problems of Drug Dependence.* Washington, D.C.: U.S. Government Printing Office.

Bauman, L. J., and Adair, E. G. (1989) Use of ethnographic interviewing to inform questionnaire construction. Presented at the Annual Meeting of the American Association for Public Opinion Research, St. Petersburg, Fla., May.

Beck, C., Ward, C., Mendelson, M., Mock, J., and Erbaugh, J. (1961) An inventory measuring depression. *Archives of General Psychiatry* 4:561–571.

Beniger, J. R. (1984) Mass media, contraceptive behavior, and attitudes on abortion: Toward a comprehensive model of subjective social change. In C. F. Turner and E. Martin, eds., *Surveying Subjective Phenomena.* Vol. 2. New York: Russell Sage.

Benney, M., Riesman, D., and Star, S. A. (1956) Age and sex in the interview. *American Journal of Sociology* 62:143–152.

Bentler, P. M. (1968a) Heterosexual behaviour assessment. I. Males. *Behaviour Research and Therapy* 6:21–25.

Bentler, P. M. (1968b) Heterosexual behaviour assessment. II. Females. *Behaviour Research and Therapy* 6:27–30.

Benus, J., and Ackerman, J. C. (1971) The problem of nonresponse in sample surveys. In J. B. Lansing, S. B. Withey, A. C. Wolfe et al., eds., *Working Papers on Survey Research in Poverty Areas,* Ann Arbor: Survey Research Center, Institute for Social Research, University of Michigan.

Ben-Yehuda, N. (1980) Are addicts' self-reports to be trusted? *International Journal of the Addictions* 15:1265–1270.

Bernard, H. R. (1988) *Research Methods in Cultural Anthropology.* Newbury Park, Calif.: Sage.

Biderman, A. D., and Lynch, J. P. (1981) Recency bias in data on self-reported victimization. *Proceedings of the American Statistical Association (Social Statistics Section)* 1981:31–40.

Biderman, A. D., and Moore, J. C. (1980) Report of the workshop on applying cognitive psychology to recall problems of the National Crime Survey. Unpublished manuscript. Bureau of Social Science Research, Washington, D.C.

Bihari, B., and Ottomanelli, G. (1989) Defense mechanisms and HIV risk related behaviors in substance abusers. Presented at the Fifth International Conference on AIDS, Montreal, June 4–9.

Billy, J. O. G., and Udry, J. R. (1985) Patterns of adolescent friendship and effects on sexual behavior. *Social Psychology Quarterly* 48:27–41.

Bishop, Y. M. M., Fienberg, S., and Holland, P. W. (1975) *Discrete Multivariate Analysis.* Cambridge, Mass.: Massachusetts Institute of Technology Press.

Bledsoe, C. (1990) The politics of AIDS and condoms for stable heterosexual relations in Africa: Recent evidence from the local print media. In W. P. Handwerker, ed., *Births and Power: The Politics of Reproduction.* Boulder, Colo.: Westview Press.

Blumstein, P., and Schwartz, P. (1977) Bisexuality: Some social psychological issues. *Journal of Social Issues* 33:30–45.

Blumstein, P. W., and Schwartz, P. (1983) *American Couples: Money, Work, and Sex.* New York: Morrow.

Bonito, A. J., Nurco, D. N., and Shaffer, J. W. (1976) The veridicality of addicts' self-reports in social research. *International Journal of the Addictions* 11:719–724.

Borgatta, E. F., Blumstein, P., and Schwartz, P. (1987) Research Methodologies for Sensitive Data Collection: Final Report submitted to the Centers for Disease Control. Department of Sociology, University of Washington, Seattle.

Boruch, R. F. (1989) Resolving privacy problems in AIDS research: A primer. In L. Sechrest, H. Freeman, and A. Mulley, eds., *Health Services Research Methodology: A Focus on AIDS*. Conference Proceedings. Rockville, Md.: National Center for Health Services Research and Health Care Technology Assessment.

Bradburn, N. W., Rips, L. J., and Shevell, S. K. (1987) Answering autobiographical questions: The impact of memory and inference on surveys. *Science* 236:157–161.

Bradburn, N. M., Sudman, S., and Associates (1979) *Improving Interview Method and Questionnaire Design*. San Francisco: Jossey Bass.

Brady, J. P., and Levitt, E. E. (1965) The scalability of sexual experiences. *Psychological Record* 15:275–279.

Brewer, M. B., Dull, V. T., and Jobe, J. B. (1989) Social cognition approach to reporting chronic health conditions. *Vital and Health Statistics*, Series 6, Whole No. 3.

Brooks, C. A., and Bailar, B. (1978) *An Error Profile: Employment as Measured by the Current Population Survey*. Statistical Policy Working Paper 3. Washington, D.C.: U.S. Department of Commerce.

Brown, L. S., Phillips, R., Ajulchukwu, D., Battjes, R., Primm, B. J., and Nemoto, T. (1989) Demographic and behavioral features of HIV infection in intravenous drug users in New York City drug treatment programs: 1985–1988. Presented at the Fifth International Conference on AIDS, Montreal, June 4–9.

Cain, V. S., and Baldwin, W. (1989) The national study of health and sexual behavior. Presented at the Fifth International Conference on AIDS, Montreal, June 4–9.

Campbell, A. A. (1987) Randomized response technique (letter). *Science* 236:1049.

Cannell, C. F., Fisher, G., and Bakker, T. (1965) Reporting of hospitalization in the Health Interview Survey. *Vital and Health Statistics*, Series 2, Whole No. 6.

Cannell, C. F., Marquis, K. H., and Laurent, A. (1977) A summary of studies of interviewing methodology. *Vital and Health Statistics*, Series 2, Whole No. 69.

Cannell, C. F., Miller, P. V., and Oksenberg, L. (1981) Research on interviewing techniques. In S. Leinhardt, ed., *Sociological Methodology 1981*. San Francisco: Jossey-Bass.

Cannell, C., Oksenberg, L., Kalton, G., Bischoping, K., and Fowler, F. J. (1989) New techniques for pretesting survey questions. Final Report to the National Center for Health Services Research and Health Care Technology Assessment. Survey Research Center, University of Michigan, Ann Arbor, Mich.

Carrier, J. M. (1989) Sexual behavior and the spread of AIDS in Mexico. *Medical Anthropology* 10:129–142.

Carrier, J. M., and Magana, J. R. (n.d.) Applied anthropology and AIDS in a health care agency. Unpublished manuscript. Orange County Health Care Agency, Orange County, Calif.

Cassidy, C. M., and Porter, R. W. (1989) *Ethnographic Perspectives on Nonpenetrative Sexual Behavior*. Research Triangle Park, N.C.: AIDSCOM, Family Health International.

Castro, K. G., Lieb, S., Jaffe, H. W., Narkonas, J. P., Calisher, C. H., et al. (1988) Transmission of HIV in Belle Glade, Florida: Lessons for other communities in the United States. *Science* 239:193–197.

Catania, J. A., McDermott, L. J., and Pollack, L. M. (1986) Questionnaire response bias and face-to-face interview sample bias in sexuality research. *Journal of Sex Research* 22:52–72.

Catania, J. A., Gibson, D. R., Chitwood, D. D., and Coates, T. J. (1990a) Methodological problems in AIDS behavioral research: Influences on measurement error and participation bias in studies of sexual behavior. *Psychological Bulletin* 108:339-362.

Catania, J. A., Gibson, D. R., Marin, B., Coates, T. J., and Greenblatt, R. M. (1990b) Response bias in assessing sexual behaviors relevant to HIV transmission. *Evaluation and Program Planning* 13:19-29.

Centers for Disease Control (CDC). (1988) HIV-related beliefs, knowledge, and behaviors among high school students. *Morbidity and Mortality Weekly Report* 37:717–721.

Chaisson, R. E., Osmond, D., Moss, A. R., Feldman, H. W., and Bernacki, P. (1987) HIV, bleach, and needle sharing. *Lancet* 20 June:1430.

Chaisson, R. E., Osmond, D., Bacchetti, P., Brodie, B., Sande, M. A., and Moss, A. R. (1988) Cocaine, race and HIV infection in IV drug users. Presented at the Fourth International Conference on AIDS, Stockholm, June 12–16.

Chaisson, R. E., Bacchetti, P., Osmond, D., Brodie, B., Sande, M. A., and Moss, A. R. (1989) Cocaine use and HIV infection in intravenous drug users. *Journal of the American Medical Association* 261:561–609.

Cisin, I. H., and Parry, H. L. (1979) Sensitivity of survey techniques in measuring illicit drug use. In J. D. Rittenhouse, ed., *Developmental Papers: Attempts to Improve the Measurement of Heroin Use in the National Survey.* Washington, D.C.: National Institute on Drug Abuse.

Citro, C. F., and Cohen, M. L. (1985) *The Bicentennial Census: New Directions for Methodology in 1990.* Report of the National Research Council Panel on Decennial Census Methodology. Washington, D.C.: National Academy Press.

Clark, A. L. and Wallin, P. (1964) The accuracy of husbands' and wives' reports of the frequency of marital coitus. *Population Studies* 18:165–173.

Clark, J. P., and Tifft, L. L. (1966) Polygraph and interview validation of self-reported deviant behavior. *American Sociological Review* 31:516–523.

Coates, R. A., Soskolne, C. L., Calzavara, L., Read, S. E., Fanning, M. M., et al. (1986) The reliability of sexual histories in AIDS-related research: Evaluation of an interview-administered questionnaire. *Canadian Journal of Public Health* 77:343–348.

Coates, R. A., Calzavara, L. M., Soskolne, C. L., Read, S. E., Fanning, M. M., et al. (1988) Validity of sexual histories in a prospective study of male sexual contacts of men with AIDS or an AIDS-related condition. *American Journal of Epidemiology* 128:719–728.

Cochran, W. G., Mosteller, F., and Tukey, J. W. (1953) Statistical problems of the Kinsey report. *Journal of the American Statistical Association* 48:673–716.

Communication Technologies, Inc. (1987) *A Report on Designing an Effective AIDS Prevention Campaign Strategy for San Francisco: Results from the Fourth Probability Sample of an Urban Gay Male Community.* San Francisco: Communication Technologies, Inc., July 31, 1987.

Communication Technologies, Inc. (1988) *A Report on Planning for the AIDS Epidemic in California: A Population-Based Assessment of Knowledge, Attitudes, and Behavior.* San Francisco: Communication Technologies, Inc., June 30, 1988.

Conant, F. P. (1989) AIDS and beyond: The need, and a design, for a targeted cultural information management system. Unpublished manuscript. Department of Anthropology, Hunter College, City University of New York.

Connors, M. (1989) Perception of risk and HIV infection among intravenous drug users (IVDUs) in Worcester, Mass. Unpublished manuscript. Department of Anthropology, University of Massachusetts, Amherst.

Conte, H. R. (1983) Development and use of self-report techniques for assessing sexual functioning: A review and critique. *Archives of Sexual Behavior* 12:555–576.

Converse, J. M., and Schuman, H. (1974) *Conversations at Random: Survey Research as Interviewers See It.* New York: Wiley.

Coombs, L. C. (1977) Levels of reliability in fertility survey data. *Studies in Family Planning* 8:218–232.

Council of American Survey Research Organizations (CASRO) (1982) *On the Definition of Response Rates. A Special Report of the CASRO Task Force on Completion Rates.* Port Jefferson, N.Y.

Cox, T. J., and Longwell, B. (1974) Reliability of interview data concerning current heroin use from heroin addicts on methadone. *International Journal of the Addictions* 9:161–165.

Coxon, A. P. M. (1986) Report of a Pilot Study: Project on Sexual Lifestyles of Non-Heterosexual Males. Unpublished manuscript. Social Research Unit, University College, Cardiff, Wales.

Coxon, A. P. M. (1988) Something sensational: The sexual diary as a tool for mapping detailed sexual behavior. *Sociological Review* 35:353–367.

Coxon, A. P. M., and Carballo M. (1989) Editorial Review: Research on AIDS: Behavioral perspectives. *AIDS* 3:191–197.

Coxon, A. P. M., and Davies, P. M. (1989) Using structured sexual diaries data to estimate rates, predictors and context of high-risk sexual behaviour. Presented at the Fifth International Conference on AIDS, Montreal, June 4–9.

Crider, R. A. (1985) Heroin incidence: A trend comparison between National Household Survey data and indicator data. In B. A. Rouse, N. J. Kozel, and L. G. Richards, eds., *Self-Report Methods of Estimating Drug Use: Meeting Current Challenges to Validity.* DHHS Publication No. (ADM) 85–1402. National Institute on Drug Abuse Research Monograph No. 57. Washington, D.C.: U.S. Government Printing Office.

Criqui, M. H. (1979) Response bias and risk ratios in epidemiologic studies. *American Journal of Epidemiology* 109:394–399.

Cronbach, L. J., and Gleser, G. C. (1965) *Psychological Tests and Personnel Decisions.* 2nd ed. Urbana: University of Illinois Press.

Cynamon, M. L. (1989) The national survey of health and sexual behavior: The pretest experience. Presented at the Fifth International Conference on AIDS, Montreal, June 4–9.

Czaja, R. (1987–88) Asking sensitive behavioral questions in telephone surveys. *Applied Research and Evaluation* 8:23–32.

Daniel, W. W. (1975) Nonresponse in sociological surveys. *Sociological Methods and Research* 3:291–307.

Darrow, W. W., Jaffe, H. W., Thomas, P. A., Haverkos, H. W., Rogers, M. F., et al. (1986) Sex of interviewer, place of interview, and responses of homosexual men to sensitive questions. *Archives of Sexual Behavior* 15:79–88.

Davies, P. M. (1986) Some problems in defining and sampling non-heterosexual males. Working Paper No. 21. Social Research Unit, University College, Cardiff, Wales.

Davis, K. H., Hawks, R. L., and Blanke, R. V. (1988) Assessment of laboratory quality in urine drug testing. *Journal of the American Medical Association* 260:1749–1754.

Day, N., Houston-Hamilton, A., Taylor, D., Lemp, G., and Rutherford, G. (1989) Tracking survey of AIDS knowledge, attitudes and behaviors in San Francisco's Black communities. Presented at the Fifth International Conference on AIDS, Montreal, June 4–9.

De Gruttola, V., and Fineberg, H. V. (1989) Estimating prevalence of HIV infection. Considerations in the design and analysis of a national seroprevalence survey. *Journal of Acquired Immune Deficiency Syndromes* 2:472–480.

DeLamater, J. D. (1974) Methodological issues in the study of premarital sexuality. *Sociological Methods and Research* 3:30–61.

DeLamater, J., and MacCorquodale, P. (1975) The effects of interview schedule variations on reported sexual behavior. *Sociological Methods and Research* 4:215–236.

DeLamater, J., and MacCorquodale, P. (1979) *Premarital Sexuality: Attitudes, Relationships, Behavior.* Madison, Wisc.: University of Wisconsin Press.

DeMaio, T. J., ed. (1984) *Approaches to Developing Questionnaires.* Statistical Policy Working Paper No. 10. Washington, D.C.: Office of Management and Budget.

DeMaio, T. J. (1984) Social desirability and survey measurement: A review. In C. F. Turner and E. Martin, eds., *Surveying Subjective Phenomena.* Vol. 2. New York: Russell Sage.

Derogatis, L. R. (1980) Psychological assessment of psychosexual functioning. *Psychiatric Clinics of North America* 3:113–131.

Derogatis, L. R., and Melisaratos, N. (1979) The DSFI: A multidimensional measure of sexual functioning. *Journal of Sex and Marital Therapy* 5:244–281.

Des Jarlais, D. C., and Friedman, S. R. (1988a) Intravenous cocaine, crack, and HIV infection. *Journal of the American Medical Association* 259:1945–1946.

Des Jarlais, D. C., and Friedman, S. R. (1988b) Needle sharing among IVDUs at risk for AIDS. *American Journal of Public Health* 78:1498.

Des Jarlais, D. C., and Friedman, S. R. (1988c) The psychology of preventing AIDS among intravenous drug users: A social learning conceptualization. *American Psychologist* 43:865–870.

Des Jarlais, D. C., Friedman, S. R., and Stoneburner, R. L. (1988) HIV infection and intravenous drug use: Critical issues in transmission dynamics, infection outcomes, and prevention. *Reviews of Infectious Diseases* 10:151–158.

Des Jarlais, D. C., Friedman, S. R., Sotheran, J. L., and Stoneburner, R. (1988) The sharing of drug injection equipment and the AIDS epidemic in New York City: The first decade. In R. J. Battjes and R. W. Pickens, eds., *Needle Sharing Among Intravenous Drug Abusers: National and International Perspectives.* National Institute on Drug Abuse Research Monograph 80. Washington, D.C.: U.S. Government Printing Office.

Des Jarlais, D. C., Tross, S., Abdul-Quader, A., Kouzi, A., and Friedman, S. R. (1989a) Intravenous drug users and maintenance of behavior change. Presented at the Fifth International Conference on AIDS, Montreal, June 4–9.

Des Jarlais, D. C., Hagen, H., Purchase, D., Reid, T., and Friedman, S. R. (1989b) Safer injection among participants in the first North American syringe exchange program. Presented at the Fifth International Conference on AIDS, Montreal, June 4–9.

Dougherty, J. A. (1988) Prevention of HIV transmission in IV drug users. Presented at the IV International Conference on AIDS, Stockholm, June 12–16.

Drug Enforcement Administration (DEA). (1988) *Crack Cocaine Availability and Trafficking in the United States.* Washington, D.C.: U.S. Department of Justice. January.

Eckerman, W. C., Bates, J. D., Rachal, J. V., and Poole, W. K. (1971) *Drug Usage and Arrest Charges.* Washington, D.C.: Bureau of Narcotics and Dangerous Drugs.

Eisenberg, D. (1981) A scientific gold rush. *Science* 213:1104–1105.

Ericsson, K. A., and Simon, H. A. (1980) Verbal reports as data. *Psychological Review* 87:215–251.

Exner, T. M., Meyer-Bahlburg, H. F. L., Gruen, R. S., Ehrhardt, A. A., and Gorman, J. M. (1989) Peer norms for safer sex as a predictor of sexual risk behaviors in a cohort of gay men. Presented at the Fifth International Conference on AIDS, Montreal, June 4–9.

Eyre, S. L. (1989) Metaphors of AIDS: Social and existential function. Presented at the Annual Meeting of the American Anthropological Association, Washington, D.C., November 16–19.

Farmer, P. (1990) Sending sickness: Sorcery, politics, and changing concepts of AIDS in rural Haiti. *Medical Anthropology Quarterly* 4:6–27.

Farmer, P., and Kleinman, A. (1989) AIDS as human suffering. *Daedalus* 118:135–160.

Fay, R. E., Turner, C. F., Klassen, A. D., and Gagnon, J. H. (1989) Prevalence and patterns of same-gender sexual contact among men. *Science* 243:338–348.

Feldman, H. F., and Biernacki, P. (1988) The ethnography of needle sharing among intravenous drug users and implications for public policies and intervention strategies. In R. J. Battjes and R. W. Pickens, eds., *Needle Sharing Among Intravenous Drug Abusers: National and International Perspectives.* DHHS Publication No. (ADM) 88–1567. National Institute on Drug Abuse Research Monograph 80. Washington, D.C.: U.S. Government Printing Office.

Ferber, R. (1966) *The Reliability of Consumer Reports of Financial Assets and Debts.* Bureau of Economic and Business Research, University of Illinois, Urbana.

Fineberg, H. (1988) Education to prevent AIDS: Prospects and obstacles. *Science* 239:592–596.

Flaskerud, J. H., and Nyamathi, A. M. (1989) An AIDS education program for black and Latina women. Presented at the Fifth International AIDS Conference, Montreal, June 4–9.

Fowler, F. J., and Mangione, T. W. (1990) *Standardized Survey Interviewing.* Newbury Park, Calif: Sage.

Fox, J. A., and Tracy, P. E. (1986) *Randomized Response: A Method for Sensitive Surveys.* Beverly Hills, Calif: Sage Publications.

Franks, F. (1981) *Polywater.* Cambridge, Mass.: Massachusetts Institute of Technology Press.

Friedman, S. R., and Des Jarlais, D. C. (1989) *Measurement of Intravenous Drug Use Behaviors that Risk HIV Transmission.* Unpublished manuscript. Narcotic and Drug Research, Inc., New York.

Friedman, S. R., Sotheran, J. L., Abdul-Quader, A., Primm, B. J., Des Jarlais, D. C., et al. (1987a) The AIDS epidemic among blacks and Hispanics. *The Milbank Quarterly* 65:455–499.

Friedman, S. R., Des Jarlais, D. C., Sotheran, J. L., Garber, J., Cohen, H., and Smith, D. (1987b) AIDS and self-organization among intravenous drug users. *International Journal of the Addictions* 22:201–219.

Friedman, S. R., Dozier, C., Sterk, C., Williams, T., Sotheran, J. L., et al. (1988) Crack use puts women at risk for heterosexual transmission of HIV from intravenous drug users. Presented at the Fourth International Conference on AIDS, Stockholm, June 12–16.

Friedman, S. R., Rosenblum, A., Goldsmith, D., Des Jarlais, D. C., Sufian, M. , et al. (1989) Risk factors for HIV-1 infection among street-recruited intravenous drug users in New York City. Presented at the Fifth International Conference on AIDS, Montreal, June 4–9.

Fullilove, R. E. III, Fullilove, M. T., Bowser, B., and Gross, S. A. (1989) Crack use and risk for AIDS among black adolescents. Presented at the Fifth International Conference on AIDS, Montreal, June 4–9.

Fullilove, R. E., Fullilove, M. T., Bowser, B., and Gross, S. (1990) Crack users: The new AIDS risk group? *Journal of Cancer Prevention and Detection* 14:363-368.

Gagnon, J. H. (1988) Sex research and sexual conduct in the era of AIDS. *Journal on AIDS* 1:593–601.

Gawin, F. H., and Ellinwood, E. H., Jr. (1988) Cocaine and other stimulants: Actions, abuse, and treatment. *New England Journal of Medicine* 318:1173–1182.

Gebhard, P. H. (1972) Incidence of overt homosexuality in the United States and Western Europe. In National Institute of Mental Health Task Force on Homosexuality, *Final Report and Background Papers*. Washington, D.C.: U.S. Government Printing Office.

Gebhard, P. H., and Johnson, A. B. (1979) *The Kinsey Data: Marginal Tabulations of 1938–1963 Interviews Conducted by the Institute for Sex Research*. Philadelphia: W. B. Saunders.

Gelmon, K., Schechter, M. T., Sheps, S. B., Hershler, R., and Craib, K. J. P. (1989) Recall bias and memory failure: An empiric demonstration in persons with acquired immune deficiency syndrome. Presented at the Fifth International Conference on AIDS, Montreal, June 4–9.

Gibson, D., Wermuth, L., Sorensen, J. L., Menicucci, L., and Bernal, G. (1987) Approval need in self-reports of addicts and family members. *International Journal of the Addictions* 22:895–903.

Gibson, D. R., Sorensen, J. L., Lovelle-Drache, J., Catania, J., Kegeles, S., and Young, M. (1988) Psychosocial predictors of AIDS high risk behavior among intravenous drug users and their sexual partners. Presented at the Fourth International Conference on AIDS, Stockholm, June 12–16.

Gibson, D. R., Lovelle-Drache, J., Derby, S., Garcia-Soto, M., Sorensen, J. L., and Melese-d'Hospital, I. (1989) Brief counseling to reduce AIDS risk in IV drug users: Update. Presented at the Fifth International Conference on AIDS, Montreal, June 4–9.

Gonzalez, M., Ogus, J., Shapiro, G., and Tepping, B. (1975) Standards for discussion and presentation of errors in survey and census data. *Journal of the American Statistical Association* 70(351, whole pt. 2).

Goodstadt, M. S., and Gruson, V. (1975) The randomized response technique: A test on drug use. *Journal of the American Statistical Association* 70:814–818.

Goodstadt, M. S., Cook, G., and Gruson, V. (1978) The validity of reported drug use: The randomized response technique. *International Journal of the Addictions* 13:359–367.

Goyder, J. (1987) *The Silent Minority: Nonrespondents on Sample Surveys.* Cambridge, U.K.: Polity Press.

Groves, R. M., and Kahn, R. L. (1979) *Surveys by Telephone: A National Comparison with Personal Interviews.* New York: Academic Press.

Gulliksen, H. (1950) *Theory of Mental Tests.* New York: Wiley.

Haberman, P. W., Josephson, E., Zanes, A., and Ellinson, J. (1972) High school drug behavior: A methodological report on pilot studies. In S. Einstein and S. Allen, eds., *Proceedings of First International Conference on Student Drug Surveys.* New York: Baywood Publishing.

Hamid, A. (1990) The political economy of crack-related violence. *Contemporary Drug Problems* Spring 1990.

Hamilton, M. (1960) A rating scale for depression. *Journal of Neurological and Neurosurgical Psychiatry* 23:56–61.

Harbison, J. J. M., Graham, P. J., Quinn, J. T., McAllister, H., and Woodward, R. (1974) A questionnaire measure of sexual interest. *Archives of Sexual Behavior* 3:357–366.

Harrell, A. V. (1985) Validation of self-report: The research record. In B. A. Rouse, N. J. Kozel, and L. G. Richards, eds., *Self-Report Methods of Estimating Drug Use: Meeting Current Challenges to Validity.* National Institute on Drug Abuse Research Monograph No. 57. Washington, D.C.: U.S. Government Printing Office.

Heckert, K., Shultz, J., and Salem, N. (1989) The Minnesota general public AIDS survey: A behavioral risk factor survey supplement. Presented at the Fifth International Conference on AIDS, Montreal, June 4–9.

Heitzman, C. A., Sorensen, J. L., Gibson, D. R., Morales, E. R., Costantin, M., et al. (1989) AIDS prevention among IV drug users: Behaviors changes. Presented at the Annual Meeting of the Society of Behavioral Medicine, San Francisco, Calif.

Henson, R., Cannell, C. F., and Lawson, S. (1973) *Effects of Interviewer Style and Question Form on Reporting of Automobile Accidents.* Ann Arbor: Survey Research Center, University of Michigan.

Herb, F., Watters, J. K., Case, P., and Petitti, D. (1989) Endocarditis, subcutaneous abscesses, and other bacterial infections in intravenous drug users and their association with skin-cleaning at drug injection sites. Presented at the Fifth International Conference on AIDS, Montreal, June 4–9.

Herold, E. S., and Way, L. (1988) Sexual self-disclosure among university women. *Journal of Sex Research* 24:1–14.

Hesselbrock, M., Babor, T. F., Hesselbrock, V., Meyer, R. E., and Workman, K. (1983) Never believe an alcoholic? On the validity of self-report measures of alcohol dependence and related constructs. *International Journal of the Addictions* 18:593–609.

Himmelweit, H. T., and Turner, C. F. (1982) Social and psychological antecedents of depression. In P. Baltes and O. Brim, eds. *Life-span Development and Behavior.* New York: Academic Press.

Ho, C. Y., Powell, R. W., and Liley, P. E. (1974) Thermal conductivity of the elements: A comprehensive review. *Journal of Physical and Chemical Reference Data* 3:1–244.

Hochhauser, M. (1987) Readability of AIDS educational materials. Presented at the Annual Meeting of the American Psychological Association, New York, August.

Hofferth, S. L., Kahn, J. R., and Baldwin, W. (1987) Premarital sexual activity among U.S. teenage women over the past three decades. *Family Planning Perspectives* 19:46–53.

Hoon, E. F., Hoon P. W., and Wincze, J. P. (1976) An inventory for the measurement of female sexual arousability: The SAI. *Archives of Sexual Behavior* 5:291–300.

Huang, K. H. C., Watters, J. K., and Case, P. (1988) Psychological assessment and AIDS research with intravenous drug users: Challenges in measurement. *Journal of Psychoactive Drugs* 20:191–195.

Huang, K. H. C., Watters, J., and Case, P. (1989) Compliance with AIDS prevention measures among intravenous drug users: Health beliefs or social/environmental factors? Presented at the Fifth International Conference on AIDS, Montreal, June 4–9.

Hubbard, R. L, Marsden, M. E., and Allison, M. (1984) *Reliability and Validity of TOPS Data.* Research Triangle Park, N.C.: Research Triangle Institute.

Hubbard, R. L., Eckerman, W. C., Rachal, J. V. and Williams, J. R. (1977) Factors affecting the validity of self-reports of drug use: An overview. *Proceedings of the American Statistical Association (Social Statistics Section)* 1977:360–365. Chicago, Ill., August 15–18.

Hunter, J. S. (1977) Quality assessment of measurement methods. In National Research Council, *Environmental Monitoring,* Vol. 4a. Washington, D.C.: National Academy of Sciences.

Hunter, J. S. (1980) The national system of scientific measurement. *Science* 210:869–874.

Hyman, H. H., Cobb, W. J., Feldman, J. J., Hart, C. W., and Stember, C. H. (1954) *Interviewing in Social Research.* Chicago: University of Chicago Press.

Jabine, T. B., Straf, M. L., Tanur, J. M., Tourangeau, R., eds. (1985) *Cognitive Aspects of Survey Methodology.* Washington, D.C.: National Academy Press.

Jackson, D. D., Lee, W. B., and Liu, C. (1980) Aseismic uplift in southern California: An alternative interpretation. *Science* 210:534–536.

Jacobson, N. S., and Moore, D. (1981) Spouses as observers of the events in their relationship. *Consulting and Clinical Psychology* 49:269–277.

Johnson, A., Wadsworth, J., Elliot, P., Prior, L., Wallace, P., et al. (1989) A pilot study of sexual lifestyle in a random sample of the population of Great Britain. *AIDS* 3:135–141.

Johnston, L. D., and O'Malley, P. M. (1985) Issues of validity and population coverage in student surveys of drug use. In B. A. Rouse, N. J. Kozel, and L. G. Richards, eds., *Self-report methods of estimating drug use: Meeting current challenges to validity.* DHHS Publication No. (ADM) 85–1402. National Institute on Drug Abuse Research Monograph No. 57. Washington, D.C.: U.S. Government Printing Office.

Josephson, E. (1970) Resistance to community surveys. *Social Problems* 18:117–129.

Kahn, J. R., Kalsbeek, W. D., and Hofferth, S. L. (1988) National estimates of teenage sexual activity: Evaluating the comparability of three national surveys. *Demography* 25:189–204.

Kahn, R. L., and Cannell, C. F. (1957) *The Dynamics of Interviewing.* New York: Wiley.

Kane, S. (1989a) Heterosexuals, AIDS and the heroin subculture. Unpublished manuscript. Kane Agency, New York, N.Y.

Kane, S. (1989b) Interviews with two women: AIDS, addiction and hetero-sex on Chicago's south side. Unpublished manuscript. Kane Agency, New York, N.Y.

Kann, L., Nelson, G. D., Jones, J. T., and Kolbe, L. J. (1989) Establishing a system of complementary school-based surveys to annually assess HIV-related knowledge, beliefs, and behaviors among adolescents. *Journal of School Health* 59:55–58.

Kann, L., Nelson, G., Jones, J., and Kolbe, L. (1989) HIV-related knowledge, beliefs and behaviors among high school students in the United States. Presented at the Fifth International Conference on AIDS, Montreal, June 4–9.

Kaplan, H. B. (1989) Methodological problems in the study of psychosocial influences in the AIDS process. *Social Science and Medicine* 29:277–292.

Kaplan, H. B., Johnson, R. J., Bailey, C. A., and Simon, W. (1987) The sociological study of AIDS: A critical review of the literature and suggested research agenda. *Journal of Health and Social Behavior* 28:140–157.

Keeter, S., and Bradford, J. B. (1988) Knowledge of AIDS and related behavior change among unmarried adults in a low-prevalence city. *American Journal of Preventive Medicine* 4:146–152.

Kelly, J. A., St. Lawrence, J. S., Hood, H. V., and Brasfield, T. L. (1989) Behavioral intervention to reduce AIDS risk activities. *Journal of Consulting and Clinical Psychology* 57:60–67.

King, F. W. (1970) Psychology in action: Anonymous versus identifiable questionnaires in drug usage surveys. *American Psychologist* 25:982–985.

Kinsey, A. C., Pomeroy, W. B., and Martin, C. E. (1948) *Sexual Behavior in the Human Male.* Philadelphia: W. B. Saunders.

Kinsey, A. C., Pomeroy, W. B., Martin, C. E., and Gebhard, P. H. (1953) *Sexual Behavior in the Human Female.* Philadelphia: W. B. Saunders.

Kipke, M. D., and Drucker, E. (1988) A method for assessing needle-sharing behavior in intravenous drug users. Presented at the Fourth International Conference on AIDS, Stockholm, June 12–16.

Klassen, A. D., Williams, C. J., and Levitt, E. E. (1989) *Sex and Morality in the U.S.,* edited by H. J. O'Gorman. Middletown, Conn.: Wesleyan University Press.

Klassen, A. D., Williams, C. J., Levitt, E. E., Rudkin-Miniot L., Miller H., and Gunjal, S. (1989) Trends in premarital sexual behavior. In C. F. Turner, H. G. Miller, and L. E. Moses, eds., *AIDS, Sexual Behavior, and Intravenous Drug Use.* Washington, D.C.: National Academy Press.

Koblin, B., McCusker, J., Lewis, B., Sullivan, J., Birch, F., and Hagen, H. (1988) Racial differences in HIV infection in IVDUs. Presented at the Fourth International Conference on AIDS, Stockholm, June 12–16.

Koester, S. (1989a) The risk of HIV transmission from sharing water, drug-mixing containers and cotton filters among intravenous drug users. Unpublished manuscript. University of Colorado School of Medicine, Boulder, Colo.

Koester, S. (1989b) When push comes to shove: Poverty, law enforcement and high risk behavior. Unpublished manuscript. University of Colorado School of Medicine, Boulder, Colo.

Koss, M. P., and Gidycz, C. A. (1985) Sexual experiences survey: Reliability and validity. *Journal of Consulting and Clinical Psychology* 53:422–423.

Lange, W. R., Snyder, F. R., Lozovsky, E., Kaistha, V., Jaffe, J. H., et al. (1988) Geographic distribution of human immunodeficiency virus markers in parenteral drug abusers. *American Journal of Public Health* 78:443–446.

Leach, C., Viker, S., Kuhls, T., Parris, N., Cherry, J., and Christenson, P. (1989) Changes in sexual behavior of a cohort of female health care workers during the AIDS era. Presented at the Fifth International Conference on AIDS, Montreal, June 4–9.

Leonard, T. L. (1990) Male clients of female street prostitutes: Unseen partners in sexual disease transmission. *Medical Anthropology Quarterly* 4:41–55.

Lessler, J., Tourangeau, R., and Salter, W. (1989) Questionnaire design in the cognitive research laboratory. *Vital and Health Statistics* Series 6, Whole No. 1.

Lever, J., Rogers, W. H., Carson, S., Hertz, R., and Kanouse, D. E. (1989) Behavioral patterns of bisexual males in the U.S., 1982. Presented at the Fifth International Conference on AIDS, Montreal, June 4–9.

Levinger, G. (1966) Systematic distortion in spouses' reports of preferred and actual sexual behavior. *Sociometry* 29:291–299.

Lide, D. R., Jr. (1981) Critical data for critical needs. *Science* 212:1343–1349.

Loftus, E. F. (1975) Leading questions and the eyewitness report. *Cognitive Psychology* 7:560–572.

Loftus, E. F., and Marburger, W. (1983) Since the eruption of Mt. St. Helens, has anyone beaten you up? Improving the accuracy of retrospective reports with landmark events. *Memory and Cognition* 11:114–120.

Loftus, E. F., and Palmer, J. C. (1974) Reconstruction of automobile destruction: An example of the interaction between language and memory. *Journal of Verbal Learning and Verbal Behavior* 13:585–589.

LoPiccolo, J., and Steger, J. C. (1974) The sexual interaction inventory: A new instrument for assessment of sexual dysfunction. *Archives of Sexual Behavior* 3:585–595.

Luetgert, M. J., and Armstrong, A. H. (1973) Methodological issues in drug usage surveys: Anonymity, recency, and frequency. *International Journal of the Addictions* 8:683–689.

MacKuen, M. B. (1981) Social communication and the mass policy agenda. In M. B. MacKuen and S. L. Coombs, eds., *More than News: Media Power in Public Affairs*. Beverly Hills, Calif.: Sage.

MacKuen, M. B. (1984) Reality, the press, and citizens' political agendas. In C. F. Turner and E. Martin, eds., *Surveying Subjective Phenomena*. Vol. 2. New York: Russell Sage.

MacKuen, M. B. and Turner, C. F. (1984) The popularity of presidents: 1963–80. In C. F. Turner and E. Martin, eds., *Surveying Subjective Phenomena*. Vol. 2. New York: Russell Sage..

Maddux, J., and Desmond, D. (1975) Reliability and validity of information from chronic heroin users. *Journal of Psychiatric Research* 12:87–95.

Madow, W. G., Nisselson, H., and Olkin, I., eds. (1983) *Incomplete Data in Sample Surveys. Vol. 1, Report and Case Studies; Vol. 2, Theory and Bibliographies; Vol. 3, Proceedings of the Symposium*. New York: Academic Press.

Magura, S., Goldsmith, D., Casriel, C., Goldstein, P. J., and Lipton, D. S. (1987) The validity of methadone clients' self-reported drug use. *International Journal of the Addictions* 22:727–749.

Maisto, S. A., and O'Farrell, T. J. (1985) Comment on the validity of Watson et al.'s "Do alcoholics give valid self-reports?" *Journal of Studies on Alcohol* 46:447–453.

Maisto, S. A., Sobell, L. C., and Sobell, M. B. (1982–83) Corroboration of drug abusers' self-reports through the use of multiple data sources. *American Journal of Drug and Alcohol Abuse* 9:301–308.

Marasca, G., D'Arcangelo, E., De Candido, D., Della Giusta, G., Liseo, B., et al. (1989) Sexual behaviour and HIV related knowledge among a random sample of young population of Italy. Presented at the Fifth International Conference on AIDS, Montreal, June 4–9.

Marks, I. M., and Sartorius, N. H. (1968) A contribution to the measurement of sexual attitude. *Journal of Nervous and Mental Disease* 145:441–451.

Marshall, P., O'Keefe, J. P., Fisher, S. G., Caruso, A. J., and Surdukowski, J. (1990) Patients' fear of contracting the acquired immune deficiency syndrome from physicians. *Archives of Internal Medicine* 150:1501-1506.

Martin, J. L., and Vance, C. S. (1984) Behavioral and psychosocial factors in AIDS: Methodological and substantive issues. *American Psychologist* 39:1303–1308.

Mason, T. (1988) AIDS prevention among black IV drug users and their sexual partners in a Baltimore public housing project. Presented at the First International Symposium on Information and Education on AIDS, Ixtapa, Mexico, October 18.

Mason, T. (1989) The politics of culture: Drug users, professionals, and the meaning of needle sharing. Presented at the Annual Meeting of the Society for Applied Anthropology, Santa Fe, April.

Mason, T. (1989) A preliminary look at social and economic dynamics influencing drug markets, drug use patterns, and HIV risk behaviors among injecting drug users in two Baltimore networks. In *Proceedings of the Community Epidemiology Work Group: Chicago, Illinois, June 1989*. National Institute on Drug Abuse, Division of Epidemiology and Statistical Analysis, Rockville, Md.

May, R. M., and Anderson, R. M. (1987) Transmission dynamics of HIV infection. *Nature* 326:137–142.

May, R. M., Anderson, R. M., and Blower, S. M. (1989) The epidemiology and transmission dynamics of HIV-AIDS. *Daedalus* 118:163–201.

McCombie, S. C. (1986) The cultural impact of the AIDS test: The American experience. *Social Science and Medicine* 23:455–459.

McCombie, S. C. (1989) Rituals of infection control among health care workers. Unpublished manuscript. Annenberg School of Communications, University of Pennsylvania.

McCombie, S. C. (1990) Patterns of condom use in Trinidad and Tobago. Unpublished manuscript. Annenberg School of Communications, University of Pennsylvania.

McGlothlin, W. H., Anglin, M. D., and Wilson, B. D. (1977) *An Evaluation of the California Civil Addict Program*. Rockville, Md.: National Institute on Drug Abuse.

McLaws, M. L., McGirr, J., Croker, W., and Cooper, D. A. (1988) Risk factors for HIV and HBV infections in intravenous drug users. Presented at the Fourth International Conference on AIDS, Stockholm, June 12–16.

McNemar, Q. (1946) Opinion-attitude methodology. *Psychological Bulletin* 43:289–374.

Means, B., Nigam, A. Zarrow, M., Loftus, E. F., and Donaldson, M. S. (1989) Autobiographical memory for health related events. *Vital and Health Statistics* Series 6, Whole No. 1.

Michael, R. T., Laumann, E. O., Gagnon, J. H., and Smith, T. W. (1988) Number of sex partners and potential risk of sexual exposure to human immunodeficiency virus. *Mortality and Morbidity Weekly Report* 37:565–568.

Miller, H. G., Turner, C. F., and Moses, L. E. (1990) *AIDS: The Second Decade.* Washington, D.C.: National Academy Press.

Millstein, S., and Irwin, C. (1983) Acceptability of computer-acquired sexual histories in adolescent girls. *Journal of Pediatrics* 103:815–819.

Minkoff, H., McCalla, S., Delke, I., Feldman, J., Stevens, R., and Salwen, M. (1989) Cocaine use and sexually transmitted diseases including HIV. Presented at the Fifth International Conference on AIDS, Montreal, June 4–9.

Moatti, J. P., Tavares, J., Durbec, J. P., Bajos, N., Menard, C., and Serrand, C. (1989) Modifications of sexual behavior due to AIDS in French heterosexual "at risk" population. Presented at the Fifth International Conference on AIDS, Montreal, June 4–9.

Mooney, H. W., Pollack, B. R., and Corsa, L. (1968) Use of telephone interviewing to study human reproduction. *Public Health Reports* 83:1049–1060.

Moser, C. A., and Kalton, G. (1972) *Survey Methods in Social Investigation.* 2d ed. New York: Basic.

Moss, A. R., Bacchetti, P., Osmond, D., Meakin, R., Keffelew, A., and Gorter, R. (1989) Seroconversion for HIV in intravenous drug users in San Francisco. Presented at the Fifth International Conference on AIDS, Montreal, June 4–9.

Mukherjee, B. N. (1975) Reliability estimates of some survey data on family planning. *Population Studies* 29:127–142.

Myers, V. (1977a) Survey methods for minority populations. *The Journal of Social Issues* 33:11–19.

Myers, V. (1977b) Toward a synthesis of ethnographic and survey methods. *Human Organization* 36:244–251.

National Research Council (NRC) (1979) *Privacy and Confidentiality as Factors in Survey Response.* Washington, D.C.: National Academy of Sciences.

Needle, R. H., Jou, S., and Su, S. S. (1989) The impact of changing methods of data collection on the reliability of self-reported drug use of adolescents. *American Journal of Drug and Alcohol Abuse* 15:275–289.

Needle, R., McCubbin, H., Lorence, J., and Hochhauser, M. (1983) Reliability and validity of adolescent self-reported drug use in a family-based study: A methodological report. *International Journal of the Addictions* 18:901–912.

Neisser, U. (1981) John Dean's memory: A case study. *Cognition* 9:1–22.

Newcomer, S., and Udry, J. R. (1988) Adolescents' honesty in a survey of sexual behavior. *Journal of Adolescent Research* 3:419–423.

Newman, R. G., Cates, M., Tytun A., and Werbell, B. (1976) Reliability of self-reported age of first drug use: Analysis of New York City narcotics register data. *International Journal of the Addictions* 11:611–618.

Newmeyer, J. A. (1988) Why bleach? Development of a strategy to combat HIV contagion among San Francisco intravenous drug users. In R. J. Battjes, and R. W. Pickens, eds., *Needle Sharing Among Intravenous Drug Abusers: National and International Perspectives.* DHHS Publication No. (ADM) 88–1567. National Institute on Drug Abuse Research Monograph 80. Washington, D.C.: U.S. Government Printing Office.

Nisbett, R. E., and Wilson, T. D. (1977) Telling more than we can know: Verbal reports on mental processes. *Psychological Review* 84:231–259.

Novick, D. M., Trigg, H. L., Des Jarlais, D. C., Friedman, S. R., Vlahov, D., et al. (1989) Drug abuse patterns and ethnicity in IVDA during the early years of the HIV epidemic. Presented at the Fifth International Conference on AIDS, Montreal, June 4–9.

Nurco, D. N. (1985) A discussion of validity. In B. A. Rouse, N. J. Kozel, and L. G. Richards, eds., *Self-report Methods of Estimating Drug Use: Meeting Current Challenges to Validity.* DHHS Publication No. (ADM) 85–1402. National Institute on Drug Abuse Research Monograph No. 57. Washington, D.C.: U.S. Government Printing Office.

Oetting, E. R., Edwards, R., and Beauvais, F. (1985) Reliability and discriminant validity of the children's drug-use survey. *Psychological Reports* 56:751–756.

O'Reilly, K. R. (1989) Risk behaviors and their determinants. In R. Kulstad, ed., *AIDS 1988: American Association for the Advancement of Science Symposia Papers.* Washington, D. C.: American Association for the Advancement of Science.

Page, B. P., Chitwood, D. D., Smith, P. C., Kane, N., and McBride, D. C. (1990) Intravenous drug use and HIV infection in Miami. *Medical Anthropology Quarterly* 4:56–71.

Page, W. F., Davies, J. E., Ladner, R. A., Alfassa, J., and Tennis, H. (1977) Urinalysis screened versus verbally reported drug use: The identification of discrepant groups. *International Journal of the Addictions* 12:439–450.

Parker, R. (1987) Acquired immunodeficiency syndrome in urban Brazil. *Medical Anthropology Quarterly* 1:155–175.

Parker, R. (1989) Bodies and pleasures in the construction of erotic meaning in contemporary Brazil. *Anthropology and Humanism Quarterly* 14:58–64.

Pearson, R. W., Ross, M., and Dawes, R. (1989) A theory of personal recall and the limits of retrospection in surveys. Unpublished manuscript. Social Science Research Council, August 1, 1989.

Pelto, P., and Pelto, G. (1978) *Anthropological Research: The Structure of Enquiry.* London: Cambridge University Press.

Peterson, J. L., and Bakeman, R. (1989) AIDS and IV drug use among ethnic minorities. *Journal of Drug Issues* 19:27–37.

Petzel, T. P., Johnson, J. E., and McKillip, J. (1973) Response bias in drug surveys. *Journal of Consulting and Clinical Psychology* 40:437–439.

Podell, L., and Perkins, J. C. (1957) A Guttman scale for sexual experience—A methodological note. *Journal of Abnormal and Social Psychology* 54:420-422.

Poti, S. J., Chakraborti, B., and Malaker, C. R. (1960) Reliability of data relating to contraceptive practices. In C. V. Kiser, ed., *Research In Family Planning.* Princeton: Princeton University Press.

Public Health Service (PHS). (1988) Report of the Second Public Health Service AIDS Prevention and Control Conference. *Public Health Reports* 103, Supplement No. 1.

Quart, A. M., Small, C. B., and Klein, R. S. (1989) Local destruction of labial surface of mandibular teeth by direct application of cocaine in drug users with AIDS. Presented at the Fifth International Conference on AIDS, Montreal, June 4–9.

Reining, P. (1989) Male circumcision status in relationship to seroprevalence data in Africa: A review of method. Unpublished manuscript. Department of Anthropology Catholic University.

Research Triangle Institute (RTI). (1989) *National Household Seroprevalence Survey: Pilot Study Report.* Research Triangle Park, N.C.: Research Triangle Institute.

Robertson, J. R., Skidmore, C. A., and Roberts, J. J. K. (1988) HIV infection in intravenous drug users: A follow-up study indicating changes in risk-taking behaviour. *British Journal of Addiction* 83:387–391.

Robinson, T. W., Davies, P., and Beveridge, S. (1989) Sexual practices and condom use amongst male prostitutes in London: Differences between streetworking and non-streetworking prostitutes. Presented at the Fifth International Conference on AIDS, Montreal, June 4–9.

Rodgers, J. L., Billy, J. O. G., and Udry, J. R. (1982) The rescission of behaviors: Inconsistent responses in adolescent sexuality data. *Social Science Research* 11:280–296.

Rolnick, S. J., Gross, C. R., Garrard, J., and Gibson, R. W. (1989) A comparison of response rate, data quality, and cost in the collection of data on sexual history and personal behaviors. *American Journal of Epidemiology* 129:1052–1061.

Rossi, P. H., Wright, J. D., and Anderson, A. B., eds. (1983) *Handbook of Survey Research*. New York: Academic Press.

Rounsaville, B., Kleber, H. D., Wilber, C., Rosenberger, D., and Rosenberger, P. (1981) Comparisons of opiate addicts' reports of psychiatric history with reports of significant-other informants'. *American Journal of Drug and Alcohol Abuse* 8:51–69.

Rouse, B. A., Kozel, N. J., and Richards, L. G., eds. (1985) *Self-report Methods of Estimating Drug Use: Meeting Current Challenges to Validity*. National Institute on Drug Abuse Research Monograph No. 57. Washington, D.C.: U.S. Government Printing Office.

Saltzman, S. P., Stoddard, A. M., McCusker, J., Moon, M. W., and Mayer, K. H. (1987) Reliability of self-reported sexual behavior risk factors for HIV infection in homosexual men. *Public Health Reports* 102:692–697.

Schaeffer, N. C. and Thomson, E. (1989) The discovery of grounded uncertainty: Developing standardized questions about strength of fertility motivation. Center for Demography and Ecology Working paper No. 88–19. Madison, Wisc.: Center for Demography and Ecology, University of Wisconsin.

Schiavi, R. C., Derogatis, L. R., Kuriansky, J., O'Connor, D., and Sharpe, L. (1979) The assessment of sexual function and marital interaction. *Journal of Sex and Marital Therapy* 5:169–224.

Schilling, R. F., Schinke, S. P., Nichols, S. E., Zayas, L. H., Miller, S. O., et al. (1989) Developing strategies for AIDS prevention research with black and Hispanic drug users. *Public Health Reports* 104:2–11.

Schmidt, K. W., Krasnik, A., Brendstrup, E., Zoffman, H., and Larsen, S. O. (1988) Occurrence of sexual behaviour related to the risk of HIV-infection. *Danish Medical Bulletin* 36:84–88.

Schoepf, B. G., Walu, E., Rukarangira, Wn., Payanzo, N., and Schoepf, C. (In press) Action research on AIDS with women in Central Africa. *Social Science and Medicine*.

Schofield, M. (1965) *The Sexual Behavior of Young People*. Boston: Little, Brown, and Co.

Schuman, H. and Presser, S. (1981) *Questions and Answers in Attitude Surveys: Experiments in Question Form, Wording, and Context*. New York: Academic Press.

Seage, G. R., III, Mayer, K. H., Horsburgh, C. R., Cai, B., and Lamb, G. A. (1989) Validation of sexual histories of homosexual male couples. Presented at the Fifth International Conference on AIDS, Montreal, June 4–9.

Siegel, K., and Bauman, L. J. (1986) Methodological issues in AIDS-related research. In D. A. Feldman and T. M. Johnson, eds., *The Social Dimensions of AIDS: Method and Theory.* New York: Praeger.

Single, E., Kandel, D. B., and Johnson, B. D. (1975) The reliability and validity of drug use responses in a large scale longitudinal survey. *Journal of Drug Issues* 5:426–443.

Skinner, H. A., and Allen, B. A. (1983) Does the computer make a difference? Computerized versus face-to-face self-report assessment of alcohol, drug, and tobacco use. *Journal of Consulting and Clinical Psychology* 51:267–275.

Smith, A. F., Jobe, J. B., and Mingay, D. J. (In press) Retrieval from memory of dietary information. *Applied Cognitive Psychology.*

Smith, T. W. (1988) *A Methodological Review of the Sexual Behavior Questions on the 1988 General Social Survey (GSS).* GSS Methodological Report No. 58, National Opinion Research Center: University of Chicago.

Sorensen, J. L., and Leder, D. (1978) Measuring the readability of written information for clients. In G. Landsberg, W. D. Neigher, R. J. Hammer, C. Windle, and J. R. Woy, eds., *Evaluation in Practice: A Sourcebook of Program Evaluation Studies from Mental Health Care Systems in the United States.* DHEW Publication No. (ADM) 78–763. Washington, D.C.: U.S. Government Printing Office.

Sorensen, J. L., Gibson, D., Heitzmann, C., Calvillo, A., Dumontet, R., et al. (1988) Pilot trial of small group AIDS education with IV drug abusers (abstract). In L. S. Harris, ed., *Problems of Drug Dependence 1988: Proceedings of the 50th Annual Scientific Meeting, Committee on the Problems of Drug Dependence.* National Institute on Drug Abuse, Research Monograph 90. Washington, D.C.: U.S. Government Printing Office.

Sorensen, J. L., Gibson, D. R. , Heitzmann, C., Dumontet, R., London, J., et al. (1989a) AIDS prevention: Behavioral outcomes with outpatient drug abusers. Presented at the Annual Meeting of the American Psychological Association, New Orleans, La.

Sorensen, J. L., Guydish, J., Costantini, M., and Batki, S. L. (1989b) Changes in needle sharing and syringe cleaning among San Francisco Drug Abusers. *New England Journal of Medicine* 320:807.

Sorensen, J. L., Batki, S. L., Gibson, D. R., Dumontet, R., and Purnell, S. (1989c) Methadone maintenance and behavior change in seropositive drug abusers: The San Francisco General Hospital Program for AIDS Counseling and Education (PACE). Presented at the Fifth International Conference on AIDS, Montreal, June 4–9.

Spencer, B. D. (1989) On the accuracy of current estimates of the numbers of intravenous drug users. In C. F. Turner, H. G. Miller, and L. E. Moses, eds., *AIDS, Sexual Behavior, and Intravenous Drug Use.* Washington, D.C.: National Academy Press.

Spencer, L., Faulkner, A., and Keegan, J. (1988) *Talking About Sex.* (Publication P. 5997) London: Social and Community Planning Research.

Steger, K., Comella, B., Forbes, J., McLoughlin, R., Hoff, R. A., and Craven, D. E. (1989) Use of a fingerstick paper-absorbed blood sample for HIV serosurveys in intravenous drug users. Presented at the Fifth International Conference on AIDS, Montreal, June 4–9.

Stephens, R. (1972) The truthfulness of addict respondents in research projects. *International Journal of the Addictions* 7:549–558.

Sterk, C. (1989) Fieldwork among prostitutes in the AIDS era. In C. Smith and W. Kornblum, eds., *In the Field: Readings on the Field Research Experience*. New York: Praeger.

Stimson, G. V., Donoghoe, M., Alldritt, L., and Dolan, K. (1988a) HIV transmission risk behaviours of clients attending syringe-exchange schemes in England and Scotland. *British Journal of Addiction* 83:1449–1455.

Stimson, G. V., Alldritt, L. J., Dolan, K. A., Donoghoe, M. C., and Lart, R. A. (1988b) *Injecting Equipment Exchange Schemes: Final Report*. London: Monitoring Research Group, Goldsmiths' College.

Strunin, L., and Hingson, R. (1987) Acquired immunodeficiency syndrome and adolescents: Knowledge, beliefs, attitudes, and behaviors. *Pediatrics* 79:825–828.

Sudman, S., and Bradburn, N. M. (1974) *Response Effects in Surveys*. Chicago: Aldine.

Sundet, J. M., Kvalem, I. L., Magnus, P., Grommesby, J.K., Stigum, H., and Bakketeig, L. S. (1989) The relationship between condom use and sexual behavior. Presented at the Fifth International Conference on AIDS, Montreal, June 4–9.

Tracy, P. E., and Fox, J. A. (1981) The validity of randomized response for sensitive measurements. *American Sociological Review* 46:187–200.

Traeen, B., Rise, J., and Kraft, P. (1989) Condom behavior in 17, 18 and 19 year-old Norwegians. Presented at the Fifth International Conference on AIDS, Montreal, June 4–9.

Tross, S., Abdul-Quader, A., Des Jarlais, D. C., Kouzi, A., and Friedman, S. R. (1989) Determinants of sexual risk reduction in female IV drug users recruited from the street. Presented at the Fifth International Conference on AIDS, Montreal, June 4–9.

Tucker, C., Vitrano, F., Miller, L., and Doddy, J. (1989) Cognitive issues and research on the consumer expenditure diary survey. Presented at the 1989 Annual Meetings of the American Association for Public Opinion Research, St. Petersburg, Fla., May.

Turner, C. F. (1978) Fallible indicators of the subjective state of the nation. *American Psychologist* 33:456–470.

Turner, C. F. (1984) Why do surveys disagree? Some preliminary hypotheses and some disagreeable examples. In C. F. Turner and E. Martin, eds., *Surveying Subjective Phenomena*. Vol. 2. New York: Russell Sage.

Turner, C. F. (1989) Research on sexual behaviors that transmit HIV: Progress and problems. *AIDS* 3:563–569.

Turner, C. F., and Fay, R. E. (1987/1989) Monitoring the spread of HIV infection. Background paper for ad hoc advisory group, Centers for Disease Control. Atlanta, Ga., July 7, 1987. Reprinted in C. F. Turner, H. G. Miller, and L. E. Moses, eds., (1989) *AIDS, Sexual Behavior, and Intravenous Drug Use*. Washington, D.C.: National Academy Press.

Turner, C. F., and Martin, E., eds. (1984) *Surveying Subjective Phenomena*. Two volumes. New York: Russell Sage.

Turner, C. F., Miller, H. G., and Barker, L. F. (1989) AIDS research and the behavioral and social sciences. In R. Kulsad, ed., *AIDS, 1988: AAAS Symposium Papers*. Washington, D.C.: American Association for the Advancement of Science.

Turner, C. F., Miller, H. G., and Moses, L. E., eds. (1989) *AIDS, Sexual Behavior, and Intravenous Drug Use*. Washington, D.C.: National Academy Press.

Udry, J. R., and Morris, N. M. (1967) A method for validation of reported sexual data. *Journal of Marriage and the Family* 29:442–446.

Vessey, M. P., Johnson, B., and Donnelly, J. (1974) Reliability of reporting by women taking part in a prospective contraceptive study. *British Journal of Preventive and Social Medicine* 28:104–107.

Vinokur, A., Oksenberg, L., and Cannell, C. F. (1977) Effects of feedback and reinforcement on the report of health information. In C. F. Cannell, L. Oksenberg, and J. M. Converse, eds., *Experiments in Interviewing Techniques*. Washington, D.C.: National Center for Health Surveys Research.

Wagennar, W. A. (1986) My memory: A study of autobiographical memory over six years. *Cognitive Psychology* 18:225–252.

Waterton, J. J., and Duffy, J. C. (1984) A comparison of computer interviewing techniques and traditional methods in the collection of self-report alcohol consumption data in a field survey. *International Statistical Review* 52:173–182.

Watson, C. G. (1985) More reasons for a moratorium: A reply to Maisto and O'Farrell. *Journal of Studies on Alcohol* 46:450–453.

Watters, J. K. (1989) Observations on the importance of social context in HIV transmission among intravenous drug users. *Journal of Drug Issues* 19:9–26.

Webb, E. J., Campbell, D. T., Schwartz, R. D., and Sechrest, L. (1966) *Unobtrusive Measures: Nonreactive Research in the Social Sciences*. Chicago: Rand McNally.

Weibel, W. W. (1988) Combining ethnographic and epidemiologic methods in targeted AIDS interventions: The Chicago model. In *Needle Sharing Among Intravenous Drug Abusers: National and International Perspectives*. National Institute on Drug Abuse Monograph 80. Washington, D.C.: U.S. Government Printing Office.

Wells, J. A., Wilensky, G. R., Valleron, A. J., Bond, G., Sell, R. L., and DeFilippes, P. (1989a) Population prevalence of AIDS high risk behaviors in France, the United Kingdom and the United States. Presented at the Fifth International Conference on AIDS, Montreal, June 4–9.

Wells, J. A., Sell, R. L., Will, A., and DeFilippes, P. (1989b) Readability analysis of AIDS brochures and pamphlets from the United States. Presented at the Fifth International Conference on AIDS, Montreal, June 4–9.

Wermuth, L., and Ham, J. (1989) Women don't wear condoms: Coping with AIDS risk among women partners of intravenous drug users. Presented at the Annual Meeting of the American Sociological Association, San Francisco, Calif.

Whitehead, P. C., and Smart, R. G. (1972) Validity and reliability of self-reported drug use. *Canadian Journal of Criminology and Corrections* 14:83–89.

Wigdor, A. K., and Garner, W. R., eds. (1982) *Ability Testing*. Two vols. Washington, D.C.: National Academy Press.

Wiley, J. (1989) *Studying Nonresponse in the AMEN Cohort Survey* (unpublished notes). Survey Research Center, University of California at Berkeley, July.

Winkelstein, W., Jr., Samuel, M., Padian, N. S., Wiley, J. A., Lang, W., et al. (1987a) The San Francisco Men's Health Study. III. Reduction in human immunodeficiency virus transmission among homosexual/bisexual men, 1982–1986. *American Journal of Public Health* 77:685–689.

Winkelstein, W., Jr., Samuel, M., Padian, N. S., and Wiley, J. A. (1987b) Selected sexual practices of San Francisco heterosexual men and risk of infection by the human immunodeficiency virus. *Journal of the American Medical Association* 257:1470–1471.

Winkelstein, W., Jr., Lyman, D. M., and Padian, N. S. (1987c) Sexual practices and risk of infection by the AIDS-associated retrovirus: The San Francisco Men's Health Study. *Journal of the American Medical Association* 257:321–325.

Wish, E., Johnson, B., Strug, D., Chedekel, M., and Lipton, D. (1983) *Are Urine Tests Good Indicators of the Validity of Self-Reports of Drug Use? It Depends on the Test.* New York: Narcotic and Drug Research, Inc.

Wolk, J. S., Wodak, A., and Guinan, J. (1989) The effect of a needle and syringe exchange on a methadone maintenance unit. Presented at the Fifth International Conference on AIDS, Montreal, June 4–9.

Wolk, J. S., Wodak, A., Guinan, J. J., Morlet, A., Gold, J., et al. (1988) HIV seroprevalence in syringes of intravenous drug users using syringe exchanges in Sydney, Australia, 1987. Presented at the Fourth International Conference on AIDS, Stockholm, June 12–16.

Woodward, J. A., Retka, R. L., and Nig, L. (1984) Construct validity of heroin abuse estimators. *International Journal of Addictions* 19:93–117.

World Health Organization: Global Programme on AIDS (1988) *Progress Report No. 4.* Geneva: World Health Organization.

Worth, D. (1989) Sexual decisionmaking and AIDS: Why condom promotion among vulnerable women is likely to fail. Presented at the Population Council, New York. March 7.

Wyatt, G. E., and Peters, S. D. (1986) Methodological considerations in research on the prevalence of child sexual abuse. *Child Abuse and Neglect* 10:241–251.

Youden, W. (1961) How to evaluate accuracy. *Materials Research and Standards* 1:268–271.

Youden, W., and Steiner, E., eds. (1975) *Statistical Manual of the Association of Official Analytical Chemists.* Washington, D.C.: Association of Official Analytical Chemists.

Zelnik, M., and Kantner, J. F. (1980) Sexual activity, contraceptive use and pregnancy among metropolitan-area teenagers: 1971–1979. *Family Planning Perspectives* 12:230–237.

Zeugin, P., Dubois-Arber, F., Hausser, D., and Lehmann, P. H. (1989) Sexual behaviour of young adults and the effects of AIDS-prevention campaigns in Switzerland. Presented at the Fifth International Conference on AIDS, Montreal, June 4–9 .

Zich, J., and Temoshok, L. (1986) Applied methodology: A primer of pitfalls and opportunities in AIDS research. In D. A. Feldman and T. M. Johnson, eds., *The Social Dimensions of AIDS: Method and Theory.* New York: Praeger.

Zuckerman, M. (1973) Scales for sex experience for males and females. *Journal of Consulting and Clinical Psychology* 41:27–29.

Zuckerman, M., Tushup, R., and Finner, S. (1976) Sexual attitudes and experience: Attitude and personality correlates and changes produced by a course in sexuality. *Journal of Consulting and Clinical Psychology* 44:7–19.

Zuckerman, B. S., Hingson, R. W., Morelock, S., Amaro, H., Frank, D., et al. (1985) A pilot study assessing maternal marijuana use by urine assay during pregnancy. In B. A. Rouse, N. J. Kozel, and L. G. Richards, eds., *Self-report Methods of Estimating Drug Use: Meeting Current Challenges to Validity.* DHHS Publication No. (ADM) 85–1402. National Institute on Drug Abuse Research Monograph No. 57. Washington, D.C.: U.S. Government Printing Office.

D

Sampling and Randomization:
Technical Questions about Evaluating CDC's
Three Major AIDS Prevention Programs

Following the release of the first edition of *Evaluating AIDS Prevention Programs,* CDC program personnel met with the panel and raised a number of questions about the report. This appendix deals with essentially technical matters relating to the implementation of some of the report suggestions—in particular, questions about sampling and the random assignment of treatment and control groups. Appendix E deals with the evaluation of projects that are ancillary to, emerging, or related to those discussed in Chapters 3 and 5.

The first section of this appendix treats the following technical issues related to sampling: the number of case studies to be used in a process evaluation of the counseling and testing program; the sample sizes needed to evaluate the effectiveness of all three programs; suggestions for controlling attrition; and the comparison of convenience samples and probability samples. The second section addresses two aspects of using randomized experiments to evaluate a project's effectiveness: successful experiments in the AIDS prevention arena and the ethics of no-treatment controls.

The panel's objective is to outline some of the general principles involved with sampling and randomization as part of research design. Because the panel's original task was one of developing overall evaluation strategy rather than rendering detailed technical advice, we have been reluctant to provide any kind of specificity on questions of sample size, the use of convenience samples, and so on. The panel believes strongly that technical advice of this sort is so context-driven that each set of evaluation objectives warrants its own response. Such advice is best fashioned by statistical and subject matter experts who can assess each evaluation problem on its own terms. Thus, our foremost recommendation is that CDC either develop the requisite in-house expertise among personnel responsible for evaluation research or contract for expert services when these types of questions arise. Nonetheless, we offer the following *general* information in the hopes that it will prove to be useful.

SAMPLING ISSUES

Personnel from the National AIDS Information and Education Program (NAIEP) and the Center for Prevention Services (CPS) raised questions about the optimal number of case studies and sample sizes needed for evaluating a project's effectiveness. Related to the issue of sample size is the question of how to control attrition. In addition to addressing these sampling issues, this section includes some thoughts about using convenience samples when it is not possible to carry out probability sampling.

Number of Case Studies

The purpose of conducting case studies of counseling and testing sites is to identify the variables to be considered in evaluating how well services are delivered: i.e., who is being served, do they complete the service protocol, what are the barriers, and so on. The question is simple: How many case studies need to be performed? The answer is complicated: As many as it takes to identify the relevant variables and no more. Unfortunately, it is impossible to predict how many case studies this will entail. Moreover, no "optimal number" exists, and it is impossible to recognize that a satisfactory number has been covered until that number has been exceeded. In other words, when the researcher recognizes that additional case studies are shedding no more significant light on one's understanding of service delivery, it no longer makes practical sense to continue such field research.[1]

A good sampling scheme is important in making a correct decision. The panel believes that a stratified sample of counseling and testing sites is the best method for gathering case data on service delivery variables. In Chapter 4, the panel suggested a 2 × 2 × 2 matrix (stratifying by seroprevalence rates, activity, and target group), for case studies of a

---

[1] Obviously, if the goals of service delivery or the needs of evaluation research change, new case studies will again become necessary.

sample of community-based organization (CBO) projects. This scheme would require a minimum of 8 case studies.[2] The panel believes that the sample of case studies of counseling and testing projects should be similarly laid out but will be larger because of the greater number of site variations.

A stratification scheme would probably best be planned by CDC program personnel, who are familiar with key variables in the different projects that the agency funds as well as the distribution of those variables. Nonetheless, the panel suggests the following stratification variables:

- Type of facility, e.g., health department, family planning clinic, drug treatment center, clinic for treatment of sexually transmitted disease, and so on (already the matrix is larger than that proposed for CBOs because of the diversity in types of setting);
- Seroprevalence rates or number of AIDS cases (i.e., low, middle, or high prevalence areas);
- Type of region (i.e., urban or rural).

Sites should be selected on the basis of the important service variables, not simply because they are convenient or their staffs are cooperative. The important dimensions should incorporate the diversity among counseling and testing sites.

As case studies are conducted, program staff at CDC or the staff's evaluation consultants will need to carefully assess information as it is collected from site visits to determine when it is sufficient, so that resources are not needlessly spent on gathering redundant information. Staff will also need to keep abreast of organizational and goal-related changes at the project level, so that the information does not become outdated.

Estimating Sample Sizes

In the panel's experience, sample size calculations *rarely overestimate the number of units required and quite commonly underestimate them*. To determine sample size for use in an efficacy or effectiveness trial, the investigator must first specify four factors. For the simplest possible case,[3] they are:

---

[2] As mentioned in Chapter 4, some cells in the matrix may be empty, in which case the number of case studies required would be smaller.

[3] This explication presents a *simplified* overview that omits many complications that are not treated here. Detailed treatments of this topic can be found in Lipsey (1990), Cohen (1988), and Kraemer and Thiemann (1987).

1. The kind of analysis that will be performed (e.g., t test, regression, estimation of a proportion or difference in proportions, etc.) and the statistical model that is assumed to describe the data distribution.
2. The minimum effect the experimenter wishes to detect, if indeed there is an effect. For instance, if an investigator's outcome variable is a respondent's number of sexual partners, the desired "effect size" might be a reduction by a factor of 2. There are standard ways to express the effect size, and they depend on the type of analysis that will be performed. For example, for comparing two group means, the effect size (ES) is usually defined as the difference between the two population means (μ_1, μ_2), in units of standard deviations (σ). The formula is:

$$ES = \frac{\mu_1 - \mu_2}{\sigma}$$

3. The "level of significance" (α) at which the test will be performed. The level of significance is the probability of concluding there is an effect when none really exists. Conventional values are .01 and .05.[4]
4. The desired "power" for the test. Power refers to the probability that the minimum effect specified (or a larger effect) will be detected, if it exists.

These factors are sufficient to determine the needed sample sizes, but they must be specified in light of their possible uses. Although the last three factors may be specified by a sophisticated investigator, combining the four factors to derive the implied sample size is best left to a statistician. For example, a statistician might suggest careful research designs such as blocking and matching to reduce the size of the standard deviation (σ), which in turn can either increase the size of the effect one will detect or reduce the size of the sample necessary for the study.

As intuition may suggest, the appropriate sample sizes increase as smaller effect sizes or smaller α's are chosen and/or as the desired power increases. Statistical texts can help investigators determine these various factors and then use them to find the appropriate sample size, but even these specialized texts and their reference tables require an

---

[4]It should be recognized that besides merely testing the null hypothesis (that the difference between groups is zero), one may have a particular interest in obtaining an estimate of the magnitude of the treatment effect with a given degree of precision. The texts noted in the preceding footnote will provide detailed guidance in this regard.

understanding of several statistical concepts. Moreover, tables do not exist for comparisons more complicated than t tests and analyses of variance. To resolve the matter, the panel advises that the investigator specify the desired factors (effect size, α, power level) and then consult with a statistical expert to determine the necessary sample size.

Controlling Attrition

In Chapter 6, the panel discussed attrition and a lack of compliance as potentially important detractors from a project's effectiveness, and we noted that such phenomena are useful endpoints to be studied because they can reveal whether a project is too unattractive to retain its participants. A project that cannot motivate its participants to comply or to stick with the protocol cannot be practically effective.

In some cases, however, attrition occurs for reasons unrelated to project attractiveness. The loss of data through attrition is a potentially serious source of bias, with the level of the problem depending in part on the amount of attrition and in part on other factors. Attrition becomes more serious, for example, if the outcome variable is relatively uncommon, if the treatment is causing experimental group members to drop out, or if the lack of treatment is causing control group members to drop out. Whether attrition is a problem depends on a given situation, so that no "standard appropriate attrition rate" can be advised.

The panel wishes to suggest ways to help contain attrition. In Chapter 4, the panel mentioned two ways: confidentiality guarantees and some form of compensation to respondents. We further discuss these and other suggestions below.

Confidentiality Guarantees

Assurances of confidentiality, which should be fairly easy to guarantee in any CBO study, typically have been found to decrease attrition and item nonresponse (Singer, 1978; Panel on Privacy and Confidentiality as Factors in Survey Response, 1979). Anonymity may be still more successful in reducing nonresponse (Moore, Lessler, and Caspar, 1989), but it obviously hinders follow-up. To meet this challenge, researchers involved in CDC's community demonstration projects have tried a code name system to track individuals. Under this system, media announcements summon respondents by code groups for periodic reinterviews. Return rates, however, have been modest, ranging from 50 to 80 percent of project participants, perhaps because the media approach is not sufficiently visible or persuasive. More intensive follow-up would require names and other locator information. Tanur (1982) has proposed one method for protecting the anonymity of respondents for whom this information is known; i.e., making telephone follow-ups asking respondents to anonymously call back the interviewer later.

Compensation

Under certain conditions, compensation has been shown to be an effective method of curbing attrition. Ferber and Sudman (1974) reviewed the effects of compensation on response rates in consumer surveys and found a mix of outcomes. For example, some form of compensation (cash, gifts) appeared to contribute to a higher response rate when the study conditions were burdensome to participants (e.g., when they were asked to participate in a longitudinal study, to keep records or diaries, or to come in to a study site). In less burdensome settings (such as one-time interviews with no written records), compensation was not particularly helpful in increasing response. Moreover, compensation seemed to be more effective among certain groups of respondents than others (e.g., it was more effective among participants with lower incomes and education than it was among middle class participants).

Cannell and Henson (1974) posit that survey participants must be sufficiently motivated to provide information. When the purpose of the study is perceived to be compatible with personal or social goals, compensation may not be important; however, money might motivate the respondent who feels that no other goal for participating exists.[5] In the AIDS prevention arena, few studies have been made on the impact of compensation to complete a study's protocol, but the studies that are available suggest that the goals or motivations of participants are indeed important in recruitment and attrition. For example, Fox and Jones (1989) found that participants in the Baltimore MACS study reported that prizes were not a major reason for continuing to volunteer. In fact, 74 percent of recruits returned for follow-up after a single mailed notice was sent (follow-up was even higher—84 to 90 percent—after telephone requests for return). Carballo-Dieguez and colleagues (1989) provide an example in which compensation was counterproductive. They found that a $10/hour payment appeared to be the major motivation for participation in a 5-year study on HIV disease progression among intravenous drug users and led some candidates to become what investigators characterized as aggressive and manipulative to secure enrollment.

---

[5]The most important source of motivation appeared to be the investigators' interactions with the participants (Cannell and Henson, 1974).

In an interesting contrast, Davis, Faust, and Ordentlich (1984) turned the concept of financial incentives on its head in a successful plan to reduce dropout rates in a smoking cessation program. In a randomized alternative treatments study, researchers obtained $20 deposits from volunteers who received one of four different self-help packages; their deposits were refunded only after five follow-up interviews were completed (regardless of outcome). The follow-up rate was 95 percent. Implementing this suggestion clearly would not be feasible in low-income community or outreach projects; it might, however, be possible in other types of projects, such as one that provides valuable resources like counseling activities to middle class gay males.

Stabilization Funds

To retain respondents in an intervention study, some (CDC) personnel suggested providing emergency "stabilization" funds to project participants. Such funds go beyond a token compensation and, for some participants, can mean the difference between leaving the study area or staying to receive an intervention and participate in its evaluation. The panel looked at this suggestion from two sides. On the one hand, we saw that it may at times be necessary to alter the social environment to *provide* the intervention. Conversely, however, if the purpose is to *evaluate* the intervention, it is damaging to alter the environment because it may contaminate the intervention with an "additional value" (here, the emergency funds).

One method of incorporating such incentives into a research design is to provide the additional value to the whole pool of program candidates before assigning individuals to the experimental and control groups.[6] In this way, the samples are drawn from a homogeneous population. In fact, this method could enhance the feasibility of randomization because an investigator is likely to have a larger pool of willing study participants once members of a community learn that a given evaluation will provide them additional funds. However, the provision of the additional value would change the evaluation from a study of effectiveness to a study of efficacy.[7]

Cultivating and Tracking Respondents

Other ways that have helped to avoid attrition include: familiarizing respondents at first contact with the importance and purpose of the study

---

[6]Designs that provide incentives only to participants and not to controls confound the incentive with the treatment. The results of such designs would be particularly difficult to interpret.

[7]See Chapter 3 for a full discussion of "efficacy" versus "effectiveness."

and cultivating their participation; proxy reporting (less likely but possible when sex and drug partners are recruited into a project); participant screening (described in Chapter 6); and rigorous follow-up. The last is strengthened when the researcher gathers all relevant information about all respondents (experimental and control group members alike) at the time of initial contact and, if multiple follow-ups are anticipated, every time that respondents are recontacted. "All relevant information" is meant to include locator information, characteristics of the target population, and information about variables affecting the content of the treatment that are related to the outcome.

Gathering such comprehensive information serves multiple purposes, but it is especially important for tracking respondents. In addition to routine information such as respondents' names and addresses, nontraditional identifying data, such as alternative locator information, social security number, and date of birth should be collected. Follow-up is facilitated when the researcher has the name and address of several persons who are likely to know a respondent's whereabouts; alternative locator information is especially useful in situations that involve mobile populations such as intravenous drug users or prostitutes. Access to respondents' social security numbers and birth dates also facilitates locating them through archival records such as voter registries, tax rolls, motor vehicle records, credit bureaus, marriage licenses, real estate records, death certificates, wills, and the like. Federal agencies that remain in touch with some respondents include the Veterans Administration, the Social Security Administration, and the Internal Revenue Service. Successful follow-up by mail includes the use of postal services such as forwarding and record updates. Telephone techniques include the use of directories, local and long distance operators, and reverse directories that provide numbers of former neighbors. Telephone searches may include searches made directly for the respondent, for known relatives or alternative locators, or for persons with the same last name who may be related to the respondent.

Tracking adolescents poses some particular problems. For one thing, state law sometimes prevents a researcher from gaining access to adolescents without parental consent. In some contexts, when the adolescent *comes to the researcher,* the teen is legally considered an "emancipated minor" with power to consent. For an adolescent to initiate and persist in these contacts, he or she must be strongly motivated to participate in the research. In cases such as these, compensation may be an effective motivating tool.

On the other hand, where parental consent is given, investigators can actively follow up their adolescent participants. Pirie and colleagues

(1989) report on studies for which good background data on the adolescents and their parents and guardians (names and social security numbers) was helpful, as was the cooperation of school districts in tracking students and transfers. Other public records were generally not successful sources for tracking adolescents, with the exception of driver's license records in a study centering on suburban adolescents. Telephone tracking was important, but had to be modified to focus on parents or guardians; telephone tracking was particularly important in rural areas, where listings for a given name often led to persons who knew or were related to the respondents.

Personnel for Tracking Respondents
Even with good information for tracking respondents, investigators must use sheer persistence to approach the goal of 100 percent follow-up. For maximum follow-up, the research team has to have the personnel necessary to do the tracking (which implies having the necessary resources to support such personnel). Trackers need not be research investigators, but they do need to be trained in the search techniques discussed above.

The time necessary to follow up respondents should not be underestimated. In addition to tracking participants through a paper trail of records, field work is necessary to locate many individuals. Field work involves tracking time and interview time, both of which need to be factored into each scheduled follow-up. In some cases, the tracking procedure may be more intensive than the intervention itself. For example, tracking participants from a drug treatment center may be much more labor intensive than providing the original counseling intervention.

Modeling Attrition
The second reason to get as much information about individuals in the study at intake is that, if attrition does occur, researchers will be able to estimate the characteristics of nonrespondents. Since nonrespondents differ from respondents in terms of their refusal to respond or their being untraceable, they may also differ in terms of the variable that the evaluator is trying to measure. When they do, the validity of evaluation results will be subject to question.

Where attrition occurs, there is a need to model the causes and distribution of nonresponse. Ignoring nonresponse altogether implies acceptance of a model that says that nonrespondents are distributed in the same way as respondents.[8] Alternatives to ignoring nonresponse all

---

[8]This admits to some refinement depending on the analytic strategy employed. A typical default assumption in a life-table analysis is that persons lost resemble persons followed from the time of loss onward, not from time 0.

call for estimating—or guessing—the ways in which nonrespondents may differ. One way is to assume that they resemble some specified subset of the respondents. Other ways may exploit information about the nonrespondents (e.g., demographic features, responses at initial contact, etc.) to estimate or impute their later, missing responses. (For further discussion of missing data, see, e.g., Little and Rubin, 1987.) Another approach is to locate and interview the dropouts to find out what caused attrition and thus to model self-selection bias.[9]

(As noted in Chapter 6, it should be clearly understood that attrition and noncompliance in an experiment introduce uncertainties that directly parallel those that arise in nonexperimental studies. Modeling their effects, in turn, invites inferential uncertainties parallel to those that beset modeling effects in nonrandomized studies.)

Convenience and Probability Sampling

As noted in Chapter 5, the panel has recommended that CDC conduct population surveys that include potential and actual clients of counseling and testing services. By measuring a population's experience with and desire for these services, such surveys could be used to evaluate barriers to access and provide insight into perceived availability, needs for the services, and fears about the system. In addition to community and general population surveys, the panel recommended surveys of high-risk or hard-to-reach groups using probability samples whenever possible. We recognized that it may sometimes be difficult to construct the sampling frames from which probability samples of some high-risk groups can be drawn. The numbers and demographic profiles of gay men and intravenous drug users, for example, are not known with any certainty, nor are definitions of group membership always clear.

The panel observed that because of the difficulty and cost involved with population-based samples, replicable convenience samples can sometimes be used. The term "convenience" sample is not meant to convey a naive or effortless assemblage of study participants. Convenience samples are simply a type of nonprobability sample and can be devised in many ways, with some designs weaker or stronger than others. For example, "accidental" samples are drawn from subjects at hand and are rather easy to implement, but are far from being representative of the general population. "Purposive" samples are more carefully constructed to reflect the researcher's best judgment about what is typical of the

---

[9]Rossi and Freeman (1982) suggest community surveys as often the only feasible means of discovering nonparticipants; the panel considers this alternative more difficult than getting the important information at intake and tracking tirelessly.

larger population; they probably have a more substantive claim to an adequate coverage of the population. Regardless of construction design, estimates of population parameters from these sorts of convenience samples have unknowable amounts of bias and variance, and results are not generalizable to the constituents of the high-risk groups.

For comparing interventions, however, convenience samples may be useful. Alternative interventions can be compared by assigning them to randomly chosen subsets of a convenience sample of persons, or clinics, or other relevant unit of analysis. The random assignment solves the question of internal validity. The main hazard to external validity arises from the possibility of qualitative interaction between treatment effects and population subgroups. This risk cannot be dismissed, but it can be typically expected to be less threatening than the risk of large direct differences between population and convenience samples.

The panel did not discuss convenience samples at much length, but the parent committee in its first report (Turner, Miller, and Moses, 1989) did review a number of nonrandom or nonprobability sample studies of gay and bisexual men and of drug users. Briefly, the studies can be arranged along a spectrum of the strength of their sampling schemes. The panel believes that it would be helpful to highlight and update these examples here.

Sample Studies of Gay and Bisexual Men
Convenience samples recruited from narrowly circumscribed or "accidental" sources (e.g., STD clinics or gay bars) are frequently used, but their potential for inferring effects to the whole population is seriously flawed. For example, gay men recruited from an STD clinic (e.g., Swarthout et al., 1989) will quite likely have different information needs as well as a different awareness of available testing facilities than the gay population at large; if they are seropositive they may have different medical referral needs as well.

Samples that recruit volunteers through public notices (e.g., the Baltimore MACS sample[10]) are somewhat more useful. Although still a form of accidental sampling, such kinds of nonprobability samples are improved by casting a wider net, and the volunteers will probably have a more diverse base of needs for and concerns about counseling and testing services. Nevertheless, data derived from such a design will be biased by the self-selection of respondents into the sample.

Nonprobability samples and probability samples of narrow universes can be purposively enlarged to ensure differences among respondents by

[10]MACS—the Multicenter AIDS Cohort Studies—are described in Chapter 6.

including presumably representative groups in a sample. An example of such a purposive sample is a cohort assembled by Martin (1986). The design began with a probability sample of men belonging to at least one gay organization; the sample was supplemented with self-selected volunteers, recruits from a Gay Pride festival, respondents from a public health clinic, and a snowball sampling from persons already enrolled in the study.[11] This purposive sampling example is only illustrative—not definitive—as it likely overselects respondents with reasonably high knowledge of available services. For the purpose of measuring barriers to counseling and testing, it might be more helpful to diversify the sample, e.g., by supplementing the base probability sample with patrons of gay bars rather than users of health clinics.

Finally, a probability sample of gay and bisexual men is not impossible and of course would produce the most defensible data. One such sample was drawn by the San Francisco Men's Health Study from the Castro district of San Francisco, an area highly populated by gay men and having the highest incidence of AIDS cases in the city (see Winkelstein et al., 1987). The sample was representative of that community, and such a design might be quite appropriate in other high-profile gay communities for evaluating the accessibility of testing services.[12]

Sample Studies of Intravenous Drug Users

Intravenous drug users are a difficult population to survey because of the clandestine nature of drug use activities and the difficulty of defining who is or has been a user at risk of HIV from needle-sharing. Nonetheless, the spectrum of sampling done among intravenous drug users is similar to that done among gay men. Surveys have been largely limited to accidental convenience samples of subpopulations, but purposive and probability sampling have been possible.

Members of drug treatment centers constitute the most accessible populations for convenience samples, and numerous examples exist of research samples drawn from methadone and detoxification clinics. Assignment to treatment, however, is nonrandom, and results are not representative of the general drug-using population. Researchers would face

---

[11] A snowball sample is a sampling method in which each person interviewed is asked to suggest additional people for interviewing.

[12] The design was a clustered probability sampling of single men aged 25 to 55 in the 19 San Francisco census tracts that comprised the area of the city with the highest AIDS incidence rate. Note, however, that despite its scientific sampling plan, the representativeness of the survey could have been flawed by a fairly high nonresponse rate (41 percent), although investigators judged differences between respondents and nonrespondents to be "insufficient" to warrant that conclusion.

similar problems getting information about testing and counseling services from such a sample: treatment clientele are likely to have different testing needs and different perceptions about the availability of services than persons who choose to continue using drugs or cannot get into treatment. Other frequently used convenience samples include drug users in hospitals, emergency rooms, and health clinics.

A more varied but still accidental population is arrestees, of whom some 15-50 percent can be identified as drug users (Eckerman et al., 1976). Using a sample of arrestees would probably result in a more diverse group than a sample of clinic clients in terms of individuals' awareness of counseling and testing services and barriers to access. Because self-reports of drug use by arrestees may be unreliable, however, screening such as urinalysis may be necessary, making this design more difficult to implement because researchers cannot be sure of the individuals' consent. Moreover, arrestees may constitute a more desperate class of drug users—those who resort to crime to support their habit—than is representative of the population.

Purposive, nonprobability samples using street outreach to recruit IV drug users often attempt to draw on a broader cross-section and be more representative of the drug-using population than samples drawn from arrestees. For example, several studies have sampled IV drug users recruited from the streets of neighborhoods where drug use prevalence is high (e.g., Abdul-Quader et al., 1989; Inciardi et al., 1989; Wiebel et al., 1989). As with gay study recruits, street user recruits are probably more representative of the broader population than are institutional populations and, because they are active users and vulnerable to health problems, would likely have a variety of needs for counseling and testing services. Still, the conclusions from these samples cannot be generalized to the total population.

Some researchers have purposively enlarged nonprobability samples to ensure differences among respondents. Such purposive sampling cohorts have been assembled by researchers in Portland, Oregon (Sibthorpe et al., 1989, recruited from a corrections facility, county health clinics, private welfare organizations, and street outreach), at Johns Hopkins in Baltimore (e.g., Nelson et al., 1989, recruited from street outreach, clinics for sexually transmitted disease, emergency rooms, and drug treatment centers), and New York (Carballo-Dieguez et al., 1989, recruited from a poster campaign, methadone clinics, and inpatient wards). Depending on their final composition, these samples may provide some good results. Nonetheless, they are not substitutes for probability sampling and will never provide wholly representative results.

Finally, a probability sample is possible, at least of street drug users. Such a sample can be drawn from a systematic mapping of drug-related activity that includes the enumeration of activities and individuals as well as the selection of potential informants (such as ex-users) to identify active users (e.g., McAuliffe et al. [1987] used this method to deliver AIDS education to randomized neighborhoods of intravenous drug users). This sort of probability sampling could provide good data for analyzing access and barriers to counseling and testing services on the part of noninstitutionalized IV drug users.

RANDOMIZATION

CDC staff members expressed interest in learning more about successfully randomized samples in the AIDS prevention arena. This section provides some additional examples of such samples, including examples of experiments with no-treatment control groups. The section also readdresses the ethics of implementing randomized trials with no-treatment controls.

Examples of Randomized Experiments

In Chapter 4, the panel recommended a strategy of evaluating health education/risk reduction through randomized experiments in the context of street outreach. Although few evaluation studies of this sort have been published, the strategy is certainly feasible. One example is the sample drawn by McAuliffe and colleagues (1987), who used ex-addicts to deliver AIDS health education to intravenous drug users in randomly assigned neighborhoods of Baltimore; the experimental group had significantly more knowledge at follow-up than did control group members who did not receive the intervention, although there were no significant behavioral differences.

Few formal examples of randomized evaluation of street outreach studies are available in the literature; however, anecdotal reports and discussions with community-based providers indicate substantial opportunities and support for systematically testing various strategies. Community-based studies offer multiple units that can be randomized, such as street corners, street blocks, public housing communities, and less well-defined neighborhoods. Because of limited resources, outreach efforts in these communities sometimes have to be employed in a delayed implementation design. Alternative methods of outreach, such as comparing indigenous outreach workers with health professionals, may also be possible.

It may be possible that only a handful of street outreach projects will meet the criteria, discussed in Chapter 4, for randomizing to no-treatment. Similarly, the possibilities in other community-based settings may be few, but where they occur they should be creatively used. As an example of the latter, Bellingham and Gillies (1989) recently reported on a successful randomized control trial in Great Britain, in which six youth training centers were randomly assigned to receive an AIDS education comic book. No differences between the groups were detected at pretest, but at posttest the knowledge scores of the experimental group were significantly higher.

Randomizing alternative treatments may be easier still. A recent example of a "natural" experiment where student classes were randomly assigned to alternative treatments was reported by Ziffer and Ziffer (1989). Investigators administered pretests and posttests to students enrolled in parallel one-semester courses on AIDS. The class that received a values and attitudes component in addition to a basic "facts" course showed significant attitudinal change compared with the class who received facts only.

The experience of the panelists indicates that the research community is well aware of most of the steps that lead to a well-controlled experiment. We wish to emphasize, however, a sometimes neglected step, which is to involve project practitioners in the development of the research protocol. Such involvement, we believe, ought to facilitate cooperation and active participation in experimental studies. By designating a particular program to help in the development of the protocol and to serve as the test site, a prototype is created for the experimental trials. Staff of the prototype project could also assist in the training of new randomly selected sites in the controlled experiment.

The Ethics of No-treatment Controls

Although in Chapter 5 the panel does not recommend randomized studies with no-treatment controls for evaluating counseling and testing, the panel does recommend such a design in Chapter 4 for evaluating new CBO projects. Panelists debated this issue long and hard. In not recommending the design for counseling and testing, the panel's conclusion is based on an ethical consideration that needs to be made more explicit, especially because it may sometimes apply to certain CBO projects: *the panel believes that efficacious patient care is essential and, on ethical grounds, should not be withheld for purposes of evaluation.* This aspect should be considered along with the other justifications listed in Chapter 4 for no-treatment control conditions: scarce resources with which to provide a service; interventions that are of unproven value; and availability of related services elsewhere.

The panel notes an important difference between many CBO interventions and CDC's larger counseling and testing program. Despite

CDC's characterization of counseling and testing as an AIDS prevention program, the services can and should be distinguished. Unlike other projects, *it is not simply a behavioral intervention.* Rather, it is a program that offers HIV testing. Although testing can provide important information to be used in decisions about sexuality, contraceptive use, and needle-sharing, the test itself is a diagnostic tool and is an important aspect of patient care that the panel believes should be available to all who seek it. Because of this distinction, HIV testing should never be withheld for purposes of evaluating its effectiveness. Similarly, although counseling alone might be considered an intervention to encourage behavioral change, *when it is joined to testing* it becomes part of an effective medical care procedure (as a means of explaining test results and as a psychological and social support). Thus, counseling (in the context of counseling and HIV testing) also should not be withheld for purposes of evaluation. The panel therefore recommends an evaluation strategy for counseling and testing in which alternative counseling treatments are randomized and their relative effectiveness assessed. This strategy retains the essential parts of the service: the diagnostic technology of HIV testing and the counseling that is part of patient care.[13] At the same time, it allows for the evaluation of alternative counseling methodologies that may be found to have superior value in promoting behavioral change.

In deciding whether to withhold a given CBO service, care must be taken to distinguish whether the service offered is an integral aspect of patient care or is an intervention of unproven worth that is available elsewhere. Consider, for example, a CBO project that provides bleach to intravenous drug users. Bleach is known to be an effective agent for reducing HIV transmission; thus, information about the utility of bleach as a preventive tool should not be withheld. It is not known, however, whether *providing* a supply of bleach is effective in getting people to use it. Assuming that bleach is otherwise readily accessible, it would be ethical to randomly assign the provision of bleach samples across communities or organizations.

REFERENCES

Abdul-Quader, A., Tross, S., Des Jarlais, D. C., Kouzi, A., Friedman, S. R., and McCoy, E. (1989) Predictors of Attempted Sexual Behavior Change in a Street Sample of Active Male IV Drug Users in New York City. Presented at the Fifth International Conference on AIDS, Montreal, June 4-9.

Bellingham, K. and Gillies, P. (1989) AIDS Education for Youth - A Randomised Controlled Trial. Presented at the Fifth International Conference on AIDS, Montreal, June 4-9.

---

[13] Although the panel believes it would be unethical not to *offer* counseling as a part of patient care, it is important to recognize that patients have the prerogative to refuse counseling.

Cannell, C. F., and Henson, R. (1974) Incentives, motives, and response bias. *Annals of Economic and Social Measurement* 3(2):307-317.

Carballo-Dieguez, A., El-Sadr, W., Gorman, J., Joseph, M., McKinnon, J., and Sorrell, S. (1989) Research with Intravenous Drug Users: Problems and Practical Recommendations. Presented at the Fifth International Conference on AIDS, Montreal, June 4-9.

Cohen, J. (1988) *Statistical Power Analysis for the Behavioral Sciences.* Rev. ed. Hillsdale, N.J.: Lawrence Erlbaum Associates.

Cook, T. D., and Campbell, D. T. (1979) *Quasi-Experimentation: Design & Analysis Issues for Field Settings.* Boston: Houghton Mifflin.

Davis, A. L., Faust, R., and Ordentlich, M. (1984) Self-help smoking cessation and maintenance programs: A comparative study with 12-month follow-up by the American Lung Association. *American Journal of Public Health* 74(11):1212-1217.

Eckerman, W. C., Rachal, J. V., Hubbard, R. L., and Poole, W. K. (1976) Methodological issues in identifying drug users. In *Drug Use and Crime.* Report of the Panel on Drug Use and Criminal Behavior (Appendix). Research Triangle Park, N. C.: Research Triangle Institute.

Ferber, R., and Sudman, S. (1974) Effects of compensation in consumer expenditure studies. *Annals of Economic and Social Measurement* 3(2):319-331.

Fox, R., and Jones, L. T. (1989) Maintaining followup in prospective epidemiologic studies of HIV infection: Experience in the Baltimore MACS study. Presented at the Fifth International Conference on AIDS, Montreal, June 4-9.

Inciardi, J. A., Chitwood, D., McCoy, C. B., and McBride, D. C. (1989) Needle sharing behaviors and HIV serostatus in Miami, Florida. Presented at the Fifth International Conference on AIDS, Montreal, June 4-9.

Kraemer, H. C., and Thiemann, S. (1987) *How Many Subjects? Statistical Power Analysis in Research.* Newbury Park, Calif.: Sage Publications.

Lipsey, M. W. (1990) *Design Sensitivity: Statistical Power for Experimental Research.* Newbury Park, Calif.: Sage Publications.

Little, R. J. A., and Rubin, D. B. (1987) *Statistical Analysis with Missing Data.* New York: Wiley.

Martin, J. L. (1986) AIDS risk reduction recommendations and sexual behavior patterns among gay men: A multifactorial categorical approach to assessing change. *Health Education Quarterly* 13(4):347-358.

McAuliffe, W. E., Doering, S., Breer, P., Silverman, H., Branson, B., and Williams, K. (1987) An evaluation of using ex-addict outreach workers to educate intravenous drug users about AIDS prevention. Presented at the Third International Conference on AIDS, Washington, D.C., June 1-5.

Moore, R. P., Lessler, J. T., Caspar, R. A. (1989) *Technical Report: Results of Intensive Interviews to Study Nonresponse in the National Household Seroprevalence Survey.* Research Triangle Park, N.C.: Research Triangle Institute.

Nelson, K. E., Vlahov, D., Solomon, L., Lindsay, A., and Chowdhury, N. (1989) Clinical symptoms and medical histories of a cohort of IV drug users: Correlation with HIV seroprevalence. Presented at the Fifth International Conference on AIDS, Montreal, June 4-9.

Panel on Privacy and Confidentiality as Factors in Survey Response (1979) *Privacy and Confidentiality as Factors in Survey Response.* Report of the NRC Committee on National Statistics. Washington, D.C.: National Academy Press.

Pirie, P. L., Thomson, S. J., Mann, S. L., Peterson, A. V., Murray, D. M., Flay, B. R., and Best, J. A. (1989) Tracking and attrition in longitudinal school-based smoking prevention research. *Preventive Medicine* 18:249-256.

Rossi, P. H., and Freeman, H. E. (1982) *Evaluation: A Systematic Approach.* 2nd ed. Beverly Hills, Calif.: Sage Publications.

Sibthorpe, B. M., Fleming, D., McAlister, R., Klockner, R., and Gould, J. (1989) Needle sharing among IVDU's where needles are available without prescription. Presented at the Fifth International Conference on AIDS, Montreal, June 4-9.

Singer, E. (1978) Informed consent: Consequences for response rate and response quality in social surveys. *American Sociological Review* 43:144-162.

Swarthout, D., Gonsiorek, J., Simpson, M., and Henry, K. (1989) A behavioral approach to HIV prevention among sero-negative or untested gay/bisexual men with a history of unsafe behavior. Presented at the Fifth International Conference on AIDS, Montreal, June 4-9.

Tanur, J. M. (1982) Advances in methods for large-scale surveys and experiments. In R. M. Adams, N. J. Smelser, and D. J. Treiman, eds., *Behavioral and Social Science Research: A National Resource.* Part II. Report of the NRC Committee on Basic Research in the Behavioral and Social Sciences. Washington, D.C.: National Academy Press.

Turner, C. F., Miller, H. G., and Moses, L. E., eds. (1989) *AIDS, Sexual Behavior, and Intravenous Drug Use.* Washington, D.C.: National Academy Press.

Wiebel, W., Altman, N., Chene, D., and Fritz, R. (1989) Risk taking and risk reduction among IV drug users in 4 US cities. Presented at the Fifth International Conference on AIDS, Montreal, June 4-9.

Winkelstein, W., Samuel, M., Padian, N. S., Wiley, J. A., Lang, W., Anderson, R. E., and Levy, J. A. (1987) The San Francisco Men's Health Study: III. Reduction in human immunodeficiency virus transmission among homosexual/bisexual men, 1982-86. *American Journal of Public Health* 76(9):685-689.

Ziffer, A., and Ziffer, J. (1989) The need for psychosocial emphasis in academic courses on AIDS. Presented at the Fifth International Conference on AIDS, Montreal, June 4-9.

E

Ancillary, Emerging, and Related Projects

The second type of question raised by CDC program personnel following the release of the first edition of the panel's report involved ancillary, emerging, or related projects of the National AIDS Information and Education Program (NAIEP) and the Center for Prevention Services (CPS). These projects include: (1) evaluating materials distributed through the National AIDS Information Clearinghouse, (2) evaluating referral services for individuals testing HIV antibody positive in CPS's nationwide counseling and testing program, and (3) monitoring counseling and testing services provided in private (non-CDC funded) sites. (See Appendix D for a discussion of technical matters relating to some of the report's suggestions.)

Evaluating Clearinghouse Materials

In Chapter 3, the panel focused on evaluation strategies for the most prominent intervention of the NAIEP—the multiphase *America Responds to AIDS* campaign of public service announcements (PSAs). The panel noted that NAIEP, which oversees the media campaign, also has funded several other media projects, such as the mass mailing of AIDS informational brochures to households nationwide and the national AIDS hotline. An important NAIEP project not mentioned in Chapter 3 is the National AIDS Information Clearinghouse (NAIC), which has been sponsored since October 1987. The panel considered a simple strategy for evaluating the Clearinghouse materials.

Background and Objectives

NAIC acts as a centralized resource for information about AIDS-related organizations and educational materials. Its three main services include:

(1) two online information data bases—one for resources and one for educational materials—that are each supplemented with technical and reference assistance by staff specialists; (2) outreach services, in which staff members provide conference support and program building; and (3) direct distribution of selected educational materials.

According to its March 1989 *User Guide,* NAIC "evaluates its services and resources on an ongoing basis" and assists in "the development and assessment of resources." The "evaluation" and "assessment" activities refer not to the impact of services and resources but rather to their quality (quality being measured subjectively as well as objectively). Much of the assessment is done by internal staff, although external reviewers may sometimes be used. For example, projects and organizations are entered into the Resources Database only after they "meet NAIC criteria" and undergo "a rigorous process of internal validation." In addition, national organizations and state HIV coordinators are sometimes asked to provide a measure of external review. In-house staff also review publications, software, and audiovisuals before they are entered into the Educational Materials Database; like resources, educational materials are "indexed according to stringent guidelines" and undergo "a thorough quality control review" (*User Guide,* March 1989). Finally, NAIC has an internal review board that recommends the materials for direct distribution by the Clearinghouse, although CDC makes the final decision on these materials. The internal board bases its recommendations on judgments about the materials' accuracy, appropriateness to target audience, and currency.

CDC has proposed that, in addition to the internal review board, NAIC form an external review committee to review publications listed in the Educational Materials Database (except certain publications such as meeting proceedings and directories). The external board would look at materials on a regularly scheduled basis to assure their currency and to identify gaps in needed materials.

Because materials can become outdated, periodic reviews are needed to ensure currency. Similarly valuable is the need for NAIC to ensure quality control in the validation process and to assess the accuracy and appropriateness of educational materials. Although these activities frequently entail subjective judgment, they contribute to an assessment of how well services are delivered. They do not, however, answer the questions, "Does it work?" or "What works better?"

Does It Work?

As discussed in Chapter 1, the panel believes that the most efficient way to answer "Does it work?" is with a randomized field experiment that compares a group that receives an intervention with a control group that does not receive it. In Chapter 4, the panel discusses conditions under which having a no-treatment control is appropriate: scarce resources with which to provide a service; interventions that are of unproven value; and availability of related services elsewhere. (This subject is further elaborated in Appendix D.) In the case of the Clearinghouse services and resources, scarcity is not an issue, and availability of alternative services is questionable; therefore, the panel believes that having a no-treatment control group is inappropriate. What can be answered, however, is "What works better?"

What Works Better?

This question is appropriate for evaluating those materials in the Clearinghouse that NAIC recommends or intends to recommend to CDC for direct distribution. To answer the question of "What works better?," the panel recommends a small-scale strategy similar to the copy testing that was proposed for a formative evaluation of the media campaign. A simple experiment can be set up to randomly assign groups to receive different treatments and then compare the results. To contain costs and personnel resources, focus groups or convenience samples of certain risk groups[1] can be randomly assigned to receive different informational brochures about a given subject matter (e.g., needle use). Self-administered questionnaires of knowledge, attitudes, and beliefs can be designed to center on particular subject matters and on general AIDS information; results can then be analyzed for cognitive differences between groups. (A more elaborate experiment would follow up the groups at a fixed later date (2 weeks, 4 weeks) to analyze differences in self-reported behavior.)

Several comparative tests can be made. One test might compare the effect of different levels of readability on cognition—for example, brochures written at the 7th and the 10th grade levels.[2] Another test might compare materials containing different amounts of information. For example, one brochure might discuss risks and risk reduction involving needle use, while another provides the same information along with additional information related only peripherally to the central theme, such as morbidity and mortality data. Another type of test might compare the effects of bilingual publications and English-only materials.

The panel also considered the possibility of comparing NAIC outreach services (conference planning and program building). Ultimately

---

[1] Convenience sampling is discussed in Appendix D.

[2] Hochhauser (1987) analyzed 16 AIDS prevention brochures written for the general population and found that, on average, they were written at a 14th grade level (second year of college). This level may be too high to foster a good understanding of recommended material.

we decided that the measurement of success is tenuous (e.g., attendance at a conference may be excellent, but the conference may be poor) and cannot be well controlled (e.g., weather can affect attendance at different sites). For these reasons, the panel believes that evaluation efforts should be confined to materials recommended for direct distribution by NAIC.

Evaluating Referral Services of the Counseling and Testing Program

In Chapter 5, the panel noted that "the purpose of the counseling and testing program has evolved and may still be evolving," in part because "advances in the treatment of asymptomatic HIV-infected individuals may increase the demand for testing and counseling services." Shortly after the report was issued, representatives from the CPS stated that the program's purpose indeed is shifting. Just as it had once evolved from screening the nation's blood supply to disease prevention, it is now moving to the provision of follow-up referral services for seropositive individuals.[3] This shift raises two questions: "What is the quality of follow-up referral services?" and "Are these services available?"

These concerns fall within the context of the original question posed in Chapter 5, "How well are services delivered?" Out of the five aspects of service delivery that were identified to gather answers to this question, two are relevant to the new questions: the adequacy of the referrals that are actually provided and the accessibility of referral services. The panel recognizes that both adequacy and accessibility are subjective terms that call for judgment on the part of the evaluator. At the same time, the panel also believes that some standards can be agreed upon as essential, so that an evaluation can determine if those standards have been met.

In Chapter 5, the panel described "adequacy" as correspondence with client needs, such as the need for confidentiality. The needs of seropositive clients were briefly discussed and were said to include information and counseling about the medical and psychological management of infection and partner notification. To these requirements, the panel now adds the need for information about financial management (given the enormous cost of medical treatment for HIV disease), legal rights, contraception, and drug treatment, when applicable. Depending on individual circumstances, such information might include facts about insurance, referrals to Medicaid, the welfare system, gynecological services, drug treatment facilities, and, if discrimination is an issue, legal aid. As a useful first step to developing standards by which to judge the quality of

---

[3]Indeed, provision of case management services is likely to be another important component in the continuity and success of the counseling and testing program's essential prevention messages.

referrals, the panel suggests that CDC identify and draw up a checklist of appropriate referral services, just as the agency has identified and prescribed checklists for pretest and posttest counseling.

Judgment about accessibility is also somewhat subjective, but a basis can be constructed that will help answer the question "How well are services delivered?" To evaluate the accessibility of counseling and testing services, the panel recommended four sources of information. Three of the sources (client surveys, site inventories, case studies) are useful for determining accessibility to referral services as well; a fourth (population surveys) could be useful, but the return on investment is not likely to be as high as the others.

- *Client Surveys.* Surveys of the clients of HIV testing sites can reveal whether clients returned for referral services, whether such services were offered, and what the referral needs were. Client surveys can elicit information about referrals made for specific populations as well as about the scope and relevance of the referrals. In fact, a client survey at a pilot stage is warranted to help establish client needs and to identify the types of referrals that should appear on a checklist of potential services.

- *Site Service Inventories.* Information about the accessibility of referral services can be gathered in the site service inventories recommended in Chapter 5. These inventories can monitor the services that sites provide to persons testing positive for HIV. They can also demonstrate whether clients returned for referrals and whether and what referrals were made, using the checklist recommended above. The inventories can be analyzed according to site types, risk factors, local variations, and so on. If socioeconomic status were also collected (see footnote 4, Chapter 5), referral needs might be further illuminated.

- *Case Studies.* The panel recommends using independent observers of clinician-client interactions to gather information about the accessibility of referral services. The panel does not recommend the use of "professional customers," as we did for the direct observation of counseling and testing services. The distinction is made because the relevant population of referees (seropositive individuals) would require "professional seropositives" to evaluate the referral services. Although adding the HIV rates of a handful of professional customers should not overly disturb a facility's surveillance counts, the introduction of only seropositive individuals as professional customers could inflate the counts.

The panel notes that CDC is currently funding a few confidential test sites to ask case managers to follow up on the services offered seropositive individuals. Such case studies ought to be important sources of information not only about HIV medical and legal referrals but also about indirectly related services, such as drug treatment or contraceptive services, that may be eclipsed by HIV services.

- *Population group surveys of high-risk individuals.* The panel believes that these types of surveys should be given the lowest priority. Although they might shed light on the accessibility of referral services for seropositive individuals, the number of persons actually infected is too small for population surveys to be recommended. Nonetheless, if this approach is considered, the panel hopes that the discussion in Appendix D on probability-based surveys and convenience sampling will be helpful.

Monitoring Services at Non-CDC Testing Sites

Surveillance information from test labs indicates that some people are being tested for HIV in private sector sites, but CDC does not know who or how many people are doing so and what services they obtain. To learn about counseling and testing services provided at non-CDC-funded sites, CDC can build on the *population group surveys* previously recommended as evaluation sources. The panel suggested this type of survey in Chapter 5 to evaluate site accessibility and barriers to using counseling and testing services, but items on such surveys can be readily modified or added to determine whether, what, and where services are being obtained elsewhere. Because survey respondents may not know whether the test site they visit is funded by CDC, one item should ask the site location so that it can later be cross-checked by CDC program personnel.

As discussed in Chapter 5, population surveys can be targeted to particular communities or high-risk populations, although sampling frames for some high-risk groups may be difficult to construct. Alternatively, a survey of the general population would be helpful. As with research to evaluate CDC-funded sites, such general population surveys would help identify the services people desire and how available they perceive them to be. Either a new survey could be launched—which would be expensive—or questions could be added to the National Health Interview Survey (NHIS) about the reasons people seek or avoid testing.

The panel notes that CDC has had problems with timely access to the NHIS data in the past. Both the National Center for Health Statistics and the Office of Management and Budget have lengthy approval processes for items to be added to their surveys. In addition, there are delays in sharing data once they are collected. As we did in Chapter 6, the panel wishes to register its concern about both of these problems and express its hope that, at least in the latter case, a greater cooperation between NCHS and other divisions within CDC can be effected.

Finally, the panel considered, but decided not to recommend, *client surveys* of non-CDC-funded sites. The panel felt that it would be too difficult to induce cooperation with a representative sample of private sites to conduct confidential client surveys. The panel recognized, however, that such research could potentially shed light on the adequacy and completion rates of private counseling and testing services and could provide a useful comparison with services provided by CDC-funded sites.

REFERENCES

Hochhauser, M. (1987) Readability of AIDS education materials. Presented at the Annual Meeting of the American Psychological Association, New York, August 30.

National AIDS Information Clearinghouse (1989) *User Guide.* March.

F

The Use of Selection Modeling to Evaluate AIDS Interventions with Observational Data

Robert Moffitt

I. INTRODUCTION

This paper considers the potential applicability to AIDS interventions of nonexperimental evaluation methods developed by econometricians in the evaluation of social programs. Econometric methods for program evaluation have been studied by economists over the past twenty years and are by now quite well-developed. To give the discussion a focus, two types of interventions are considered: AIDS counseling and testing (C&T) programs, and AIDS programs run by community-based organizations (CBOs). While both C&T programs and CBOs are quite diverse, especially the CBOs, many are designed to encourage the adoption of sexual prevention behaviors and to encourage risk reduction behaviors more generally. It is this outcome that will be the focus of the analysis here.

This paper was presented at the Conference on Nonexperimental Approaches to Evaluating AIDS Prevention Programs convened on January 12-13, 1990 by the Panel on the Evaluation of AIDS Interventions of the National Research Council. The views expressed in this paper are those of the author; they should not be attributed to the Panel or to the NRC. Comments on an earlier version of the paper from James Heckman, V. Joseph Hotz, Roderick Little, Charles Manski, and Lincoln Moses are appreciated. A version of this paper is to appear in *Evaluation Review.*

In the next section of the paper, a brief historical overview of the development of econometric methods for program evaluation is given. Following that, in Section III, a more formal statistical exposition of those methods is given. This section constitutes the major part of the paper. The conclusion of the discussion is that nonexperimental evaluation in general requires either adequate data on the behavioral histories of participants and non-participants in the interventions, or the availability of identifying variables ("Z's") that affect the availability of the treatment to different individuals but not their behavior directly. Whether either of these conditions can be met in the evaluation of AIDS interventions is then discussed in Section IV for C&T and CBO programs. A summary and conclusion is provided in Section V.

II. HISTORICAL DEVELOPMENT OF ECONOMETRIC METHODS FOR PROGRAM EVALUATION

Most of the econometric methods for program evaluation have been designed to evaluate government-sponsored manpower training programs, where the major issue has been whether such programs increase individual earnings and other indicators of labor market performance. Such programs began to appear in the early 1960s with the Manpower Development and Training Act (MDTA) of 1962, and grew more extensive in the late 1960s as part of the War on Poverty. They became a fixture in the 1970s and 1980s, though changing in name and form from, for example, the Comprehensive Employment and Training Act (CETA) program in the 1970s to the Job Training and Partnership Act (JTPA) program in the 1980s. However, economists have also conducted extensive studies of welfare programs of other types, of health and education programs, and many others.

One of the earliest studies (Ashenfelter, 1978) presented an econometric model for the estimation of the effect of the MDTA program on earnings using observational data. Many studies were later conducted of the CETA program and have been surveyed by Barnow (1987). No major evaluation studies of the JTPA program have been completed, although one is currently underway. A recent study of an experimental training program called Supported Work has been published by Heckman and Hotz (1989), and will be discussed further below.

The econometric literature on program evaluation underwent a major alteration in its formal framework after the separate development of "selectivity bias" techniques in the mid-1970s. Originally, the selectivity bias issue in economics concerned a missing-data problem that arises in the study of individual labor market behavior, namely, the inherent unobservability of the potential market earnings of individuals who are not working. The development of techniques for properly estimating such potential earnings (Gronau, 1974; Lewis, 1974; Heckman, 1974) was quickly realized to have relevance to the estimation of the effects of public programs on economic behavior. As will be discussed extensively in the next section, a similar selectivity bias problem arises in observational evaluation studies through the inherent unobservability of what would have happened to program participants had they not received the treatment, and of what would have happened to non-participants had they undergone the treatment. The connecting link was first explicitly made by Barnow, Cain, and Goldberger (1980), which included a comparison of the new technique with earlier techniques. A textbook treatment of the applicability of selectivity bias methods to program evaluation became available shortly thereafter (Maddala, 1983), as well as a survey of the applicability of those methods to health interventions in particular (Maddala, 1985).

The recent work of Heckman and Robb (1985a, 1985b) represents the most complete and general statement of the selectivity bias problem in program evaluation using observational data, and provides the most thorough analysis of the conditions under which the methods will yield good estimates and of the estimation methods available to obtain such estimates. The analysis in the next section of this paper is heavily influenced by the work of Heckman and Robb, which is itself built upon the almost twenty years of work on econometric methods for program evaluation.

III. THE STATISTICS OF PROGRAM EVALUATION WITH OBSERVATIONAL DATA

Although the statistical methods exposited in this section are applicable to any program in principle and will be developed fairly abstractly, it may help for specificity to consider the evaluation of C&T programs. Such programs have many goals but, for present purposes, it will be assumed that the major goal is to encourage those who receive the services of the program to adopt risk reduction activities and sexual prevention behaviors to reduce the likelihood of HIV infection to themselves and to others. The aim of the evaluation is to determine whether such programs do indeed have such effects and, if so, to provide an estimate of their magnitude.

To begin the formal analysis, let Y be the outcome variable (e.g., level of prevention behavior) and make the following definitions:

$Y_{it}^* =$ Level of outcome variable for individual i at time t, assuming he has not received the "treatment" (i.e., the services of a C&T program)

Y_{it}^{**} = Level of outcome variable for individual i at time t, assuming he has received the treatment at some prior date

The difference between these two quantities is the effect of the treatment, denoted α:

$$Y_{it}^{**} = Y_{it}^* + \alpha \tag{1}$$

or

$$\alpha = Y_{it}^{**} - Y_{it}^* \tag{2}$$

The aim of the evaluation is to obtain an estimate of the value of α, the treatment effect, from whatever data are available.[1] The easiest way to think about what we seek in an estimate of α is to consider individuals who have gone through a C&T program and therefore have received the treatment, and for whom we later measure their value of Y_{it}^{**}. Ideally, we wish to know the level of Y_{it}^* for such individuals—we would like to know what their level of prevention behaviors, for example, would have been had they not gone through the program. If Y_{it}^* could be known, the difference between it and Y_{it}^{**} would be a satisfactory estimate[2] of α.

The difficulty that arises is that we do not observe Y_{it}^* directly but only the values of Y_{it}^* for non-participants. Define a dummy variable for whether an individual has or has not received the treatment:

$d_i = 1$ if individual i has received the treatment

$d_i = 0$ if individual i has not received the treatment

Then a satisfactory estimate of α could be obtained by estimating the difference between Y_{it}^{**} and Y_{it}^* for those who went through the program:

$$\hat{\alpha} = E(Y_{it}^{**}|d_i = 1) - E(Y_{it}^*|d_i = 1) \tag{3}$$

where E is the expectation operator.

The estimate $\hat{\alpha}$ in (3) is, in fact, the estimate that would be obtained if we had administered a randomized trial for the evaluation. For example, as individuals come in through the door of a C&T program, they could be randomly assigned to treatment status or control status, where the latter would involve receiving none of the services of the program. At some later date we could measure the levels of Y for the two groups and calculate (3) to obtain an estimate of the effect of the program.

---

[1] For simplicity, the treatment effect, α, is assumed to be constant over time and across individuals, and to be non-random. Random treatment effects across individuals have been incorporated by Bjorklund and Moffitt (1987) and are discussed by Heckman and Robb (1985a, 1985b).

[2] In standard econometric practice, Y_{it}^* is set equal to $X\beta + \epsilon$, where X is a vector of observed variables, β is its coefficient vector, and ϵ is an error term.

The Problem

The first key point of the statistical literature on evaluation is that observational, nonexperimental data do not allow us to calculate (3) and therefore do not allow us to compute the estimate that could be obtained with a randomized trial. This is simply because we generally do not observe in such data any individuals who would have taken the treatment but do not; we only generally observe individuals who did not take the treatment at all.[3] What we can estimate with nonexperimental data is an effect denoted here as $\tilde{\alpha}$:

$$\tilde{\alpha} = E(Y_{it}^{**}|d_i = 1) - E(Y_{it}^*|d_i = 0) \qquad (4)$$

which is just the difference between mean Y for participants, those who did take the treatment ($d_i = 1$) and the mean Y for non-participants, those who did not undergo the treatment ($d_i = 0$).

When will the estimate we are able to calculate, $\tilde{\alpha}$, equal the estimate we would have obtained with a randomized trial, $\hat{\alpha}$? Comparison of (3) and (4) shows that the two will be equal if and only if the following condition is true:

$$E(Y_{it}^*|d_i = 1) = E(Y_{it}^*|d_i = 0) \qquad (5)$$

In words, the two estimates of α are equal only if the value of Y_{it}^* for those who did not take the treatment equals the value of Y_{it}^* that those who did take the treatment would have had, had they not gone through the program.

The heart of the nonexperimental evaluation problem is reflected in equation (5), and an understanding of that equation is necessary to understand the pervasiveness and unavoidability of what is termed the "selection bias" problem when observational data are employed. The equation will fail to hold under many plausible circumstances. For example, if those who go through a C&T program are concerned with their health and have already begun adopting prevention behaviors even before entering the program, they will be quite different from those who do not go through the program even prior to receiving any program services. Hence equation (5) will fail to hold because those who go through the program have different levels of Y_{it}^*, that is, different levels of prevention behavior even in the absence of receiving any program services. Our estimate of α will be too high relative to $\hat{\alpha}$, for the

---

[3] Some evaluation designs make use of individuals on waiting lists as controls. Unfortunately, these individuals may not be randomly selected from the applicant pool; if they are not, their Y values will not be an accurate proxy for those of participants.

greater level of prevention behaviors observed for the treatment group subsequent to receiving services was present even prior to the treatment, and is therefore not a result of the treatment itself. Those who are observed to have actually gone through the program are therefore a "self-selected" group out of the pre-treatment population, and the estimate of $\tilde{\alpha}$ is contaminated by "selectivity bias" because of such self-selection.

The unavoidability of the potential for selectivity bias arises because the validity of equation (5) cannot be tested, even in principle, for the left-hand side of that equation is inherently unobservable. It is impossible in principle to know what the level of Y_{it}^* for those who went through the program would have been had they not gone through it, for that level of Y_{it}^* is a "counterfactual" that can never be observed. We may know, as discussed further below, the pre-treatment level of Y_{it} for those who later undergo treatment, but this is not the same as the Y_{it}^* we seek—for the left-hand side of (5), we need to know the level of Y_{it}^* for program participants that they would have had at exactly the same time as they went through the treatment, not at some previous time.[4]

Solutions

There are three general classes of potential solutions to the selection bias problem (Heckman and Robb, 1985a, 1985b). None guarantees the elimination of the problem altogether, but rather each seeks to determine possible circumstances under which the problem could be eliminated. The question is then whether those circumstances hold. At the outset, it is important to note that two of the three solution methods have important implications for evaluation design because they require the collection of certain types of data. Whether those data can be collected for AIDS programs then becomes the most important question, which is discussed in detail in Section IV.

Solution 1: Identifying Variables ("Z's")

The selection bias problem can be solved if a variable Z_i is available, or one can be found, that (1) affects the probability that an individual receives the treatment but which (2) has no direct relationship to Y_{it}^* (e.g., no direct relationship to individual prevention behavior). What is an example of such a Z_i? A Z_i could be constructed if, for example, a C&T program were funded by CDC in one city and not in another for political

---

[4]It may be noted that Manski (1990) has pointed out that if Y_{it}^* is bounded (e.g., between 0 and 1), a worst-case/best-case analysis can be conducted in which the unobserved counterfactual is taken to equal each of the bounds in turn. This gives a range in which the true effect must lie instead of a point estimate.

or bureaucratic reasons unrelated to the needs of the populations in the two cities, and therefore unrelated to the likelihood that the individuals in the two cities practice prevention behaviors. If a random sample of the relevant subpopulations were conducted in the two cities and data on Y were collected—the data would include both participants and non-participants in the city where the C&T program was funded—a comparison of the mean values of Y in the two could form the basis for a valid estimate[5] of α. The variable Z_i in this case should be thought of as a dummy variable equal to 1 in the C&T city and 0 in the other. The variable satisfies the two conditions given above—it obviously affects whether individuals in the two cities receive the treatment, since if $Z_i = 0$ no C&T treatment is available, and it is unrelated to the level of Y_{it}^* in the two cities because the funding decision was made for reasons unrelated to sexual prevention behavior.[6] This estimation method is known in econometrics as an "instrumental-variable" method and Z_i is termed an "instrument." It is an instrument in the sense that it is used to proxy the treatment variable itself.

What is an example of an illegitimate Z_i? The same dummy variable defined in the previous example would be illegitimate if the CDC funding decision were based not on political or bureaucratic decisions but on the relative level of need in the two cities. For example, if the C&T program were placed in the city with the higher rate of HIV infection, then Z_i would not be independent of Y_{it}^*—the presence of the C&T program would be associated with lower levels of prevention behavior not because of a negative causal effect of the program but because of the reason for its placement.

Further examples of legitimate and illegitimate "Z's" will be discussed in Section IV.

Solution 2: Parametric Distributional Assumptions on Y_{it}^*

A second solution to the selection bias problem arises if a parametric distributional assumption on Y_{it}^* can be safely made or determined with reasonable certainty (Heckman and Robb, 1985a, 1985b). For example, if Y_{it}^* follows a normal, logistic, or some other distribution with a finite set of parameters, identification of a program effect free of selection bias

---

[5]For example, if $\overline{Y}_1$ is the mean value of the outcome variable in the city with the program and $\overline{Y}_0$ is the mean value in the city without one, and if p is the fraction of the relevant subpopulation in the first city that participated in the program, the impact estimate would be calculated as $(\overline{Y}_1 - \overline{Y}_0)/p$.

[6]Essentially, this is a case of what is often termed a "natural" experiment. It is similar to an experiment inasmuch as the probability of having the treatment available is random with respect to the outcome variable under study.

is possible. The reasons are relatively technical and difficult to explain in simple terms. However, this method will not be especially useful for the AIDS interventions because very little is known about the distribution of sexual prevention behaviors, for example, in the total population or even the high-risk population. Consequently, this method will not be considered further.

Solution 3: Availability of Cohort Data

A third solution method requires the availability of "cohort," "longitudinal," or "panel" data, that is, data on the same individuals at several points in time before and after some of them have undergone the treatment. In the simplest case, data on Y_{it} are available not only after the treatment but also before, giving a data set with one pre-treatment observation and one post-treatment observation for each individual, both participants and non-participants. In the more general case, three or more points in time may be available in the data.

The use of such cohort data is sufficiently important to warrant an extended discussion. To illustrate this method, first consider the situation that would arise if data at two points in time were available, one before the treatment and one after it. Let "t" denote the post-treatment point and "$t-1$" denote the pre-treatment point. Then, analogously with the cross-section case considered previously,

$Y_{it}^{*} - Y_{i,t-1}^{*}$ = Change in Y_{it}^{*} from $t-1$ to t in the absence of having undergone the treatment

$Y_{it}^{**} - Y_{i,t-1}^{*}$ = Change in Y_{it}^{*} from $t-1$ to t if having undergone the treatment

Then the effect of the treatment is α, and

$$Y_{it}^{**} - Y_{i,t-1}^{*} = (Y_{it}^{*} - Y_{i,t-1}^{*}) + \alpha \qquad (6)$$

Since $Y_{i,t-1}^{*}$ cancels out on both sides of (6), (6) is the same as (1) and therefore the true effect, α, is the same.

As before, a preferred estimate of the effect of the program could be obtained by a randomized trial in which those wishing to undergo the treatment ($d_i = 1$) are randomly assigned to participation or non-participation status. With data on both pre-treatment and post-treatment status, the estimate of the program effect could be calculated as:

$$\hat{\alpha} = E(Y_{it}^{**} - Y_{i,t-1}^{*} | d_i = 1) - E(Y_{it}^{*} - Y_{i,t-1}^{*} | d_i = 1) \qquad (7)$$

However, with observational data the second term on the right-hand side of (7) is not measurable since, once again, we cannot measure Y_{it}^{*} for those who undergo the treatment. We can instead only use the data on Y_{it}^* available from non-participants to estimate the program effect as follows:

$$\tilde{\alpha} = E(Y_{it}^{**} - Y_{i,t-1}^* | d_i = 1) - E(Y_{it}^* - Y_{i,t-1}^* | d_i = 0) \qquad (8)$$

The estimate $\tilde{\alpha}$ is often called a "differences" estimate because it is computed by comparing the first-differenced values of Y for participants and non-participants.

The estimate we are able to obtain in (8) will equal that we could have obtained in the randomized trial, (7), if and only if

$$E(Y_{it}^* - Y_{i,t-1}^* | d_i = 1) = E(Y_{it}^* - Y_{i,t-1}^* | d_i = 0) \qquad (9)$$

Equation (9) is the key equation for the two data-point case and is the analogue to equation (5) in the single post-treatment data case. The equation shows that a data set with a pre-treatment and post-treatment observation will yield a good estimate of α if the *change* in Y_{it}^* from pre to post would have been the same for participants, had they not undergone the treatment, as it actually was for non-participants. Sometimes the change in Y_{it}^* is referred to as the "growth rate" of Y_{it}^*, in which case we may say that our nonexperimental estimate requires that the growth rate of participants and non-participants be the same in the absence of the treatment.

Perhaps the most important point is that this condition may hold even though the condition in (5) does not. Equation (5), the condition that must hold for the nonexperimental estimate in a single post-treatment cross-section to be correct, requires that the *levels* of Y_{it} be the same for participants and non-participants in the absence of the treatment. Equation (9), on the other hand, only requires that the *growth rates* of Y_{it} be the same for participants and non-participants in the absence of the treatment, even though the levels may differ. The latter is a much weaker condition and will more plausibly hold.

The nature of the condition is illustrated in panels (a) and (b) of Figure 1. In panel (a), the pre-treatment levels of non-participants and participants, A and A', respectively, are quite different—participants have a higher level of Y, as would be the case, for example, if those who later undergo C&T have higher prevention behaviors in the first place. From t-1 to t, the level of Y for non-participants grows from A to B, as might occur if everyone in the population under consideration (e.g., homosexual men) were increasing their degree of risk reduction behaviors even without participating in a C&T program. The figure shows, for illustration, a growth rate of Y for participants from A'

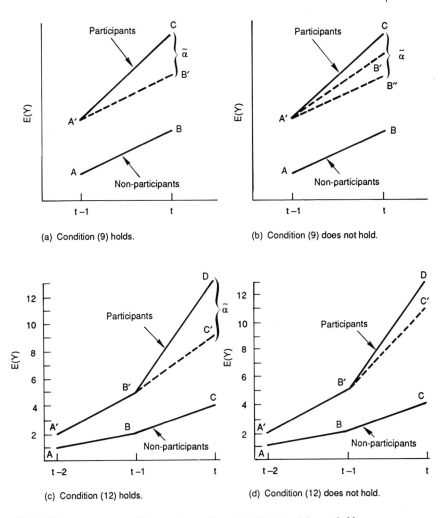

(a) Condition (9) holds.

(b) Condition (9) does not hold.

(c) Condition (12) holds.

(d) Condition (12) does not hold.

FIGURE F-1 Examples in which conditions (9) and (12) hold and do not hold.

to C, which is a larger rate of growth than for non-participants. The estimate of the treatment effect, $\tilde{\alpha}$, is also shown in the figure and is based on the assumption that, in the absence of undergoing C&T, the Y of participants would have grown from A' to B'—in other words, by the same amount as the Y of non-participants grew. Of course, this assumption cannot be verified because point B' is not observed; it is only a "counterfactual." But clearly the estimate in the figure would be a much better estimate than that obtained from a single post-treatment cross-section, which would take the vertical distance between B and C as the treatment estimate. This would be invalid because equation (5) does not hold.

Panel (b) in Figure 1 shows a case where condition (9) breaks down. In that panel, a case is shown in which the Y of participants would have grown faster than that for non-participants even in the absence of the treatment (A' to B' is greater than A to B). This might arise, for example, if those individuals who choose to undergo C&T are adopting risk reduction behaviors more quickly than non-participants. In this case, our estimate of $\tilde{\alpha}$ is too high, since it measures the vertical distance between B'' and C instead of between B' and C. Neither B' nor B'' is observed, so we cannot know which case holds.

The primary conclusion to be drawn from this discussion is that we may be able to do better in our estimate of program effect with *more data*. Adding a single pre-treatment data point permits us to compute an estimate of the treatment effect—the differences estimator in (8)—that may be correct in circumstances in which the estimator using a single post-treatment is not. The importance of having additional data on the histories of Y, or the sexual behavior histories of C&T participants and non-participants, for example, stands in contrast to the situation faced when conducting a randomized trial where, strictly speaking, only a single post-treatment cross section is required. Thus we conclude that more data may be required for valid inference in nonexperimental evaluations than in experimental evaluations.

This point extends to the availability of additional pre-treatment observations.[7] Suppose, for example, that an additional pre-treatment observation is available at time *t-2*. The estimate calculable in a randomized trial is

$$\hat{\alpha} = E[(Y_{it}^{**} - Y_{i,t-1}^*) - (Y_{i,t-1}^* - Y_{i,t-2}^*)|d_i = 1]$$
$$- E[(Y_{it}^* - Y_{i,t-1}^*) - (Y_{i,t-1}^* - Y_{i,t-2}^*)|d_i = 1] \quad (10)$$

while the estimate permitted in an observational study is

$$\tilde{\alpha} = E[(Y_{it}^{**} - Y_{i,t-1}^*) - (Y_{i,t-1}^* - Y_{i,t-2}^*)|d_i = 1]$$
$$- E[(Y_{it}^* - Y_{i,t-1}^*) - (Y_{i,t-1}^* - Y_{i,t-2}^*)|d_i = 0] \quad (11)$$

---

[7] Gathering data from additional post-treatment observations is easier but does not serve the appropriate control function. Prior to the treatment, it is known with certainty that the program could have no true effect; after the treatment, it cannot be known with certainty what the pattern of the effect is, assuming it has an effect. Consequently, participant/non-participant differences in Y_{it} after the treatment can never be treated with absolute certainty as reflecting selection bias rather than a true effect.

This estimator is often termed a "differences-in-differences" estimator because it computes the treatment effect by comparing the "change in the change" of Y for participants and non-participants.

The two estimates will be equal if and only if

$$E[(Y_{it}^* - Y_{i,t-1}^*) - (Y_{i,t-1}^* - Y_{i,t-2}^*)|d_i = 1]$$
$$= E[(Y_{it}^* - Y_{i,t-1}^*) - (Y_{i,t-1}^* - Y_{i,t-2}^*)|d_i = 0] \quad (12)$$

Equation (12) shows that a correct program impact estimate will be obtained only if the *change* in the growth rate of Y would have been the same for program participants in the absence of their having undergone treatment as it actually was for non-participants. Panel (c) of Figure 1 illustrates the situation when this condition holds. For both participants and non-participants, Y is growing at an increasing rate over time as, for example, would occur if the adoption of prevention behaviors were accelerating in the population. For non-participants, Y grows by 1 from *t-2* to *t-1* (*A* to *B*) and by 2 from *t-1* to *t* (*B* to *C*). For participants, Y grows by 3 from *t-2* to *t-1* (*A'* to *B'*) and by 8 from *t-1* to *t* (*B'* to *D*). The estimate of program effect, shown in the figure, is therefore 4 since it is assumed that the growth rate of Y for participants in the absence of the treatment would have accelerated by the same amount as it did for non-participants, namely, by 1—from a growth rate of 3 between *t-2* and *t-1* to a growth rate of 4 between *t-1* and *t* (*B'* to *C''*). Panel (d) shows a case where condition (12) does not hold—there, the growth rate of Y for participants accelerates by more even in the absence of the treatment than it did for non-participants (*B'* to *C'* is greater than *B* to *C*).

The major point to be drawn from this discussion is that the availability of three points of data permits us to obtain an estimate of program effect that may be valid in circumstances in which the estimate possible with two points of data is incorrect. For example, the application of the differences estimator in (8) to the data shown in panel (c) would give an incorrect estimate of program effect, for, in the absence of the treatment, the growth rates of Y for participants and non-participants between *t-1* and *t* (*B'* to *C'* and *B* to *C*, respectively) are *not* equal. We have before us the case illustrated in panel (b), where the differences method gives an incorrect estimate. Thus, once again, the conclusion to be drawn is that more data permit the calculation of program effects that may be valid in circumstances in which the estimate available with less data is not.

An analogous implication holds if we consider four, five, or many points of data. More periods of data make possible estimates of treatment effects which are equal to those obtainable from a randomized trial under weaker and weaker conditions, thereby strengthening the reliability of the nonexperimental estimator. In the general case, a slight modification in the model allows us to write the estimate of the treatment effect as the following:[8]

$$\tilde{\alpha} = E(Y_{it}^{**}|d_i = 1, Y_{i,t-1}^*, Y_{i,t-2}^*, \ldots, Y_{i,t-k}^*)$$
$$- E(Y_{it}^*|d_i = 0, Y_{i,t-1}^*, Y_{i,t-2}^*, \ldots, Y_{i,t-k}^*) \qquad (13)$$

assuming that data are available for k pre-treatment periods. This estimator will equal that obtainable in a randomized trial if and only if the following condition holds:

$$E(Y_{it}^*|d_i = 1, Y_{i,t-1}^*, \ldots, Y_{i,t-k}^*) = E(Y_{it}^*|d_i = 0, Y_{i,t-1}^*, \ldots, Y_{i,t-k}^*) \quad (14)$$

This condition can be interpreted as requiring that the values of d_i and Y_{it}^* must be independent of one another conditional upon the history of Y_{it}^* up to t-1. Put differently, it must be the case that it if we observe two individuals at time t-1 who have exactly the same history of Y_{it}^* up to that time (e.g., the exact same history of sexual prevention behaviors)—and who therefore look exactly alike to the investigators—they must have the same value of Y_{it}^* in the next time period regardless of whether they do or do not undergo the treatment. If, on the other hand, the probability of entering a C&T program is related to the value of Y_{it}^* they would have had if the treatment were not available, the condition in equation (14) will not hold and the nonexperimental estimate will be inaccurate.

The Relationship between Data
Availability and Testing of Assumptions

The discussion thus far has demonstrated that the availability of certain types of data—information on legitimate "Z" variables, or on individual histories—is related to the conditions that must hold, and the assumptions that must be made, in order to obtain an estimate of program effect similar to that obtainable in a randomized trial. A natural question is whether any of the assumptions can be tested, and whether it can be determined if the conditions do or do not hold. The answer to this question once again is related to data availability.

The technical answer to the question is that "overidentifying" assumptions can be tested but that "just identifying" assumptions cannot

---

[8]This autoregressive model was estimated in an early economic study by Ashenfelter (1978). A simpler model but one more focused on the evaluation question was also analyzed by Goldberger (1972) in a study of methods of evaluating the effect of compensatory education programs on test scores when the treatment group is selected, in part, on the basis of a pretest score.

Model I

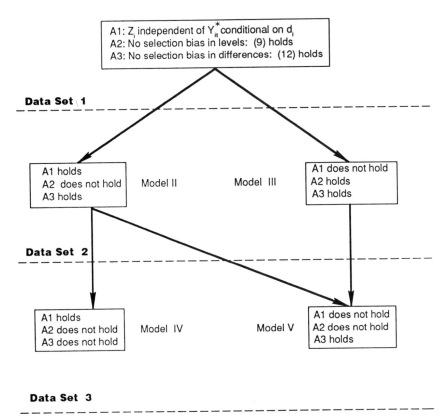

FIGURE F-2 Estimable models with different data sets. Data set 1: Single post-program, no Z_i. Data set 2: Single post-program, Z_i. Data set 3: Pre-program and post-program, Z_i.

be (Heckman and Hotz, 1989). For present purposes, a less technical answer is that assumptions can be tested if the data available are a bit more than are actually needed to estimate the model in question. This is illustrated in Figure 2, which shows five different models that can be estimated on different data sets. The model at the top of the figure can be estimated on Data Set 1, while the two models below can be estimated on a richer data set, Data Set 2, and the two models below that can be estimated on a yet richer data set, Data Set 3. At the top of the figure, it is presumed that the evaluator has a data set (Data Set 1) consisting of a single post-treatment data point with Y_{it} information, but no other variables at all—in particular, no Z_i variable is in the data set. The best the analyst can do in this circumstance is to compare the Y_{it} means of participants and non-participants to calculate $\tilde{\alpha}$ as in equation (4) above.

This estimate will equal that obtainable from a randomized trial under the three assumptions shown in the box for Model I in the figure: that the missing Z_i is independent of Y_{it}^* conditional on d_i, and that there is no selection bias in either levels or first differences. The first assumption is necessary to avoid "omitted-variable" bias, the bias generated by leaving out of the model an important variable that is correlated with both the probability of receiving the treatment and Y_{it}^*. Suppose, for example, that Z_i is a dummy for city location, as before. If city location is an important determinant of sexual behavior, and if the probability of treatment also varies across cities, then not having a variable for city location in the data set will lead to bias because the estimate of program impact (the difference in mean Y between participants and non-participants) reflects, in part, intercity differences in sexual behavior that are not the result of the treatment but were there to begin with. The second and third assumptions are necessary in order for the value of Y_{it}^* for non-participants to be the proper counterfactual, that is, for it to equal the value that participants would have had, had they not undergone the treatment.[9]

Models II and III in the Figure can be estimated if the data set contains information on a potential Z_i, like city location, but still only a single post-treatment observation on Y_{it} (Data Set 2). Each of these models requires only two assumptions instead of three, as in Model I, but each model drops a different assumption. Model II drops the assumption that there is no selection bias in levels—that is, it drops the assumption that (5) holds. This assumption can be dropped because a Z_i is now available and the instrumental-variable technique described above as Solution 1 is now available. In this method, the values of Y_{it} for participants and non-participants in a given city are not compared to one another to obtain a treatment estimate—that estimate would be faulty because participants are a self-selected group. Instead, mean values of Y_{it} across cities are compared to one another, where the cities differ in the availability of the treatment and therefore have different treatment proportions (e.g., a proportion of 0 if the city has no program at all, as in the example given previously). For the treatment-effect estimate from this model to be accurate still requires the assumption that the Z_i is a legitimate instrument—that the differential availability of the program across cities is not related to the basic levels of prevention behavior in each city (i.e., that Z_i and Y_{it}^* are independent).

---

[9] In this case, the third assumption is technically redundant because there will be no selection bias in differences if there is none in levels. This will not be true in other sets of three assumptions. Note too that, of course, more than three assumptions must be made, but these three are focused on for illustration because they are the three relevant to the richest data set considered, Data Set 3. With yet richer data sets, additional assumptions could be examined.

Not only does Model II require one less assumption than does Model I, it also permits the testing of that assumption and therefore the testing of the validity of Model I. The test of the dropped assumption—that there is no selection bias in levels—is based upon a comparison of impact estimates obtained from the two models. If the two are the same or close to one another, then it must be the case that there is, in fact, no selection bias in levels—because the impact estimate in Model I is based upon participant/non-participant comparisons whereas that in Model II is not. If the two are different, then there must be selection bias—if the participant/nonparticipant differences within cities do not generate the same impact estimate as that generated by the differences in Y_{it} across different cities, the former must be biased since the latter is accurate (under the assumption that the Z_i available is legitimate).

Model III takes the opposite tack and drops the assumption that Z_i is legitimate but maintains the assumption that there is no selection bias in levels. The model estimates the treatment effect by making participant-non-participant comparisons only within cities, that is, conditional on Z_i. If there are cities where the program is not present at all, data on Y_{it} from those cities are not utilized at all, unlike the method in Model II. The Model III impact estimate will be accurate if there is no selection bias into participation but it will also be accurate even if intercity variation is not a legitimate Z_i (e.g., if program placement were based upon need). In this case, a comparison of the impact estimate with that obtained from Model I—where participants and non-participants across cities were pooled into one data set and city location was not controlled for because the variable was not available—provides a test for whether intercity variation is a legitimate Z_i. If it is not (e.g., if program placement across cities is based on need)—then Models I and III will produce quite different treatment estimates, for Model I does not control for city location but Model III does (Model III eliminates cross-city variation entirely by examining only participant/non-participant differences within cities). On the other hand, if city location is a legitimate Z_i (e.g., if program placement is independent of need) then the two estimates should be close to one another.

The implication of this discussion is that Data Set 2 makes it possible to reject Model I by finding its assumptions to be invalid. This testing of Model I is possible because Data Set 2 provides more data than is actually necessary to estimate the model. Unfortunately, this data set does not allow the evaluator to test the assumptions of Models II and III necessary to assure their validity. Each makes a different assumption—Model II assumes that Z_i is legitimate, while Model III assumes no selection bias to be present—and the estimates from the two need not be the same. If they are different, the evaluator must gather additional information.

Such additional information may come from detailed institutional knowledge—for example, of whether Z_i is really legitimate (e.g., detailed knowledge of how programs are placed across cities). But another source of additional information is additional data, for example, information on a pre-program measure of Y_{it}. For example, if Data Set 2 is expanded by adding a pre-program measure of Y (Data Set 3) the assumptions of Models II and III can be tested by estimating Models IV and V shown in the Figure. Each of these models drops yet another assumption, although a different one in each case. Model IV drops the assumption that there is no selection bias in differences but continues to make the assumption that Z_i is a legitimate instrument. The impact estimate is obtained by the instrumental-variable technique, as in Model II, but in this case by comparing the means of $(\overline{Y}_t - \overline{Y}_{t-1})$ across cities, thereby eliminating selection bias in levels if there is any. Model V drops the assumption that there is no selection bias in levels by applying the difference estimate in (8) but still assumes that there is no selection bias in differences.

Once again, the richer data set permits the testing of the assumptions that went into Models II and III and therefore permits their rejection as invalid. The arrows in the Figure between Models show which models can be tested against one another. A comparison of the estimates of Model IV to those of Model II provides a test of the third assumption (that there is no selection bias in differences); a comparison of the estimates of Model V and Model II provides a test of the first assumption (that Z_i is a legitimate instrument); a comparison of the estimates of Model V and Model III provides a test of whether the second assumption holds (that there is no selection bias in levels). If each comparison indicates estimates that are similar to one another, the relevant assumption in the more restricted model (Model II or Model III) should be taken to be valid; when estimates differ, however, the assumption involved should be taken as invalid and the more restricted model should be rejected. Thus Models II and III may be discarded.

As before, Models IV and V now require certain assumptions in order for their impact estimates to be valid. The estimates required for each are different, but neither can be tested unless more information or more data were available. An additional pre-program data point or an additional Z_i variable would enrich the data set and permit the assumptions of the two models to be tested. New models made possible by increasing the richness of the data set permit the evaluator to discard more and more assumptions and therefore obtain impact estimates that are more and more reliable. This strategy can be pursued until models are found that are not rejected by richer data sets.[10]

IV. APPLICATION TO AIDS INTERVENTIONS

Two of the interventions being considered are C&T and CBO programs. In 1989, the CDC funded from 1,600 to 2,000 C&T programs across the country. The programs offer HIV testing and some pre-test and post-test counseling to individual clients, and sometimes partner notification and referral as well. The programs are often offered in local health departments or other local health facilities. The HIV testing and counseling are confidential and often also anonymous. There is considerable diversity across programs in the exact types of services offered, for local operators have considerable discretion in designing the type of program offered.

The CBO programs under consideration here are those which conduct local community health education and risk reduction projects. The types of programs offered are more diverse than those offered in the C&T programs, ranging from educational seminars for AIDS educators to the establishment of focus groups, conducting counseling, educating high-risk groups about risk reduction strategies, and the sponsoring of street fairs and performing arts activities in support of education and risk reduction. The organizations conducting the activities are often small and have close ties to the community, and usually target their activities on specific high-risk groups or other subsegments of the community. At present there is little systematic knowledge of the types of activities sponsored by CBOs on a nationwide basis.

Although C&T and CBO programs are quite distinct in their missions, they pose similar evaluation problems since both are generally aimed at altering sexual behavior in a target population.[11] To evaluate whether the various programs have any impact at all, and to estimate the magnitude of the impact of different types of programs, systematic and careful evaluation strategies are required.

The Panel on the Evaluation of AIDS Interventions recommends randomized trials wherever possible to evaluate these programs.[12] Unfortunately, randomization will be difficult to apply in many cases. First

---

[10]Nevertheless, as I have stressed elsewhere (Moffitt, 1989), at least one untested assumption must, by definition, always be made in any nonexperimental evaluation. It is only in a randomized trial that such an assumption is no longer necessary for valid impact estimates to be obtained.

[11]Of course, this is not the only goal of these programs and there are many other important ones as well. The techniques discussed in Section III will often be applicable to the evaluation of program impact on other goals, albeit with appropriate modification.

[12]The panel qualifies this recommendation in several respects. First, it recommends evaluation of only new CBO projects in order not to disrupt the operations of on-going ones. Second, for ethical

and foremost are the ethical issues involved in denying treatment at all, or denying a particular type of treatment, to individuals in the target population. The ethics in this case are not always a clear-cut issue. It is often argued, for example, that the ethical issues are less serious if individuals are not assigned to a zero-treatment cell but only to different types of treatments, each of which represents a gain over the individual's alternatives outside the experiment. However, even here there are ethical issues involved in any alteration of the natural order of priority in treatment assignment that would occur in the absence of randomization, especially if those operating the program believe that individuals are already being assigned to the "best" treatment for each individual. Second, there are likely to be serious political difficulties as well, for AIDS treatment has already become a highly politicized issue in local communities, and popular resistance to randomization will no doubt be even more difficult to overcome than it already is for other programs. Third, more than in most randomized trials, those in the AIDS context require a high degree of cooperation from the indigenous staff operating the programs, both to elicit accurate responses from the subjects, to reduce attrition, and in light of confidentiality requirements that often make it difficult for outside evaluators to be integrally involved in the operation and data collection of the experiment. Such cooperation may be difficult to achieve if randomization is taking place.

In any case, it is clear that observational, nonexperimental evaluation techniques must be given serious consideration in the evaluation of AIDS interventions. The techniques outlined in Section III are of potential applicability to such interventions. It is no doubt obvious that in both C&T and CBO programs selectivity bias is likely to be a problem—that those who choose to voluntarily make use of the services are likely to be quite different from those who do not, even if they had not received any program services.

The techniques outlined in Section III for addressing the selectivity bias problem point in very specific directions for a solution to the problem, namely, (1) the search for appropriate "Z's," and (2) the collection of sexual behavior histories. In addition, although it has not been heavily emphasized thus far, those techniques implicitly require the collection of data on non-participants as well as participants. If data on only participants are available, and therefore only a before-and-after study can be conducted, it will be very difficult to identify the effects of the treatment on behavior given the rapid increases in AIDS knowledge in the

---

reasons, it recommends against randomization for C&T evaluations if a zero-treatment cell is involved, preferring that all cells involve some type of treatment.

general population and the presumed steady change in sexual prevention behaviors that are occurring independently of these programs.

The Search for Z's

First, consider the issue of whether appropriate Z's can be found for AIDS interventions. It is likely to be difficult to locate such Z's, but not necessarily impossible. It is much easier, in fact, to identify variables that are inappropriate as Z's than variables that are appropriate. For example, it is extremely unlikely that any sociodemographic or health characteristic of individuals themselves would be appropriate. Health status, education level, prior sexual history, and other such characteristics no doubt affect the probability that an individual enrolls in a C&T or CBO program but also unquestionably are independently related to prevention behavior as well. Indeed, to use the language of economics, it is probably not possible to locate appropriate Z variables on the "demand" side of the market—that is, among those individuals who are availing themselves of the programs—and it would be more fruitful to look on the "supply" side, where availability of programs is determined in the first place.

On the availability side, the C&T and CBO programs are indeed differentially placed across neighborhoods within cities, between cities and suburbs, across metropolitan areas, and across states and regions. Unfortunately for the evaluation effort, however, differential availability in most cases is certain to be closely related to need. Those cities most likely to have an extensive set of programs are those with large subsegments of the high-risk population and those where HIV incidence has already been determined to be high. Within cities, it is no doubt also the case that programs are more likely to be located in neighborhoods close to high-risk populations than in neighborhoods far from them. With this process of program placement, differential availability will not constitute an appropriate Z_i.

If appropriate Z's are to be identified, it will require a more detailed investigation than is possible here but there are several directions in which such an investigation could be pursued. First, a detailed examination of the funding rules of CDC and other federal agencies would be warranted. Grants are made to applying C&T and CBO sponsors, and no doubt the need of the population to be served is a criterion in the funding decision. But the availability of a Z_i does not require that need not be used at all in the decision, only that it not be the sole criterion. To the extent that other criteria are used to make funding decisions, criteria unrelated to HIV incidence in the area, Z's may be identified. In addition, it is rarely the case that federal funding decisions are as rational and clear-cut as published funding formulas and formal points criteria suggest. It is almost always the case that some agency discretion, political factors, or bureaucratic forces come into play in some fraction of the decisions. To the extent that they are, appropriate Z's will be available.

Second, a detailed study of several large cities may result in the identification of other Z's. For example, it has been estimated that 60 percent of the male homosexual population in San Francisco has not been tested for HIV infection and has, therefore, almost certainly also not enrolled in a C&T or CBO program.[13] Why this percent is so high could be investigated. Perhaps the 60 percent who have not been tested are those with low probabilities of HIV in the first place, or those who are already practicing prevention behaviors—in this case, no appropriate Z_i would be available. On the other hand, some of the non-participants may be located in areas where no C&T or CBO program is present—for example, if they do not live in particular neighborhoods that have been targeted. If so, differential access to a program could serve as the basis for a Z.

Collection of Histories

The collection of data in general, and histories in particular, is likely to be difficult for the evaluation of AIDS interventions. The confidentiality of the testing and counseling process as well as the inherently sensitive nature of the questions that must be asked to obtain information on the necessary behaviors makes the prospect of obtaining reliable data highly uncertain at our present state of knowledge. Obtaining informed consent from those receiving the treatment as well as others may be problematical, and may result in self-selected samples that threaten the integrity of the design and consequently the validity of any impact estimates obtained. These considerations make difficult the prospect of obtaining even a single wave of post-program data, much less multiple periods of pre-program data.[14] Randomized trials have the advantage of requiring less data collection than observational studies, as noted in Section III, and hence are relatively favored in this respect.

Nevertheless, cohort studies in this area have been undertaken and have often been successful in retaining individuals in the sample, and more cohort collection efforts are underway. For example, Kaslow and colleagues (1987) report the results of a survey of sexual behavior of

---

[13] *Washington Post,* January 9, 1990.

[14] Histories can be collected from retrospective questions as well as reinterviews. For example, one or two pre-program interviews could be conducted, with the earliest one also containing a retrospective battery.

5000 asymptomatic homosexual men in which a baseline survey and lab tests were followed by reinterviews and tests at six-month intervals. As of the latest (10th) wave, about 5 years into the study, from 76 percent to 97 percent of the individuals (across areas and risk groups) are still in the sample, a very high percentage. The success of the cohort is partly a result of solid confidentiality measures as well as the heavy involvement of local gay community leaders and trained local staff from the beginning of the study.

Other cohort collection efforts include the CDC cross-city study of O'Reilly, involving both homosexual men as well as IV drug users; the study of seven CBOs headed by Vincent Mor at Brown University; the San Francisco city clinic cohort and Hepatitis B cohort; and the upcoming Westat cohort sponsored by NCHSR. How successful these efforts will be remains to be seen, but there is no question that serious cohort studies are being undertaken in increasing number. If they are successful, and if the histories described in Section III can be obtained, program evaluation designs will be greatly enhanced and impact estimates will be obtainable with much greater reliability.

V. SUMMARY AND CONCLUSIONS

The evaluation of AIDS interventions poses difficult conceptual and practical issues. Since randomized trials are unlikely to be feasible in many circumstances, evaluation methods for observational, nonexperimental data must be applied. Statistical methods developed by economists for the evaluation of the impact of social and economic programs over the past twenty years are applicable to this problem and have several important lessons for AIDS evaluations. The most important are that accurate estimates of program impact require (1) a systematic search for identifying "Z" variables, variables that affect the availability of program services to different populations but which are not direct determinants of HIV incidence or the adoption of prevention behaviors; or (2) the collection of sufficiently lengthy sexual histories from participants and non-participants in the programs that can be used to reduce the selection bias attendant upon participant/non-participant comparisons. Both of these implications are quite concrete and should provide funding agencies and program evaluators with specific directions to search for and in which to pursue evaluation designs that will yield reliable estimates of program impact.

REFERENCES

Ashenfelter, O. (1978) Estimating the effect of training programs on earnings. *Review of Economics and Statistics* 60:47-57.

Barnow, B. (1987) The impact of CETA programs on earnings: A review of the literature. *Journal of Human Resources* 22:157-193.

Barnow, B. Cain, G. and Goldberger, A. (1980) Issues in the analysis of selectivity bias. In E. Stromsdorfer and G. Farkas, eds., *Evaluation Studies Review Annual, Volume 5.* Beverly Hills, Calif.: Sage.

Bjorklund, A. and Moffitt, R. (1987) Estimation of wage gains and welfare gains in self-selection models. *Review of Economics and Statistics* 69:42-49.

Goldberger, A. (1972) Selection bias in evaluating treatment effects: Some formal illustrations. Discussion paper 123-72. Madison, Wisconsin: Institute for Research on Poverty.

Gronau, R. (1974) Wage comparisons—a selectivity bias. *Journal of Political Economy* 82:1119-1143.

Heckman, J. J. (1974) Shadow prices, market wages, and labor supply. *Econometrica* 42:679-694.

Heckman, J. J. and Hotz, V. J. (1989) Choosing among alternative nonexperimental methods for estimating the impact of social programs: The case of manpower training. *Journal of the American Statistical Association* 84:862-874.

Heckman, J. J. and Robb, R. (1985a) Alternative methods for evaluating the impact of interventions: An overview. *Journal of Econometrics* 30:239-267.

Heckman, J. J. and Robb, R. (1985b) Alternative methods for evaluating the impact of interventions. In J. Heckman and B. Singer, eds., *Longitudinal Analysis of Labor Market Data.* Cambridge: Cambridge University Press, 1985b.

Kaslow, R. W. Ostrow, D. G. Detels, R., Phair, J. P. Polk, B. F. and Rinaldo, C. R. (1987) The Multicenter AIDS cohort study: Rationale, organization, and selected characteristics of the participants. *American Journal of Epidemiology* 126:310-318.

Lewis, H. G. (1974) Comments on Selectivity Biases in Wage Comparisons. *Journal of Political Economy* 82:1145-1155.

Maddala, G. S. (1983) *Limited-Dependent Variable and Qualitative Variables in Econometrics.* Cambridge: Cambridge University Press, 1983.

Maddala, G. S. (1985) A survey of the literature on selectivity bias as it pertains to health care markets. In R. M. Scheffler, Ed., *Advances in Health Economics and Health Services Research,* Vol. 6. Greenwich, Conn.: JAI Press.

Manski, C. (1990) Nonparametric bounds for treatment effects. *American Economic Review* 80:319-323.

Moffitt, R. (1989) Comment on Heckman and Hotz. *Journal of the American Statistical Association* 84:877-878.

Index

A

Abstinence, as a health education outcome, 38, 52, 63, 78

Academic researchers, 98, 198, 203

Accessibility of services. *See* Counseling and testing projects

Accidental samples, 327, 328, 329

Adequacy of services. *See* Counseling and testing projects

Administrative records, 17, 88–90, 91–92, 105–106, 111

Advertising, paid, 64

Aggregate analysis of effectiveness, 75

AIDS (Acquired Immune Deficiency Syndrome). *See also* Ethnographic studies; Natural history studies

attitudes toward, 53, 80, 154, 158

demonstration projects, 91–92, 142, 167

epidemiology of, 166, 207, 213

incubation period of, 37

knowledge about, 44–45, 62, 65, 73, 154, 158

news coverage about, 76

prevalence rates, 80, 106n.4, 164, 165, 287n.67

research, 98, 149, 165, 198, 201, 213, 251, 268, 274, 290–291, 293

treatment, 80, 122, 338

AIDS hotline, 25, 62, 66–67, 68–69, 70–71, 74, 75–76, 78, 80

Alcohol

and reporting bias, 243–244, 263

compliance with treatment for alcoholism, 136

ALIVE, cohort of drug users, 167

Allegheny County, Pa., seroprevalence survey, 233, 235–236

American Social Health Association, 66, 80

America Responds to AIDS, 50, 51, 59, 60, 61, 63, 72, 73, 74, 76, 78, 79, 335

Anal intercourse

reporting bias, 242, 243, 244–245, 248, 282

Anonymity

HIV testing, 111, 120, 146, 161

in surveys, 217, 232, 236, 296, 321–322

Antabuse and treatment compliance, 136

Antismoking, program evaluation of, 15, 323

Archival data, 74, 78, 153

Arrestees, as sampling frame, 329

Assumptions

covariance analysis, 169–170

interrupted time series analysis, 146–147

matching studies, 163–164

modeling techniques, 175–179, 180

natural experiments, 161

nonrandomized studies, 126, 186–187

randomized experiments, 125

regression designs, 149–150, 152

survey measures, 244–245

Attrition, 23, 98, 120, 125, 129n.10, 131–132, 186

365

Outreach services, 89, 136, 330–331,
337–338
Oversight, 28, 29–30, 121, 200–205

P

Participant screening, 324
Partner notification, 42–43, 103, 104
Partner reports, 249–254
Personal interviews, 217, 222, 226, 227, 228,
231, 238
Physical evidence, 278
Pilot studies, 229–230, 235–236, 280,
281–283, 296
Pneumocystis carinii pneumonia, 115
Polio, and experimental trials, 26
Polygraph validation, 254–255
Population size, 164, 165
Population surveys, 109–110, 114, 326, 340
Positioning statement, 57
Pregnancy rates, 38–39, 41–42, 44, 78, 154,
155
Pretesting, 281n.63, 283–284, 296
Primary prevention behaviors, 41–42, 43
Private sector testing sites, 340
Probability sampling, 111, 157, 214–216,
224, 228, 232, 234–235, 242, 317,
318, 326–330
Probes, 284
Process evaluation, 16, 17, 137–138
community-based organizations, 84, 86–93,
99n.11
counseling and testing projects, 18,
103–114, 317
media campaign, 18, 66–71
research design, 18–19
Project Review Team, 121, 200–205
Prospective nonrandomized matching, 162
Protective behaviors, 42, 44, 119
Proxy reporting, 324
Psychological counseling, 119
Psychological outcomes, 35, 38, 44–45
Psychometric validation, 246–249
Public education, 102
Public Health Service, 45, 159, 179, 189,
296

Public Health Service Act, 120
Public service announcements, 50, 51–52,
53–54, 57–58, 61, 64, 66–71, 72, 74,
75–76
Purposive samples, 327, 328, 329–330

Q

Quasi-experimental studies, 19, 20–21, 94,
126, 127n.6, 137, 144–145, 183, 184,
185
assumptions, 187
covariance analysis, 168
data sources, 153–159
interrupted time series, 145–149
media campaign, 59
regression designs, 149–153

R

Race, 106n.4, 154, 169–170
Random-digit dialing, 227, 230
Random errors, 240, 241, 279
Randomized experiments, 21–26, 27, 124,
125–126, 128–129, 145n.24, 172, 189,
317, 330–331
appropriateness and feasibility of, 127,
137–144, 184, 323
attrition in, 125, 131–132
community-based organizations, 94–97, 98,
100, 200, 330–331, 332
compromised studies, 129–130, 131–136
costs of, 31–32, 50–51, 138–139
counseling and testing projects, 102,
114–115, 116, 117–120, 121, 204
interpretation of results, 186–189
matching in, 161
media campaign, 50–51, 61–63, 64, 66,
71–74, 76–77, 79, 80
outcome evaluation, 19, 21–26, 336–337
replication of, 175–176, 182
response techniques, 280–281
sample studies, 330–332
specialists, 30
threshold conditions, 23
Recommendations
community-based organizations, 91

counseling and testing services, 104, 112, 118

data collection, 159, 189

evaluation funding, 139, 142, 182

evaluation management, 27, 28, 29–30

formative evaluation, 22

media campaign, 54, 64, 74, 159

methodological research, 30, 136, 142, 182

outcome evaluation, 22, 27, 28

program objectives, 35, 36, 46

randomized experiments, 22, 136, 142

selection modeling, 182

Record keeping, 18, 113. *See also* Administrative records

Referral services, 335, 338–340

Regional comparisons, 80, 292

Regression discontinuity/regression displacement, 145, 149–153, 155–157, 158, 159–160

Regression toward the mean, 164–165

Relapse prevention, 119

Reliability, 44, 47, 111, 240, 262, 276

Replicability, 27–28, 96, 257–263, 275

Reporting bias, 45, 47, 111, 237, 243–245, 248, 255, 268–275

Research administration, 28–31

Research consent forms, 277

Research design, 18–27, 144, 320, 323

Resources and aspirations

community-based organizations, 92–93, 98–99

counseling and testing evaluation, 113–114, 121–122

media campaign, 59–61, 65–66, 70–71, 79–81

Response rates, 215, 216, 217–231, 235–236, 275, 322

Retrolental fibroplasia, observational and randomized studies of, 130, 138

Retrospective nonrandomized matching, 162–163

Return rates, 322

Reverse telephone directories, 229n.13

Risk prevention behaviors. *See* Complementary prevention behaviors; Primary prevention behaviors

Rolling panel design, 68

"Running-in" period, 135–136

S

Salk vaccine, and experimental trials, 26

Sampling issues

controlling attrition, 321–326

convenience and probability sampling, 326–330

drug users, 328–330

error, 140

gay and bisexual men, 327–328

number of case studies, 318–319

sample sizes, 25–26, 128–129n.9, 317, 318, 319–321

San Francisco, Calif.

ethnographic study, 292–293

Home Health Survey, 221, 233, 234–235

Men's Health Study, 167, 220, 233–234, 328

telephone survey, 219, 228–229

Schools, 94

media campaign and, 52–53

Seattle, Wash.

telephone survey, 219, 228, 229–230

Selection bias, 26, 75, 125, 129–130, 153

attrition, 131–132

comparability design, 144, 159

matching, 127, 161

modeling, 124, 126–127, 168, 169, 173–182, 187

regression designs, 149–150

in surveys, 215, 222–223, 236–239

Self-administered questionnaire (SAQ), 217, 222, 224–225, 228, 233, 235, 236, 238, 337

Self-reports, 296

alternatives, 277–278

drug use, 209, 234, 245n.25, 267–275, 276, 277, 278

sexual behavior, 37, 44, 244–249, 249–257, 276

Sensitivity analysis, 182n.50

Service delivery, 111, 118–119, 318–319, 338, 339

Television, 148, 159
  advertising, 58
  markets, 68, 69, 76–77, 79
Test marketing, media campaign, 62–63, 64–66
Timeliness, 45, 46, 137–138
Time series analysis, 72, 77, 158, 159–160, 184
  interrupted, 144, 145–149
  multiple, 146, 147n.26, 149–150, 162
Treatment
  alternative, 116, 117–119, 331, 332
  compliance with, 131, 132–133, 135–136, 321
  delayed, 22, 115, 141
  effects, 133, 168
  withholding, 22, 95, 102, 114–115, 141–142, 184, 317, 321, 330, 331–332
Treatment Outcome Prospective Study, 167

U

Understanding AIDS, 52, 73
Unit of assignment, 25–26, 117–118, 134
United Kingdom
  Health Education Authority, 32n.11
  Social and Community Planning Research, 281–283
United States
  AIDS in, 50
  ethnographic research in, 291
  prostitution in, 293
United States Congress, 90–91, 145–146
United States Conference of Mayors, 83, 84, 85, 95

Universities, 198, 203
Urinalysis, 255–256, 269–270, 274, 276

V

Validation, self-reports, 37, 241–242, 245–257
Validity, 44, 46, 361
  attrition and, 325–326
  client surveys, 111
  coefficients, 248
  criterion, 247
  differential, 47
  drug use measures, 274
  face, 247
  improving, 276–286
  randomized studies, 186
  systematic errors, 240–241

W

Wait-list controls, 71, 141. *See also* Delayed treatment
Women, 39, 283n.65, 295
  media campaign and, 52
  pregnancy, 41–42, 154, 155
  self-reporting, 251, 255–256, 258–259, 275, 276
  sexual behavior surveys, 225–226
  and survey interviews, 282

Y

Youth Incentive Entitlement Pilot Projects, program evaluation of, 162n.38

Z

Zelnik and Kantner survey, 257, 259